International Differences in Mortality at Older Ages

DIMENSIONS AND SOURCES

Eileen M. Crimmins, Samuel H. Preston, and Barney Cohen, *Editors*

Panel on Understanding Divergent Trends in
Longevity in High-Income Countries

Committee on Population
Division of Behavioral and Social Sciences and Education

NATIONAL RESEARCH COUNCIL
OF THE NATIONAL ACADEMIES

THE NATIONAL ACADEMIES PRESS
Washington, D.C.
www.nap.edu

THE NATIONAL ACADEMIES PRESS • 500 Fifth Street, NW • Washington, DC 20001

NOTICE: The project that is the subject of this report was approved by the Governing Board of the National Research Council, whose members are drawn from the councils of the National Academy of Sciences, the National Academy of Engineering, and the Institute of Medicine. The members of the committee responsible for the report were chosen for their special competences and with regard for appropriate balance.

This study was supported by the National Institute on Aging's Division of Behavioral and Social Research through Contract No. NO1-OD-4-2139, TO#194 between the National Academy of Sciences and the U.S. Department of Health and Human Services. Any opinions, findings, conclusion, or recommendations expressed in this publication are those of the author(s) and do not necessarily reflect the views of the organization or agencies that provided support for the project.

Library of Congress Cataloging-in-Publication Data

International differences in mortality at older ages : dimensions and sources / Eileen M. Crimmins, Samuel H. Preston, and Barney Cohen, editors ; Panel on Understanding Divergent Trends in Longevity in High-Income Countries, Committee on Population, Division of Behavioral and Social Sciences and Education.
    p. ; cm.
  Includes bibliographical references.
  ISBN 978-0-309-15733-9 (book) — ISBN 978-0-309-15734-6 (pdf) 1. Longevity. 2. Mortality. I. Crimmins, Eileen M. II. Preston, Samuel H. III. Cohen, Barney, 1959- IV. National Research Council (U.S.). Panel on Understanding Divergent Trends in Longevity in High-Income Countries. V. Title.
  [DNLM: 1. Life Expectancy—United States. 2. Aged—United States. 3. Cross-Cultural Comparison—United States. 4. Developed Countries—United States. 5. Middle Aged—United States. 6. Mortality—United States. WT 116]

    HB1531.I575 2010
    304.6'4—dc22

                                            2010037982

Additional copies of this report are available from the National Academies Press, 500 Fifth Street, NW, Lockbox 285, Washington, DC 20055; (800) 624-6242 or (202) 334-3313 (in the Washington metropolitan area); http://www.nap.edu.

Copyright 2010 by the National Academy of Sciences. All rights reserved.

Printed in the United States of America

Suggested citation: National Research Council. (2010). *International Differences in Mortality at Older Ages: Dimensions and Sources*. E.M. Crimmins, S.H. Preston, and B. Cohen, Eds. Panel on Understanding Divergent Trends in Longevity in High-Income Countries. Committee on Population, Division of Behavioral and Social Sciences and Education. Washington, DC: The National Academies Press.

THE NATIONAL ACADEMIES
Advisers to the Nation on Science, Engineering, and Medicine

The **National Academy of Sciences** is a private, nonprofit, self-perpetuating society of distinguished scholars engaged in scientific and engineering research, dedicated to the furtherance of science and technology and to their use for the general welfare. Upon the authority of the charter granted to it by the Congress in 1863, the Academy has a mandate that requires it to advise the federal government on scientific and technical matters. Dr. Ralph J. Cicerone is president of the National Academy of Sciences.

The **National Academy of Engineering** was established in 1964, under the charter of the National Academy of Sciences, as a parallel organization of outstanding engineers. It is autonomous in its administration and in the selection of its members, sharing with the National Academy of Sciences the responsibility for advising the federal government. The National Academy of Engineering also sponsors engineering programs aimed at meeting national needs, encourages education and research, and recognizes the superior achievements of engineers. Dr. Charles M. Vest is president of the National Academy of Engineering.

The **Institute of Medicine** was established in 1970 by the National Academy of Sciences to secure the services of eminent members of appropriate professions in the examination of policy matters pertaining to the health of the public. The Institute acts under the responsibility given to the National Academy of Sciences by its congressional charter to be an adviser to the federal government and, upon its own initiative, to identify issues of medical care, research, and education. Dr. Harvey V. Fineberg is president of the Institute of Medicine.

The **National Research Council** was organized by the National Academy of Sciences in 1916 to associate the broad community of science and technology with the Academy's purposes of furthering knowledge and advising the federal government. Functioning in accordance with general policies determined by the Academy, the Council has become the principal operating agency of both the National Academy of Sciences and the National Academy of Engineering in providing services to the government, the public, and the scientific and engineering communities. The Council is administered jointly by both Academies and the Institute of Medicine. Dr. Ralph J. Cicerone and Dr. Charles M. Vest are chair and vice chair, respectively, of the National Research Council.

www.national-academies.org

PANEL ON UNDERSTANDING DIVERGENT TRENDS IN LONGEVITY IN HIGH-INCOME COUNTRIES

EILEEN M. CRIMMINS (*Cochair*), Davis School of Gerontology, University of Southern California

SAMUEL H. PRESTON (*Cochair*), Department of Sociology, University of Pennsylvania

JAMES BANKS, Department of Economics, University of Manchester, and Institute for Fiscal Studies, London

LISA F. BERKMAN, Department of Society, Human Development, and Health, Harvard University School of Public Health

DANA A. GLEI, Center for Population and Health, Georgetown University

NOREEN GOLDMAN, Office of Population Research and Woodrow Wilson School, Princeton University

ALAN D. LOPEZ, School of Population Health, University of Queensland, Australia

JOHAN P. MACKENBACH, Department of Public Health, Erasmus University, Netherlands

MICHAEL G. MARMOT, Department of Epidemiology and Public Health, University College London, England

DAVID MECHANIC, Institute for Health, Health Care Policy, and Aging Research, Rutgers University

CHRISTOPHER J.L. MURRAY, School of Public Health, University of Washington

JAMES P. SMITH, RAND Corporation, Santa Monica, California

JACQUES VALLIN, Institut National d'Études Démographiques, Paris, France

JAMES W. VAUPEL, Max Planck Institute for Demographic Research, Rostock, Germany

JOHN R. WILMOTH, Department of Demography, University of California, Berkeley

BARNEY COHEN, *Study Director*
ROBERT POOL, *Consultant*
JACQUELINE R. SOVDE, *Program Associate*

COMMITTEE ON POPULATION

LINDA J. WAITE (*Chair*), Department of Sociology, University of Chicago
CHRISTINE BACHRACH, Social Science Research Institute, Duke University and School of Behavioral and Social Sciences, University of Maryland
EILEEN M. CRIMMINS, Department of Sociology, University of Southern California
PETER J. DONALDSON, Population Council, New York, New York
BARBARA ENTWISLE, Department of Sociology, University of North Carolina, Chapel Hill
JOSHUA R. GOLDSTEIN, Max Planck-Institute for Demographic Research, Rostock, Germany
CHARLES HIRSCHMAN, Department of Sociology, University of Washington
BARTHÉLÉMY KUATE-DEFO, Department of Demography, University of Montreal
WOLFGANG LUTZ, World Population Program, International Institute for Applied Systems Analysis, Laxenburg, Austria
DUNCAN THOMAS, Economics Department, Duke Global Health Institute, Duke University
BARBARA B. TORREY, Independent Consultant, Washington, DC
MAXINE WEINSTEIN, Center for Population and Health, Georgetown University

BARNEY COHEN, *Director*

Acknowledgments

In 2008, the National Research Council (NRC) convened a multidisciplinary panel of experts to examine diverging trends that have been observed in longevity at older ages across high-income countries. This companion volume contains the detailed background papers that the panel commissioned to help its work.

We gratefully acknowledge the sponsor of this project, the Division of Behavioral and Social Research at the National Institute on Aging. Particular thanks go to Dr. Richard Suzman, whose foresight in recognizing the timeliness of this project made this work possible.

The papers in this volume have been reviewed in draft form by individuals chosen for their diverse perspectives and technical expertise, in accordance with procedures approved by the Report Review Committee of the NRC. The purpose of this independent review is to provide candid and critical comments that will assist the institution in making its published volume as sound as possible and to ensure that the volume meets institutional standards for objectivity, evidence, and responsiveness to the study charge. The review comments remain confidential to protect the integrity of the process.

The Committee on Population wishes to thank the following individuals for their review of these papers: Nancy Adler, Departments of Psychiatry and Pediatrics, and Center for Health & Community, University of California, San Francisco; Robert Anderson, Division of Vital Statistics, National Center for Health Statistics, Centers for Disease Control and Prevention; James Banks, Department of Economics, University College, London, and Institute for Fiscal Studies, London; Magali Barbieri, Institut National d'Études Démographiques, Paris, France; Lisa Berkman, Department of Society, Human Development, and Health, Harvard University School of Public Health, Harvard University; John Bongaarts, Population Council, New York; Allan Brandt, Graduate School of Arts and Sciences, Harvard University; Maria Danielsson, Unit for General Welfare Analysis, Department of Statistics, Monitoring and Evaluation, National Board of Health and Welfare, Stockholm, Sweden; Majid Ezzati, Department of Global Health and Population, Department of Environmental Health, Harvard School of Public Health; Dana Glei, Department of Demography, University of California, Berkeley; Dana Goldman, Leonard D. Schaeffer Center for Health Policy and Economics, University of Southern California; Mark Hayward, Population Research Center and Department of Sociology, University of Texas at Austin; Christine L. Himes, Center for Policy Research, Syracuse University; Rasmus Hoffmann, Department for Public Health, Erasmus Medical Center, Rotterdam, Netherlands; Robert A. Hummer, Department of Sociology and Population Research Center, University of Texas at Austin; Arun Karlamangla, Division of Geriatrics, David Geffen School of Medicine at University of California, Los Angeles; Niels Keiding, Department of Biostatistics Institute of Public Health, University of Copenhagen, Denmark; Alan Lopez, School of Population Health, The University of Queensland, Brisbane, Australia; Johan Mackenbach, Department of Public Health, Erasmus Medical Center, Rotterdam, Netherlands; JoAnn E. Manson, Division of Preventive Medicine, Brigham and Women's Hospital, Harvard Medical School; Linda G. Martin, RAND Corporation, Arlington, Virginia; David Mechanic, Institute for Health, Health Care Policy, and Aging Research, Rutgers, The State University of New Jersey; Pierre-Carl Michaud, Rand Corporation, Santa Monica, California; Amos Pines, Department of Medicine 'T', Ichilov Medical Center, Tel-Aviv, Israel; Richard Rogers, Department of Sociology and Population Program, IBS, University of Colorado; James Smith, RAND Corporation, Santa Monica, California; Jacques Vallin, Institut National d'Études Démographiques, Paris, France; and Frans Willekens, Netherlands Interdisciplinary Demography Institute, The Hague.

Although the reviewers listed above have provided many constructive comments and suggestions, they were not asked to endorse the content of any of the papers nor did they see the final version of any paper before this publication. The review of this volume was overseen by Jane Menken, Population Program, Department of Sociology, University of Colorado. Appointed by the NRC, she was responsible for making certain that an independent examination of the papers was carried out in accordance with institutional procedures and that all review comments were carefully considered. Responsibility for the final content of this report rests entirely with the authors.

Contents

1 Introduction and Overview 1
   Eileen M. Crimmins, Samuel H. Preston, and Barney Cohen

Part I: Levels and Trends

2 Diverging Trends in Life Expectancy at Age 50: A Look at Causes of Death 17
   Dana A. Glei, France Meslé, and Jacques Vallin
3 Are International Differences in Health Similar to International Differences in Life Expectancy? 68
   Eileen M. Crimmins, Krista Garcia, and Jung Ki Kim

Part II: Identifying Causal Explanations

4 Contribution of Smoking to International Differences in Life Expectancy 105
   Samuel H. Preston, Dana A. Glei, and John R. Wilmoth
5 Divergent Patterns of Smoking Across High-Income Nations 132
   Fred Pampel
6 Can Obesity Account for Cross-National Differences in Life Expectancy Trends? 164
   Dawn E. Alley, Jennifer Lloyd, and Michelle Shardell
7 The Contribution of Physical Activity to Divergent Trends in Longevity 193
   Andrew Steptoe and Anna Wikman

8 Do Cross-Country Variations in Social Integration and Social Interactions Explain Differences in Life Expectancy in Industrialized Countries?   217
   James Banks, Lisa Berkman, and James P. Smith with Mauricio Avendano and Maria Glymour

Part III: The U.S. Health System

9 Low Life Expectancy in the United States: Is the Health Care System at Fault?   259
   Samuel H. Preston and Jessica Ho
10 Can Hormone Therapy Account for American Women's Survival Disadvantage?   299
   Noreen Goldman

Part IV: Inequality

11 Do Americans Have Higher Mortality Than Europeans at All Levels of the Education Distribution?: A Comparison of the United States and 14 European Countries   313
   Mauricio Avendano, Renske Kok, Maria Glymour, Lisa Berkman, Ichiro Kawachi, Anton Kunst, and Johan Mackenbach with support from members of the Eurothine Consortium
12 Geographic Differences in Life Expectancy at Age 50 in the United States Compared with Other High-Income Countries   333
   John R. Wilmoth, Carl Boe, and Magali Barbieri

Part V: International Case Studies

13 Renewed Progress in Life Expectancy: The Case of the Netherlands   369
   Johan Mackenbach and Joop Garssen
14 The Divergent Life-Expectancy Trends in Denmark and Sweden—and Some Potential Explanations   385
   Kaare Christensen, Michael Davidsen, Knud Juel, Laust Mortensen, Roland Rau, and James W. Vaupel

Biographical Sketches of Contributors   409

1

Introduction and Overview

*Eileen M. Crimmins, Samuel H. Preston,
and Barney Cohen*

According to the United Nations (UN) Population Division, life expectancy at birth in the United States in 1950 for males and females combined was 68.9 years (United Nations, 2009). At that time, relative to other countries or territories for which the United Nations collects and publishes data, the United States had the 12th highest life expectancy at birth in the world. Since then, life expectancy at birth in the United States has increased by slightly more than 10 years, to 79.2 years, a remarkable achievement. Yet during the same time period, many other countries around the world have done even better. If one were to redo the analysis using the most recently available data, life expectancy at birth in the United States would be tied for 28th place, just behind Korea, Luxembourg, Malta, and the United Kingdom, and more than 2 years behind Australia, Canada, France, Iceland, Italy, Japan, and Switzerland (United Nations, 2009). The decline in the relative position of the United States cannot be easily explained by higher rates of infant mortality in the United States than in other developed countries or by higher rates of violent deaths among young adults in the United States. Although both phenomena are evident, the vast majority of Americans (94 percent) survive to at least age 50 and when one compares international levels of life expectancy only from age 50 onward, the United States still ranks only 29th in the world, behind a surprisingly long list of other countries (see Chapter 9).

What are the reasons for the relatively poor performance of the United States at older ages? Are Americans too fat? Too stressed? Is the nation's much maligned health care system to blame? Or are there other factors that can explain the country's relatively low ranking in life expectancy?

Motivated by such questions and concerns, the National Institute on Aging (NIA) requested that the National Research Council (NRC) launch a major investigation to clarify patterns in the levels and trends in international differences in life expectancy above age 50 and to identify strategic opportunities for health-related interventions. NIA was also interested in the identification of areas for future high-priority research.

Responding to this request, the NRC appointed a panel of experts to prepare a report clarifying the state of scientific knowledge in this area. In addressing its charge, the Panel on Understanding Divergent Trends in Longevity in High-Income Countries confronted a large and burgeoning theoretical and empirical literature with contributions from virtually every field within the social and health sciences. In order to make sense of the vast amount of work, the panel decided to commission a set of background papers, each dealing with a topic relevant to the panel's work. This volume contains those papers. The panel's report, *Explaining Divergent Levels of Longevity in High-Income Countries*, is being published separately.

Taken collectively, the papers in this volume provide an assessment of the plausibility of the most obvious possible explanations that have been advanced to explain the poor position of the United States in terms of life expectancy above age 50. The authors, all of whom are at the forefront of work in their fields, provide state-of-the-art assessments of the research and identify gaps in measurement, data, theory, and research design where they exist.

For some topics, there is surprisingly little direct evidence that can address the basic question. A necessary prerequisite for investigating the importance of any potential explanation of differences in levels and trends in mortality between countries is the ability to examine comparable country-level information on the potential explanatory variables under consideration. Without such information it would be difficult, if not impossible, to draw conclusions with any degree of confidence. Fortunately, thanks to the HRS (the Health and Retirement Study) in the United States, ELSA (the English Longitudinal Study of Ageing) in the United Kingdom, and SHARE (the Survey of Health, Ageing and Retirement in Europe) across Europe and Israel, there are now comparable large-scale international surveys that contain important measures of many variables of relevance. However, the empirical basis for certain conclusions is significantly stronger in some cases than in others. For example, a lot is known about international differences in smoking patterns and levels of obesity, but far less about international differences in stress, physical exercise, and social networks.

The papers in this volume offer a wide variety of disciplinary and scholarly perspectives. Many different disciplines have made theoretical and empirical contributions to the study of mortality. The current collection is to some extent an amalgamation of concepts and insights—both old and new—obtained from various disciplines, each with its own domain of interest and style of analyzing and presenting data. Some authors review research fields that use mature methodologies and standard approaches, while others report on new avenues of investigation that are in their infancies. In these latter cases, concepts, methods, and measures still need to be refined. Nevertheless, each of the papers in this volume conveys important ideas and information.

NATURE OF THE DIFFERENCES

To better understand some of the main features of the diverging trends in life expectancy across countries, the paper by Glei, Meslé, and Vallin (Chapter 2) examines mortality changes and differences in 10 countries where high-quality mortality and cause of death data are available. In some of them, life expectancy has increased rapidly in recent years; in others, progress is lagging as in the United States.

By basing their analysis on a solid foundation of high-quality statistics, the authors are able to explore a number of important empirical relationships and see whether they stand up to close scrutiny. They point out that the story for male life expectancy at age 50 (e_{50}) is somewhat different than the story for female life expectancy at age 50. For the 10 countries examined, U.S. males have consistently ranked among the lowest in terms of e_{50}. Consequently, even though they currently appear to be faring relatively poorly, the relative position of U.S. males has not deteriorated over the last 50 years.

In contrast, the relative rank of U.S. females has deteriorated over the last 30 years. Around 1980, the pace of gains in life expectancy at age 50 slowed among women in the United States as it did for women in Denmark and the Netherlands; for the other countries, the pace of gains increased. Consequently, over the last quarter-century, gains in e_{50} among U.S. women (2.4 years) were about half those in Australia, France, and Italy (4.5-5.2 years) and less than 40 percent of that of Japan (6.3). The authors identify similar important empirical relationships by examining the contributions to gains in e_{50} by age and sex over time.

The authors provide a careful examination of cause-of-death statistics for those countries for which detailed data are available. The purpose of the analysis is to identify particular causes of death that can explain the relatively poor performance in gains in e_{50} for the three countries with the least amount of progress, Denmark, the Netherlands, and the United States. Comparative analysis of cause of death is complicated by issues of variation in coding practices across countries and over time. Nevertheless, the authors are partly successful in being able to identify particular causes of death that are either contributing factors or that can be ruled out. And although it is difficult to do justice to such careful analysis in one or two sentences, it appears that differences in female mortality due to lung cancer and respiratory diseases are an important part of the story. Such a finding is clearly consistent with the hypothesis that smoking was an important factor in slowing the mortality decline among women in those three countries.

In Chapter 3, Crimmins, Garcia, and Kim consider international patterns of morbidity and disability. These patterns shed a good deal of light on the factors that may be underlying mortality differences. The paper demonstrates that, in general, people age 50 and above in the United States have higher levels of self-reported disease and disability than those in the other countries investigated. Unusually high levels of prevalence in the United States are recorded for heart disease, stroke, and diabetes. Cancer registries show that the reported incidence of prostate cancer, breast cancer, and lung cancer is also highest in the United States. Colorectal cancer is the only disease for which the United States does not rank first in reported morbidity among the countries in the analysis. The United States also ranks first in self-reported diagnoses of hypertension and high blood cholesterol levels. On the other hand, it ranks at or near the bottom in measured hypertension and high blood cholesterol. A likely explanation of this apparent paradox is that the proportion of the population age 50 and above taking drugs to control hypertension and high cholesterol is highest in the United States.

As the authors point out, the higher prevalence of morbidity in the United States is consistent either with a higher incidence of disease or with a higher level of post-diagnostic survival. A higher reported incidence of disease could be produced by a higher true incidence or by more awareness of disease on the part of physicians and patients in the United States. Because the data systems that make possible these international comparisons are very new, they cannot yet support the longitudinal studies needed to sort out these issues of causality. Comparisons of morbidity-to-mortality patterns in this paper provide some insight, but the small number of countries involved makes it very difficult to identify relationships that are statistically significant. The high level of morbidity from major conditions in the United States is consistent with the adverse longevity of the United States. Given the location of the United States on these distributions, most of the cross-national relations reported in the chapter between morbidity and mortality are positive: higher morbidity is associated with higher mortality. Japan is often at the opposite end of both the morbidity and mortality distributions from the United States, contributing to the positive association. Finally, the authors analyze micro-level data on self-reported disease and show that the poor ranking of the United States in heart disease, stroke, and diabetes is maintained even after controlling for different levels of obesity and smoking.

CAUSAL PATHWAYS

The next five papers in the volume (Chapters 4-8) summarize what is known about some of the main behavioral health factors that are commonly believed to contribute to the observed international differences in life expectancy. As many of the authors point out in their papers, the search for internationally comparable data is often a demanding task.

Through the 1960s, the United States had much higher per capita tobacco consumption than any country in Western Europe (Forey et al., 2002), so investigating the impact of differential levels of smoking was an obvious candidate for the panel to investigate. The adverse health consequences of smoking have been known for more than 50 years: smoking harms almost every internal organ and increases the risk of dying from many different causes of death. Smoking is not only associated with cancer of directly exposed organs and tissue (esophagus, larynx, lung and bronchus, mouth, and throat), it is also associated with a range of cancers in indirectly exposed organs and tissues, including the bladder, brain, intestines, kidney, liver, pancreas, rectum, stomach, and uterus. In addition, it has been linked to a host of other respiratory diseases (asthma, bronchitis, emphysema, influenza, pneumonia, pulmonary fibrosis, and pulmonary tuberculosis), cardiovascular diseases (aortic aneurysms, cerebral vascular disease, coronary heart disease, and hypertension), and others. Even so, the full impact of smoking in many of the countries under consideration is still not fully understood because there have been few studies that contain large enough numbers of representative smokers and nonsmokers who are followed over a sufficiently long period of time to calculate definitive statistics.

In Chapter 4, Preston, Glei, and Wilmoth apply a new method for estimating the portion of total mortality attributable to smoking. Using the death rate from lung cancer as an indirect measure of smoking histories, the authors use macro-level statistical relationships to model the impact of smoking on mortality (see Preston, Glei, and Wilmoth, 2009). Their method is conceptually different from the well-known Peto-Lopez model (Peto et al., 1992) yet reaches remarkably similar conclusions with respect to the impact of smoking on mortality. The authors find that male mortality has been much more heavily influenced by smoking than female mortality but that the attributable fraction for women has been rising more rapidly. In 2003, the highest percentage of male deaths attributable to smoking occurred in Hungary (30 percent); among women, the highest fraction occurred in the United States (20 percent).

Life expectancy at age 50 has been powerfully influenced by smoking in many countries. In the United States, Preston, Glei, and Wilmoth (2009) estimate that male e_{50} would be 2.5 years longer if the smoking-attributable deaths were eliminated, female e_{50} would be 2.3 years longer. Among the 21 countries that the authors examined, if one were to remove the deaths that are attributable to smoking, the relative ranking of the United States with regard to life expectancy would improve from 17th to 9th for women and from 15th to 12th for men. These results suggest that increases in smoking-attributable mortality have dampened the gains to e_{50} since 1950 among women in all 21 countries, although the impact varied: Among U.S. women, smoking reduced the gains by 1.6 years, the largest effect in any country, while the effect of smoking-attributable deaths on life expectancy in Spain and Portugal was negligible. The authors conclude that about two-thirds of the growing shortfall in life expectancy for U.S. women since 1950 can be attributed to the effects of smoking. For U.S. men since 1950, smoking has produced a modest deterioration in their position in international comparisons of life expectancy.

Given the centrality of smoking as an underlying cause of death, Pampel (Chapter 5) investigates the reasons behind the observed divergent patterns of smoking across high-income nations. Levels of smoking in 2000 varied widely between countries: from 19 percent in Sweden and the United States to 34 percent in Spain, 35 percent in Germany, and 38 percent in Greece (Cutler and Glaeser, 2006). Even larger differentials can be observed if the comparisons are restricted to males.

Pampel explores potential explanations for the current level of smoking in the United States relative to other high-income countries. In the past, researchers have stressed such factors as prices, policies, inequality, and national-level differences in beliefs about the harmfulness of tobacco (see, e.g., Cutler and Glaeser, 2006); in contrast, Pampel explores the hypothesis that international differences in smoking can best be understood from the vantage point of an epidemic that spreads from a relatively small part of a population to other parts, and then recedes, like other epidemics.

Pampel emphasizes the importance of diffusion theory to explain observed patterns of cigarette consumption by socioeconomic group. In the early stages of the epidemic, smoking emerges initially among the highest socioeconomic group. This group is most open to innovation and has the financial resources to afford to smoke. The epidemic then diffuses to lower socioeconomic groups, and it recedes first among men of high socioeconomic status. Pampel finds that cross-national comparisons of aggregate trends in prevalence and determinants of individual differences in smoking generally support the epidemic or diffusion model. A better understanding of these cross-national patterns of cigarette smoking may have important implications for researchers' ability to project future mortality trajectories across countries.

It is well known that the prevalence of obesity has increased very dramatically in the United States since the 1970s, affecting all sex, race, and socioeconomic groups (Flegal et al., 2010). Because obesity is associated with a wide variety of chronic conditions, disability, and mortality, its rapid growth in the United States, perhaps combined with a car-dominated sedentary lifestyle, is popularly perceived as a large part of the reason that people in the United States fair so poorly in cross-national health comparisons.

In Chapter 6, Alley, Lloyd, and Shardell address this popular perception by examining both international trends in obesity and the relationship between obesity and mortality. The authors conclude that although high levels of obesity in the United States are likely to be part of the explanation, they are unlikely to account for a very large fraction of the cross-national differences in life expectancy. The authors offer two reasons for reaching this conclusion. First, the obesity epidemic is not confined to the United States: rising levels of obesity are occurring in many other countries, although admittedly they lag somewhat behind the United States. Second, the association between obesity (or high body mass index) and mortality is not straightforward and relatively weak at older ages. In fact, there is a strong relationship only between mortality and very high weight levels (morbid obesity), the prevalence of which remains relatively low even in the United States. Nevertheless, the authors conclude that the importance of rising levels of obesity as a contributing factor to life expectancy is still not fully understood and likely to grow over time as obesity increases at younger ages and at higher weights.

Maintaining a certain level of physical activity as one ages is important for a variety of reasons, including the maintenance of good cardiovascular health, lower risk of falls and fractures, higher levels of cognition and positive well-being, and higher levels of social participation. Conversely, physical inactivity has been related to higher rates of mortality, to a lower quality of life, and to a higher risk of coronary heart disease, diabetes, fractures, hypertension, obesity, osteoporosis, various types of cancers, and more.

In Chapter 7, Steptoe and Wikman assess the evidence that national-level differences in physical activity contribute to observed variation in life expectancy across high-income countries. An accurate assessment of the extent to which physical activity contributes to variations in life expectancy is hard to achieve. Among other obstacles are a paucity of internationally comparable time-series data, a lack of common metrics, and questions about the relative quality of personal recall data versus data derived by objective measurement. In addition, there is no definitive theoretical framework to guide how to assess the effects of physical activity on life expectancy: this lack of a framework results in a lack of clarity about the most important variables and when and how to measure them. For example, should relatively more weight be placed on evidence about attaining the recommended level of physical activity currently or in the past? How important is a completely sedentary lifestyle? Even if these issues can be resolved, the links between physical exercise and other behaviors, such as smoking and diet, imply that multivariate analyses are necessary.

Following a review of the strengths and limitations of self-report and objective measures of physical activity, the authors present data from four different internationally comparable data sets that have recorded the frequency, duration, and intensity of physical activity. They show that the ranking of countries in terms of physical activity is only moderately consistent across studies, implying that conclusions regarding the relationship between physical activity and health outcomes must be drawn cautiously. Using data from the ELSA, HRS, and SHARE, the authors analyze the relationship between various measures of physical activity and inactivity and self-reported health and self-reported diabetes. Their results provide important, albeit rather preliminary, evidence that is consistent with the notion that physical activity contributes to cross-national variations in health. More definitive conclusions must wait for more sophisticated cross-national comparisons that use objective measures of physical activity and multivariate analyses of time trends in physical activity.

The final paper in this section, by Banks and his coauthors (Chapter 8), considers the possibility that international differences in the degree of social integration can account for international differences in health and mortality. It focuses on comparisons between England and the United States because of closely comparable and detailed longitudinal surveys that were conducted in the two countries. The authors recognize that this comparison is not ideal because the two countries share relatively similar mortality profiles.

Their analysis of the relationship between measures of social integration and health in the two countries suggests a relatively weak role for social integration in explaining national differences. Not only are measures of social integration quite similar in England and the United States, but also is the "toxicity" of different measures in the two countries. Although the authors show the significance of many cross-sectional relationships between social integration and health outcomes, the analysis of mortality shows relatively small or inconsistent links between mortality and social integration or network measures. The authors then use Gallup survey data to demonstrate that the international variation in measures of social integration is much greater than that between England and the United States, leaving open the possibility that social relations may play a larger role on other stages. The paper concludes with a set of thoughtful observations on how research in the area can be advanced.

THE U.S. HEALTH CARE SYSTEM

The low ranking of the United States in international comparisons of life expectancy is sometimes blamed on the poor performance of the U.S. health care system rather than on behavioral or social factors. The United States spends more money on health care than any other country in the world, yet the country suffers from a number of well-documented problems, including a high level of inefficiency and waste in the system; a large number of people who are uninsured or underinsured, with accompanying reductions in access to high-quality or at least good health care; and the existence of persistent disparities in health care associated with economic status, education, ethnicity, geography, and race.

In Chapter 9, Preston and Ho present evidence on the relative performance of the U.S. health care system using death avoidance as the sole criterion. As the authors point out, given that the United States has historically had high levels of cigarette consumption and obesity, it is certainly possible that the country's low longevity ranking could be compatible with a finding that the U.S. health care system is performing relatively well, at least in identifying and administering treatments for various diseases. The authors find that, by standards of other high-income countries, the United States does well in terms of screening for cancer, survival rates from cancer, survival rates after heart attacks, and medication of individuals with high blood pressure and high levels of cholesterol.

The authors consider in greater depth mortality from prostate cancer and breast cancer, diseases for which effective methods of identification and treatment have been developed and for which behavioral factors do not play a dominant role. They show that mortality reductions from prostate cancer and breast cancer have been significantly more rapid in the United States than in other high-income countries. They argue that these unusually rapid declines are attributable to wider screening and more aggressive treatment of these diseases in the United States. On the basis of their review and their detailed consideration of these two diseases, they conclude that the low longevity ranking in the United States is not likely to be the result of medical failures in the identification or treatment of the major diseases at older ages.

One important feature of the erosion of the U.S. survival advantage is that it has been pronounced for U.S. women relative both to U.S. men and to women in other high-income nations. This pattern suggests the potential importance of gender-specific explanatory factors. In Chapter 10, Goldman discusses one attractively simple but as yet unexplored hypothesis: that the widespread use of postmenopausal hormone therapy (HT) in the United States has adversely affected U.S. mortality trends. At least prior to 2002, HT had been widely prescribed to U.S. women at menopause, not only for the relief of unpleasant symptoms (e.g., hot flashes), but also for its presumed protection against cardiovascular diseases and loss of bone density. However, the author finds little evidence to support the theory that HT use has had a notable impact on all-cause mortality and presents findings questioning whether HT is a significant risk factor for coronary heart disease. Finally, although high, the prevalence of HT in the United States is not out

of line with rates of use in several other high-income countries that have experienced steady improvements in female life expectancy.

INEQUALITY

The next two papers in the volume review the extent to which various types of inequality influence mortality differentials. In Chapter 11, Avendano and his coauthors explore the hypothesis that lower life expectancy at age 50 in the United States, relative to several Western European countries, may be partly attributable to larger socioeconomic disparities in mortality in the United States. To explore this hypothesis, the authors compare U.S. mortality rates by level of education with similar mortality data for 14 European countries.

They find that at low levels of education U.S. men have higher mortality than men in Western Europe; for highly educated men, those in the United States and several other countries had comparable rates. The pattern for women was slightly different: U.S. women had higher mortality than Western European women at all levels of education, but the U.S. excess mortality was often larger among women with low levels of education. However, most Eastern European countries had higher mortality rates than the United States, particularly at the bottom of the educational distribution. In general, disparities in mortality by education in the United States were comparable to disparities in several Western European countries, including France and Norway, but smaller than inequalities in Eastern European countries. The authors conclude that a modest part of the difference between U.S. and European mortality rates for women is attributable to larger excess mortality at lower educational levels.

In Chapter 12, Wilmoth, Boe, and Barbieri consider how geographic differentials in life expectancy at age 50 have evolved in Europe, Japan, and the United States, using a variety of indicators of regional disparities. The authors consider states and counties in the United States and Europe as a whole, with and without Eastern Europe. They also study changes in the evolution of internal geographic disparities in Canada, France, Germany, and Japan. Their analysis adds valuable texture to the analysis in the rest of this volume, which is heavily focused on measures expressed as means.

One of their most informative analyses asks how different the changes in U.S. life expectancy would have been if the pace of change in the bottom half of the geographic distribution had been the same as that in the top half. Even though the United States was the only country that had a growing disparity between the top and the bottom halves of the distributions since 1980, the authors find that the growing disparity contributed little to the poor performance of U.S. women in terms of mortality: both halves of the distribution lagged relative to their European counterparts. Additional and dramatic evidence of the widespread difficulties of U.S. women is suggested by the fact that the life expectancy of the highest quintile of American women has been below that of the lowest quintile of Japanese women since 1980.

INTERNATIONAL CASE STUDIES

The United States is not the only country to have experienced a slowing in improvements in life expectancy at the oldest ages. Denmark and the Netherlands have recently experienced slowdowns in mortality decline comparable to that of the United States (Meslé and Vallin, 2006). Interestingly, however, progress in mortality decline among the elderly resumed in Denmark around 1995 and resumed in the Netherlands around 2002. In Chapter 13, Mackenbach and Garssen investigate the case of the Netherlands, searching for clues about what might account for the observed trend in mortality. A slight upturn in life expectancy at older ages was first observed in the Netherlands around 2002 and initially attributed to favorable climatic factors (milder than average winters, cooler summers). But when mortality decline continued, it became increasingly unlikely that milder temperatures could be the sole driving force.

In order to investigate this phenomenon in more detail, Mackenbach and Garssen examined evidence on causes of death. The authors find that the main contributors to the acceleration of the rise in life expectancy at age 65 were significant reductions in death from ill-defined conditions, stroke, diabetes, dementia, and pneumonia. The authors review a wide range of possible determinants of mortality to try to explain these patterns. Health care is the only category of determinants for which substantial changes appear to have occurred and for which changes are consistent with the observed pattern in mortality and changes in cause of death. A deliberate and sudden rise in health care expenditures around 2001 seems to have resulted in an increase in availability of health care for the elderly. A rapid increase in hospitalization rates and more liberal administration of life-saving treatments to elderly people appears to be the most plausible hypothesis for explaining the sudden reversal of old-age mortality trends in the Netherlands. This paper serves to reinforce the importance of examining differential access to and the quality of health care provided to older people.

Finally, Chapter 14 focuses on a more specific comparison of Denmark, one of the countries that the panel singled out as a life-expectancy laggard, to neighboring Sweden. Christensen and his colleagues show that Denmark's life expectancy at birth dropped from 3rd highest among 20 European countries in the 1950s to 17th for males and 20th for females around 2000. The deterioration stopped in the mid-1990s but no catch-up occurred. Their analysis of cause-specific mortality data suggests that the reason for the Danish deterioration was lifestyle factors, especially smoking and high alcohol consumption. The authors conclude that smoking and alcohol-related deaths accounted for virtually all of the disparity in life expectancy between Denmark and Sweden in 1997-2001, with smoking playing the larger role. There are also some indications that lower budgets for Denmark's free national health care system, in comparison with other Nordic countries, may play a role in Denmark's adverse position.

THE WAY AHEAD

Clearly, there is a need to continue to conduct research to better understand the factors underlying international differences in life expectancy at older ages. For the most part, the papers in this volume focus on the behavioral factors that are commonly believed to contribute to those differences. Because of the interaction and the multiple causal pathways between these various factors (e.g., obesity can lead to lack of physical exercise and poor health but poor health can also lead to lack of physical exercise and obesity), the exact amount that each factor contributes to the observed health differentials remains unknown. Yet one finding seems clear: having the highest level of cigarette consumption per capita in the developed world over a 40-year period (up to the mid-1980s) has left a very visible and continuing imprint on U.S. mortality.

The papers in this volume should be considered starting points. Although some questions have been answered, many others remain. Major advances in data collection have meant that high-quality cross-national research is becoming increasingly feasible. This area of research has already produced important insights, and it seems clear that its future is promising.

REFERENCES

Cutler, D.M., and Glaeser, E.L. (2006). *Why Do Europeans Smoke More Than Americans?* NBER Working Paper 12124. Cambridge, MA: National Bureau of Economic Research.

Flegal, K.M., Carroll, M.D., Ogden, C.L., and Curtin, L.R. (2010). Prevalence and trends in obesity among U.S. adults, 1999-2008. *Journal of the American Medical Association, 303*(3), 235-241.

Forey, B., Hamling, J., Lee, P., and Wald, N. (Eds.). (2002). *International Smoking Statistics* (2nd edition). Oxford: Oxford University Press.

Gruer, L., Hart, C.L., Gordon, D.S., and Watt, G.C.M. (2009). Effect of tobacco smoking on survival of men and women by social position: A 28-year cohort study. *British Medical Journal, 338*(172), b480.

Meslé, F., and Vallin, J. (2006). Diverging trends in female old-age mortality: The United States and the Netherlands versus France and Japan. *Population and Development Review, 32*(1), 123-145.

Mokdad, A.H., Marks, J.S., Stroup, D.F., and Gerberding, J.L. (2004). Actual causes of death in the United States, 2000. *Journal of the American Medical Association, 291*(10), 1238-1245.

Peto, R., Lopez, A.D., Boreham, J., Thun, M., and Heath, C. (1992). Mortality from tobacco in developed countries: Indirect estimation from national vital statistics. *Lancet, 339*(8804), 1268-1278.

Preston, S.H., Elo, I.T., Hill, M.E., and Rosenwaike, I. (2003). *The Demography of African Americans, 1930-1990.* Dordrecht, The Netherlands: Kluwer Academic.

Preston, S.H., Glei, D.A., and Wilmoth, J.R. (2009). A new method for estimating smoking-attributable mortality in high-income countries. *International Journal of Epidemiology*, doi:10.1093/ije/dyp360.

Rogers, R.G., Hummer, R.A., Krueger, P.M., and Pampel, F.C. (2005). Mortality attributable to cigarette smoking in the United States. *Population and Development Review, 31*(2), 259-292.

United Nations. (2009). *World Population Prospects: The 2008 Revision. Volume 1: Comprehensive Tables.* New York: Author.

Part I

Levels and Trends

2

Diverging Trends in Life Expectancy at Age 50: A Look at Causes of Death

Dana A. Glei, France Meslé, and Jacques Vallin

This study focuses on three main questions: (1) Why did mortality decline slow among women (but not men) after 1980 in the United States? (2) Can slowing in Danish and Dutch trends be explained by similar sources? (3) Why did Denmark and more recently the Netherlands resume progress but the United States has not? To begin to answer these questions, we explore which ages and which causes of death contributed to disparities across the 10 study countries. We mainly used the Human Mortality Database (HMD) (2009) for age-specific mortality data and the World Health Organization (WHO) database (World Health Organization, 2009) for causes of death; additional data were obtained from national sources to complete or update these two international databases. Throughout our analyses, we focus particular attention on several outliers: countries in which levels of life expectancy at age 50 (e_{50}) in 2006 among women are lowest (Denmark, the Netherlands, and the United States) and highest (France and Japan).

The chapter is organized in several sections. First, we investigate age group contributions to gains in e_{50} during the periods 1955-1980 and 1980-2004. Second, we explore trends in mortality rates by cause of death. Third, we determine the contribution of cause groups to the gains in e_{50}. Fourth, we examine the age and cause-specific components of recent progress in Denmark and the Netherlands compared with the United States. Fifth, we present more in-depth analyses comparing several of the outliers (i.e., France, Japan, the Netherlands, and United States). The paper concludes with a review of the main findings with respect to our research questions and a discussion of the implications.

INTRODUCTION

Before focusing in-depth analysis on a small number of high-income countries, we begin by showing the 35 richest countries in terms of life expectancy at age 50 relative to gross domestic product (GDP) per capita. We then proceed to the main analysis, which is based on 10 countries selected by the committee as the most relevant for understanding the position of the United States.

In 2005, among the richest countries, we see a clear relation between e_{50} (both sexes) and the GDP per capita (Figure 2-1, right graph) ($R^2 = 0.60$), which contrasts with the situation observed in 1960 (Figure 2-1, left graph) ($R^2 = 0.05$). In between, major changes occurred in the field of public health. Until the middle of the 20th century, life expectancy was still strongly dependent on the fight against infectious diseases (even above age 50), which mainly relied on antibiotics and vaccines without much link to the GDP per capita, at least among rich countries. On the contrary, by 2005, e_{50} depends mostly on the success of the fight against degenerative diseases, including circulatory diseases.

Figure 2-1 shows some geographic clustering: among these countries at the top of the world income distribution, the group of countries in the lower left corner (lowest e_{50} and lowest GDP per capita) includes Russia and most of the countries in Central and Eastern Europe, and the countries in the rest of the world are clustered in the top half of the graph (with higher e_{50} and generally higher GDP per capita). However, the general correlation between GDP per capita and e_{50} appears to be rather strong.[1] Yet under the diagonal on Figure 2-1, there are a few outliers: e_{50} in Denmark (DNK), Ireland (IRL), Russia (RUS), Singapore (SGP), and even more so Norway (NOR) and the United States (USA), are lower than one might expect given their income level. Specific explanations could certainly be given for each of these exceptions, but it seems that at least three of them were enriched rather suddenly in recent years, perhaps without sufficient time to realize the health benefits (Ireland, Norway, and Singapore). Denmark is well known for having encountered difficulties controlling some human-made diseases like tobacco-related conditions, and Russia is not a surprise at all but typical of the excess adult mortality in Eastern Europe. Above all, the United States is the most striking because e_{50} lags many other countries despite much higher levels of income, without any clear explanation. Indeed, when excluding the six exceptional cases, the correlation is even stronger ($R^2 = 0.75$).

When looking at the trends in e_{50} over the period since 1955 among the 10 study countries, the strikingly unfavorable position of the United States

---

[1]The difficulty of ensuring good and comparable income measurement is well known. This first graph is a rough indication that a few countries, including the United States, appear to be unusual.

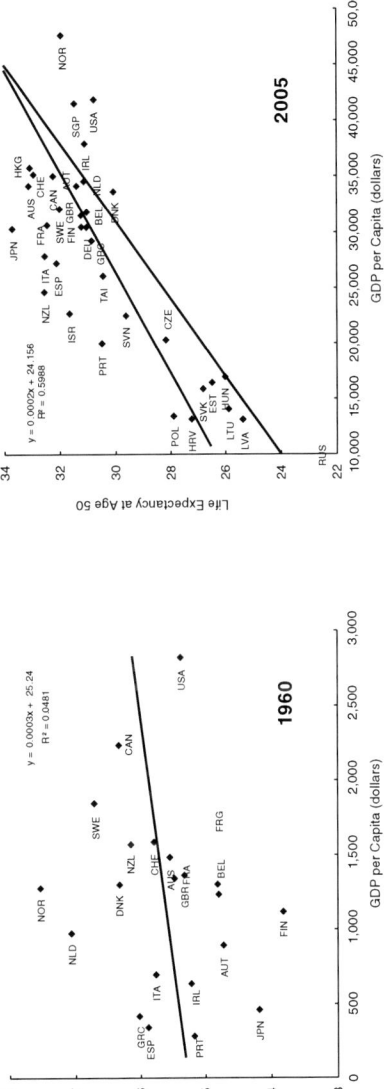

FIGURE 2-1 GDP per capita and life expectancy at age 50 in the richest countries in 1960 and 2005, both sexes.
NOTES: Countries are designated by the standard United Nations country codes (see http://unstats.un.org/unsd/methods/m49/m49alpha.htm); see the complete list below.

We define the richest countries to be those in which GDP per capita was more than 10,000 purchasing power parity dollars in 2005, excluding those in which population size is less than 1 million (i.e., Bahrain, Botswana, Brunei, Cyprus, Equatorial Guinea, Gabon, Iceland, Kuwait, Luxembourg, Macao, Malta, Oman, Qatar) or in which mortality data quality is questionable (i.e., Argentina, Chile, Malaysia, Mexico, Saudi Arabia, South Korea). In total, 35 countries are considered for the year 2005: Australia (AUS), Austria (AUT), Belgium (BEL), Canada (CAN), Croatia (HRV), Czech Republic (CZE), Denmark (DNK), Estonia (EST), Finland (FIN), France (FRA), Germany (DEU), Greece (GRC), Hong Kong (HKG), Hungary (HUN), Ireland (IRL), Israel (ISR), Italy (ITA), Japan (JPN), Latvia (LVA), Lithuania (LTU), the Netherlands (NLD), New Zealand (NZL), Norway (NOR), Poland (POL), Portugal (PRT), Russia (RUS), Singapore (SGP), Slovak Republic (SVK), Slovenia (SVN), Spain (ESP), Sweden (SWE), Switzerland (CHE), Taiwan (TAI), United Kingdom (GBR), United States (USA). For 1960, we include the same countries subject to data availability (except Germany, which is replaced by West Germany, FRG).
SOURCE: Drawn from data on Gross Domestic Product per capita from the World Bank (1976, 2008); estimates of life expectancy at age 50 from Human Mortality Database (2009 [accessed January 2009]).

appears to result from different patterns by sex (see Figures 2-2 and 2-3). Trends for U.S. men are quite similar to those of most other countries (with the exception of Denmark). It is true that U.S. men have consistently ranked among the three or four lowest positions in terms of e_{50}, but their position does not appear to have deteriorated over the past five decades.

In contrast, trends for women have strongly diverged since 1980. Until around that year, e_{50} among U.S. women stayed solidly in the middle of the group following a trend similar to the others with the exception of Japan, which started out way behind but made faster gains than the other countries throughout the period. Around 1980, the pace of gains in e_{50} slowed among women in the United States, along with Denmark and the Netherlands, while continuing at a faster pace among other countries.[2] Between 1980 and 2006, women in these three countries gained only 2.0-2.4 years in e_{50}, whereas women in most of the other countries gained 4 or more years (see Table 2-1). Yet Danish women resumed progress after the mid-1990s, and in very recent years Dutch women also began making faster gains. During the past 26 years, gains in e_{50} among U.S. women (2.4 years) were about half of those in Australia, France, and Italy (4.5-5.2 years) and less than 40 percent that of Japan (6.3 years). Not only is U.S. longevity (among both sexes combined) shorter than expected given its GDP per capita (Figure 2-1), but women appear to have fallen further behind over the last quarter of a century.

AGE GROUP CONTRIBUTIONS TO GAINS IN E_{50}

Figure 2-4 shows the contributions by age group to female gains in e_{50} during the periods 1955-1980 and 1980-2004 for Denmark, the Netherlands, and the United States compared with the 10-country mean. Detailed results for all countries are provided in Annex Tables 2A-1 and 2A-2.

Among women in the United States as well as the Netherlands and Denmark, the pace of mortality decline at ages 65-79 slowed considerably in recent years: that is, they made smaller gains in 1980-2004 compared with 1955-1980. Such a slowdown is not evident among the other countries (except Canada). In the same way, at the oldest ages (80+), the pace of mortality decline decreased somewhat in Denmark, the Netherlands, and the United States while it increased dramatically in most other countries (again, with the exception of Canada). For example, among women in France and Japan, ages 80 and older contributed 0.6-0.8 years to gains in e_{50} during the period 1955-1980 (Table 2A-1), whereas the contribution grew to 1.7-2.7

---

[2]During 1955-1980, women in the United Kingdom made the smallest gains in e_{50} (2.2 years) among these 10 countries. Yet they achieved much faster gains since 1980 (4.0 years)—far above those of the United States, Denmark, and the Netherlands. Thus, British women appear to have followed a different pattern and have not diverged in recent years.

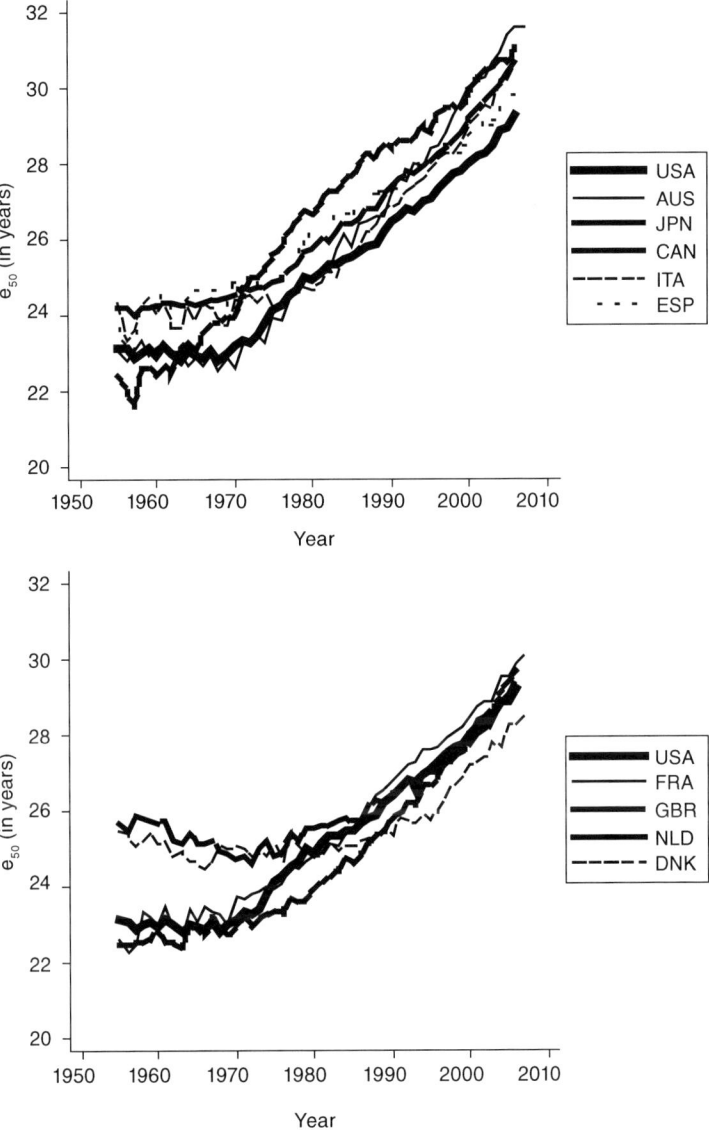

FIGURE 2-2 Annual trends in e_{50} by sex among 10 selected countries, men, 1955-2007.
NOTES: The United States is shown relative to the other countries (listed in rank order by level of e_{50} in 2006). AUS = Australia, CAN = Canada, DNK = Denmark, ESP = Spain, FRA = France, GBR = United Kingdom, ITA = Italy, JPN = Japan, NLD = the Netherlands, USA = United States.
SOURCE: Data from Human Mortality Database (2009 [accessed November 2009]).

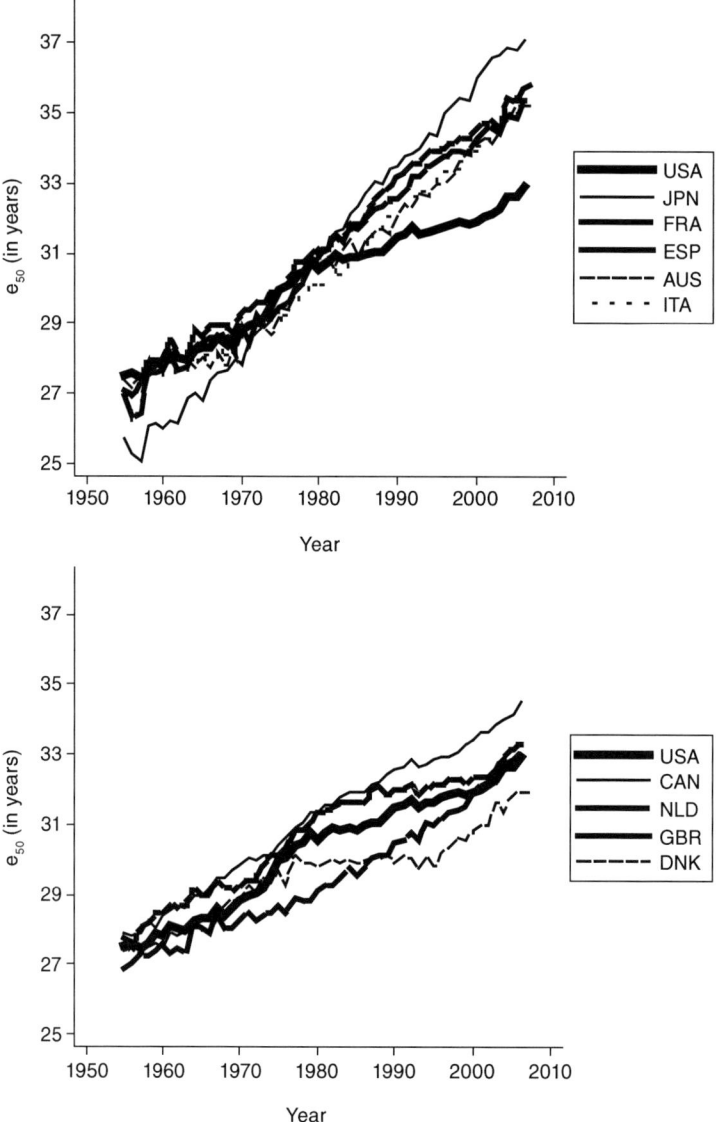

FIGURE 2-3 Annual trends in e_{50} by sex among 10 selected countries, women, 1955-2007.
NOTES: The United States is shown relative to the other countries (listed in rank order by level of e_{50} in 2006). AUS = Australia, CAN = Canada, DNK = Denmark, ESP = Spain, FRA = France, GBR = United Kingdom, ITA = Italy, JPN = Japan, NLD = the Netherlands, USA = United States.
SOURCE: Data from Human Mortality Database (2009 [accessed November 2009]).

TABLE 2-1 Life Expectancy at Age 50 (e_{50}) and Gains in e_{50}, Selected Countries, 1955-2006

	1955		1980		2006		Gain in e_{50}		
							1955-1980	1980-2006	Total (1955-2006)
	e_{50}	Rank	e_{50}	Rank	e_{50}	Rank			
Women									
AUS	27.4	5	30.7	6	35.3	4	3.3	4.6	7.9
CAN	27.9	1	31.3	1	34.5	6	3.5	3.2	6.7
DNK	27.4	4	29.8	9	31.9	10	2.4	2.1	4.5
FRA	27.1	6	31.1	3	35.7	2	4.0	4.5	8.6
ITA	27.1	7	30.0	8	35.2	5	2.9	5.2	8.1
JPN	25.7	10	30.8	5	37.1	1	5.1	6.3	11.4
NLD	27.7	2	31.3	2	33.3	7	3.6	2.0	5.6
ESP	27.0	8	31.0	4	35.4	3	4.0	4.4	8.4
GBR	26.9	9	29.1	10	33.1	8	2.2	4.0	6.2
USA	27.5	3	30.6	7	33.0	9	3.0	2.4	5.4
Mean[a] (all countries)	27.2		30.6		34.5		3.4	3.9	7.3
Excluding USA, DNK, and NLD	27.0		30.6		35.2		3.6	4.6	8.2
Composite[b] (all countries)	27.0		30.5		34.5		3.5	4.0	7.5
Excluding USA, DNK, and NLD	26.8		30.5		35.6		3.7	5.1	8.8
Men									
AUS	23.0	7	25.0	5	31.5	1	1.9	6.6	8.5
CAN	24.2	4	25.7	3	30.7	3	1.5	5.0	6.5
DNK	25.4	2	24.8	8	28.2	10	−0.7	3.5	2.8
FRA	22.6	8	24.8	7	29.9	6	2.2	5.1	7.3
ITA	24.3	3	24.7	9	30.6	4	0.3	5.9	6.2
JPN	22.4	10	26.6	1	31.0	2	4.2	4.4	8.6
NLD	25.7	1	25.5	4	29.4	8	−0.2	4.0	3.8
ESP	23.7	5	26.2	2	29.9	5	2.5	3.7	6.2
GBR	22.5	9	23.9	10	29.7	7	1.5	5.7	7.2
USA	23.1	6	24.9	6	29.2	9	1.8	4.3	6.1
Mean[a] (all countries)	23.7		25.2		30.0		1.5	4.8	6.3
Excluding USA, DNK, and NLD	23.2		25.3		30.5		2.0	5.2	7.2
Composite[b] (all countries)	23.1		25.1		30.0		2.0	4.8	6.8
Excluding USA, DNK, and NLD	23.0		25.3		30.5		2.3	5.2	7.5

[a]Based on the simple mean across countries.
[b]Data for various countries are aggregated before calculating death rates; thus, the results represent a weighted mean.
NOTE: AUS = Australia, CAN = Canada, DNK = Denmark, ESP = Spain, FRA = France, GBR = United Kingdom, ITA = Italy, JPN = Japan, NLD = the Netherlands, USA = United States.
SOURCE: Data from the Human Mortality Database, 2009 (accessed November 6, 2009).

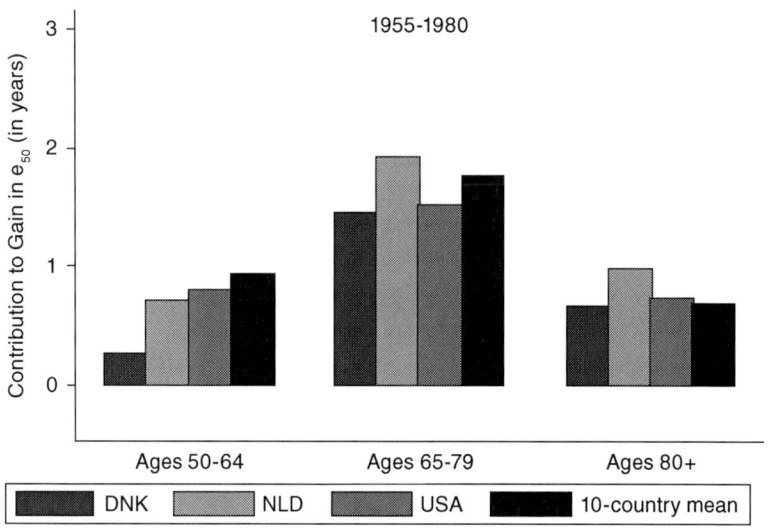

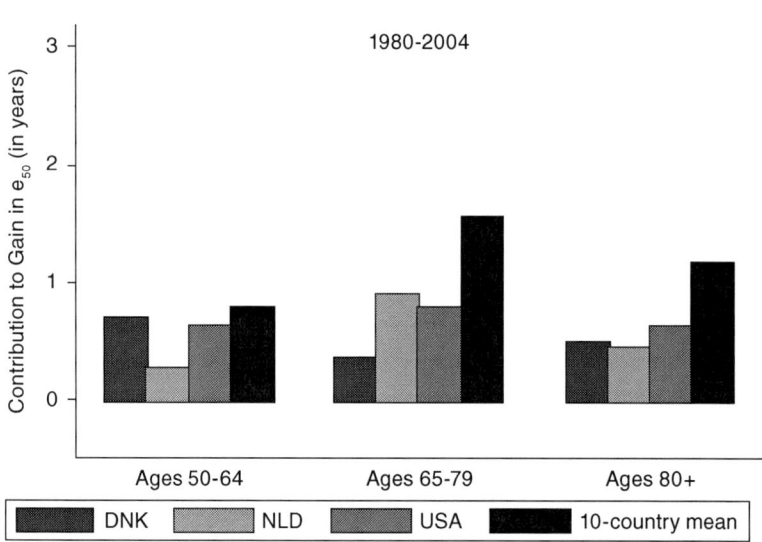

FIGURE 2-4 Age group contributions to gains in e_{50}, 1955-1980 and 1980-2004, women.
NOTE: DNK = Denmark, NLD = the Netherlands, USA = United States.
SOURCES: Calculations by authors based on data from the Human Mortality Database and the World Health Organization Mortality Database.

years during the period 1980-2004 (Table 2A-2). Thus, ages 65 and older account for the vast majority of the difference between the three laggards (Denmark, the Netherlands, United States) and the other countries: ages 65-79 because progress slowed in the former, but not the latter, and ages 80+ because the pace of mortality decline increased among the latter but not the former.

Figure 2-5 presents the corresponding results for men, who generally made faster gains in recent years across the age range in all countries. For Denmark, the Netherlands, and the United States during the period 1980-2004, the biggest sex difference occurs below age 80. For example, among these three countries, ages 50-79 contributed 2.6-3.3 years to gains in e_{50} for males during the period 1980-2004, whereas the corresponding contribution for women was only 1.1-1.4 years (Table 2A-3).

CAUSE-OF-DEATH DATA

Comparative analysis of cause-of-death trends is complicated by issues of variation in coding practice. There are two main problems: (1) accuracy of diagnosing cause of death and (2) changes in the classification system. Both can create artificial variation in cause-of-death statistics across time and place. (See the Annex for a more detailed discussion of these potential problems.) The intercountry disparities in ill-defined coding shown in Table 2A-3 could explain some of the disparities in other causes. Similarly, a shift in coding over time from ill-defined to other causes could create an artificial increase in the latter (or at least attenuate the true level of decline). Therefore, to improve comparability of the results across time and place, we have redistributed ill-defined deaths proportionately to all other cause groups. We made no other adjustments to the WHO cause-of-death data.

Trends in Mortality Rates by Cause of Death

Figures 2-6 and 2-7 show trends since 1980 in the age-standardized mortality rate (among women and men above age 50) for nine main groups of causes. One factor that might explain the slowed progress among women in the laggard countries is increased levels of smoking. Thus, we have isolated two groups of causes that are strongly associated with smoking: lung cancer and respiratory diseases.[3] If the smoking hypothesis has merit, then

---

[3]Previous research suggests that 75-90 percent of deaths from lung cancer and chronic pulmonary obstructive disease (COPD) are attributable to smoking (Royal College and Physicians of London, 2000; U.S. Department of Health and Human Services, 1989). The WHO data are not sufficiently detailed to identify COPD death for the entire period of this study. Nonetheless, among deaths at ages 50+ in 2003 in the 10-study countries, COPD comprised 38 percent of all deaths due to respiratory diseases.

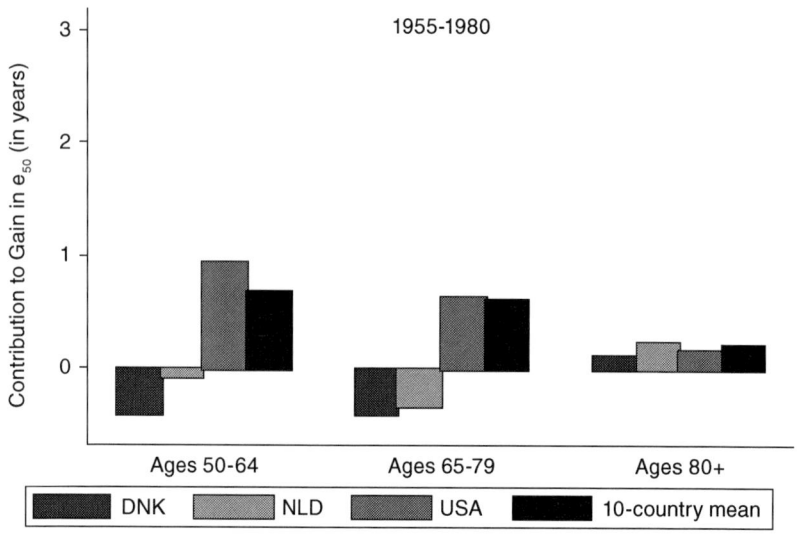
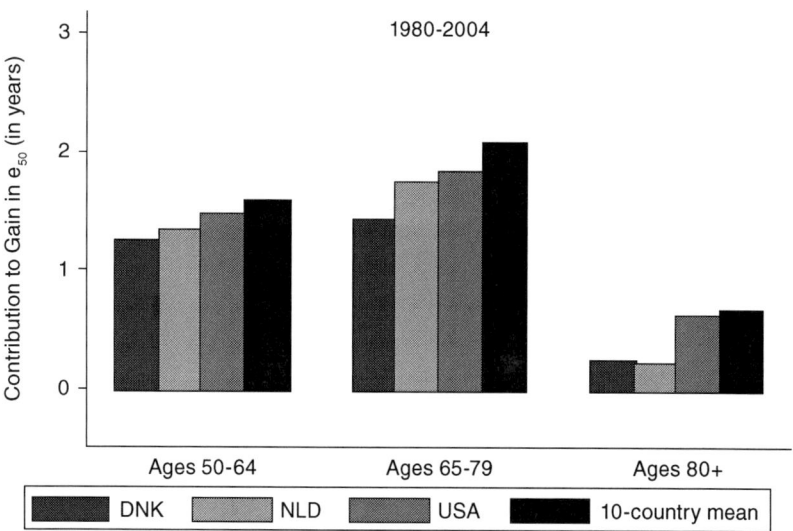

FIGURE 2-5 Age group contributions to gains in e_{50}, 1955-1980 and 1980-2004, men.
NOTE: DNK = Denmark, NLD = the Netherlands, USA = United States.
SOURCES: Calculations by authors based on data from the Human Mortality Database and the World Health Organization Mortality Database.

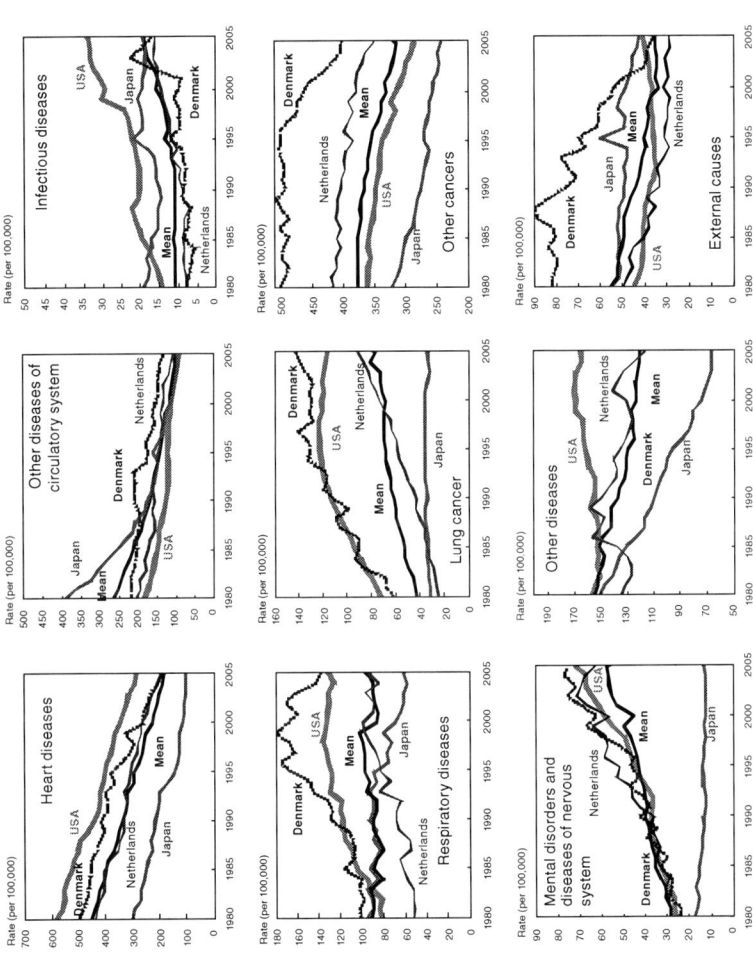

FIGURE 2-6 Age-standardized mortality rates among women ages 50 and older by cause group, United States compared with Denmark, the Netherlands, Japan, and the 10-country average, 1980-2005.
SOURCE: Calculations by authors based on data from the World Health Organization Mortality Database.

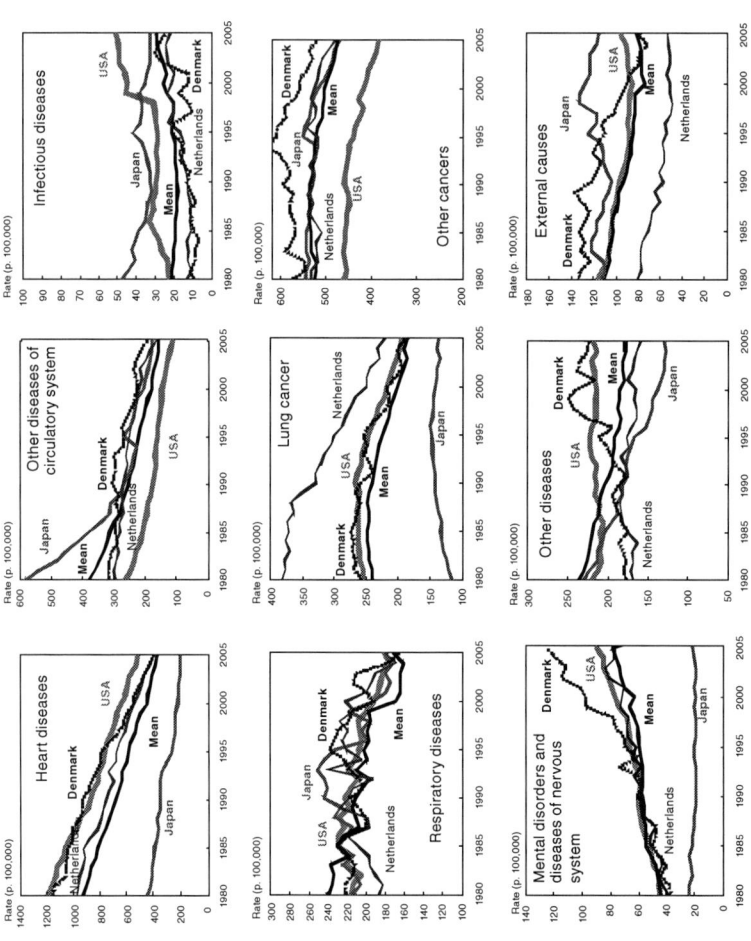

FIGURE 2-7 Age-standardized mortality rates among men ages 50 and older by cause group, United States compared with Denmark, the Netherlands, Japan, and the 10-country average, 1980-2005.
SOURCE: Calculations by authors based on data from the World Health Organization Mortality Database.

one would expect the mortality patterns for these two groups to parallel the divergence between women in the study countries. Of course, many smoking-related deaths are due to other causes. For example, research suggests that among men, 22 percent of deaths due to ischemic heart disease (IHD) are attributable to smoking. However, because IHD is one of the most common causes of death, it comprises a large number of smoking-related deaths—nearly as many as from lung cancer (Royal College of Physicians of London, 2000).

Heart diseases follow parallel trends: the United States shows the highest mortality but declines as quickly as in Denmark, Japan, the Netherlands, and the 10-country average (see Figure 2-6). Thus, heart diseases are not responsible for the diverging mortality trends among women. In contrast, women in the United States as well as the Netherlands and Denmark lost their initial advantage in terms of other circulatory diseases. Japan caught up very fast, and all four countries currently share similar levels. This is an important source of divergence. Men followed the same general pattern (see Figure 2-7).

Another shared cause of divergence among women relates to recent trends in both respiratory diseases and lung cancer. A sizeable mortality increase is observed for these two groups of causes in Denmark, the Netherlands, and the United States, whereas the 10-country mean remains more stable and trends in Japan are stable (lung cancer) or declining (respiratory diseases). Yet "other cancers" appear to follow parallel trends and thus cannot account for any diverging trends in mortality. The story is different among men. Respiratory diseases and other cancers generally follow parallel trends across countries, while lung cancer rates appear to have converged somewhat.

Prior to 2002, Denmark, the Netherlands, and the United States also shared a sharp increase in mortality due to mental disorders and diseases of the nervous system, which may have also contributed to divergence, since the corresponding increase was less pronounced for the 10-country mean and totally absent in Japan. This pattern appears to be similar in both sexes. This group of causes also clearly contributed to the recent progress among Dutch women, among whom mortality from these causes declined since 2002 while continuing to increase for their U.S. counterparts.

Finally, "other diseases" are also an important common source of divergence for Denmark, the Netherlands, and the United States (through 2002). Mortality for this mixed group of causes increased slightly in the United States and Denmark and remained relatively stable in the Netherlands, while it declined steadily for the 10-country average and even more rapidly in Japan. This group of diseases also appears to contribute to the 2002 reversal of Dutch mortality trends.

Cause-of-Death Contributions to Gains in Life Expectancy at e_{50}

Figures 2-8 and 2-9 show the contributions by cause of death to gains in e_{50} during the periods 1955-1980 and 1980-2004 for Denmark, the Netherlands, and the United States compared with the 10-country mean. We have grouped causes into seven categories.[4] Results for all countries and for more detailed causes appear in Annex Tables 2A-5 and 2A-6.

Among women, lung cancer mortality had a negative effect on e_{50} in both periods for these 10 countries on average, but especially for Denmark, the United States, and, in the later period, the Netherlands. Women in these three countries also fared worse against respiratory diseases: the 10-country mean contribution was positive in both periods, but the effect was negative in Denmark, the United States, and, since 1980, the Netherlands. Notably, although women in these countries experienced bigger losses from lung cancer since 1980, they generally fared as well or better against nonlung cancers.

Other causes have also begun to have a negative impact in many countries since 1980 (see Figure 2-9). Mortality due to mental disorders and diseases of the nervous system increased in virtually all countries between 1980 and 2004, but the biggest losses were observed among women in Canada, Denmark, the Netherlands, Spain, and the United States (see Table 2A-6). Also, since 1980, the mixed category of "other diseases" played a negative role for U.S. women and Danes of both sexes, whereas the 10-country mean was positive (see Figure 2-9).

Conversely, on the positive side, the reduction of heart disease mortality played an important role in all countries since 1980, no less so in the United States than in Japan, for example (see Table 2A-6). Nonetheless, progress against mortality from other circulatory diseases was much weaker in Denmark, the Netherlands, and the United States compared with the 10-country mean.

Within the Denmark, the Netherlands, and the United States since 1980, the most notable sex differences are for lung cancer and respiratory diseases: whereas these causes had a negative effect on e_{50} among women, the effect was positive for men (see Figure 2-9). Women in these countries also had somewhat bigger losses from mental disorders and diseases of the nervous system than their male compatriots. Although men made better progress than women against heart diseases, women did at least as well as men against other circulatory diseases and nonlung cancers.

---

[4]Two categories shown in Figures 2-6 and 2-7—infectious diseases and external causes—have been combined with the residual category of all other causes.

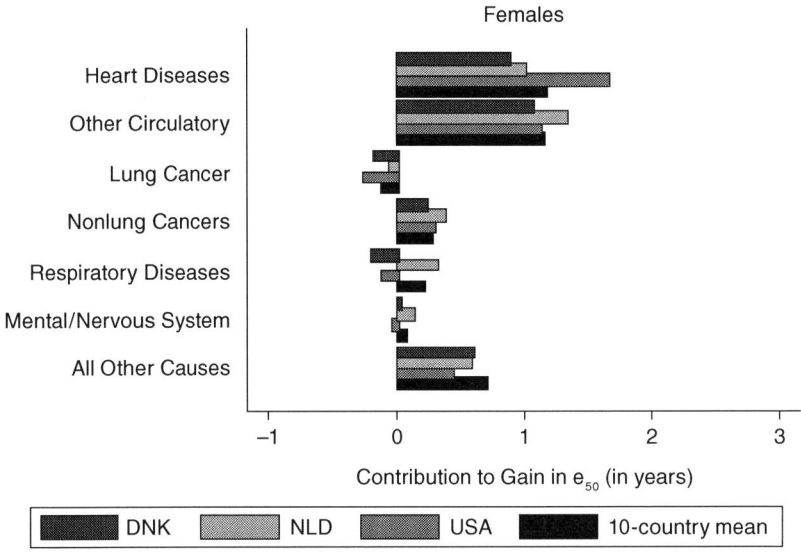
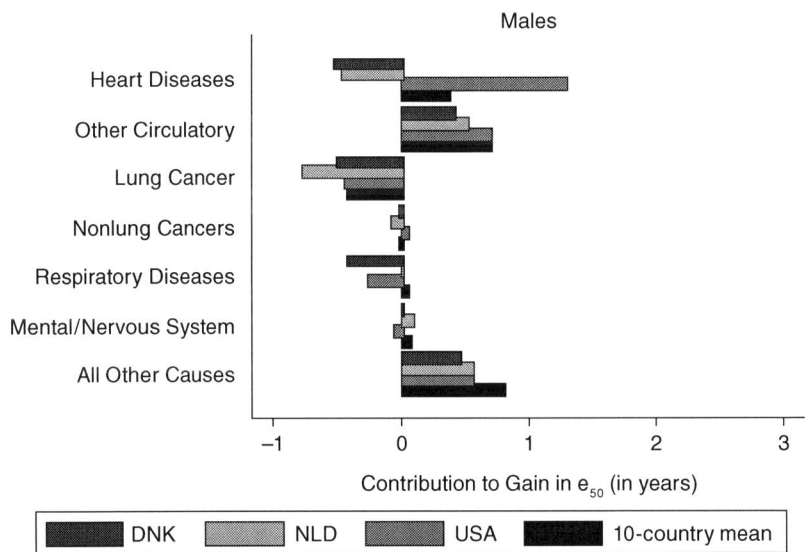

FIGURE 2-8 Contributions by cause of death to gain in e_{50}, 1955-1980.
NOTES: Deaths from ill-defined causes have been redistributed proportionately to all other categories. DNK = Denmark, NLD = the Netherlands, USA = United States.
SOURCES: Calculations by authors based on data from the Human Mortality Database and the World Health Organization Mortality Database.

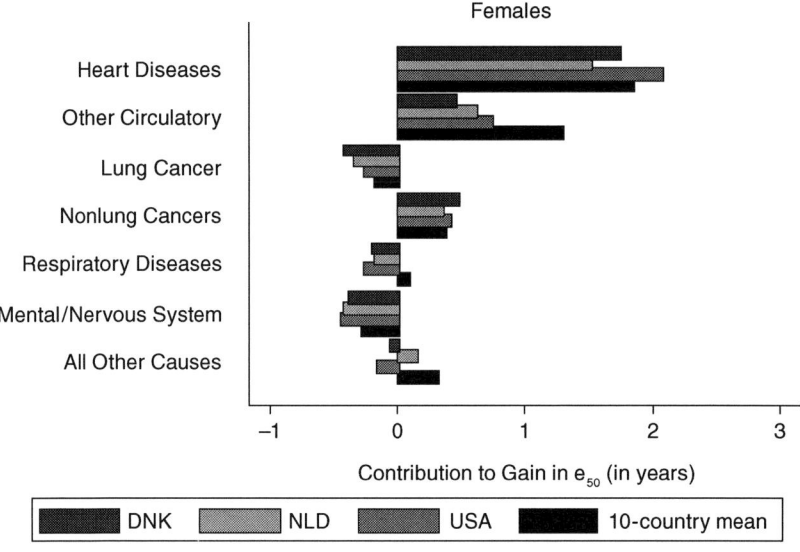
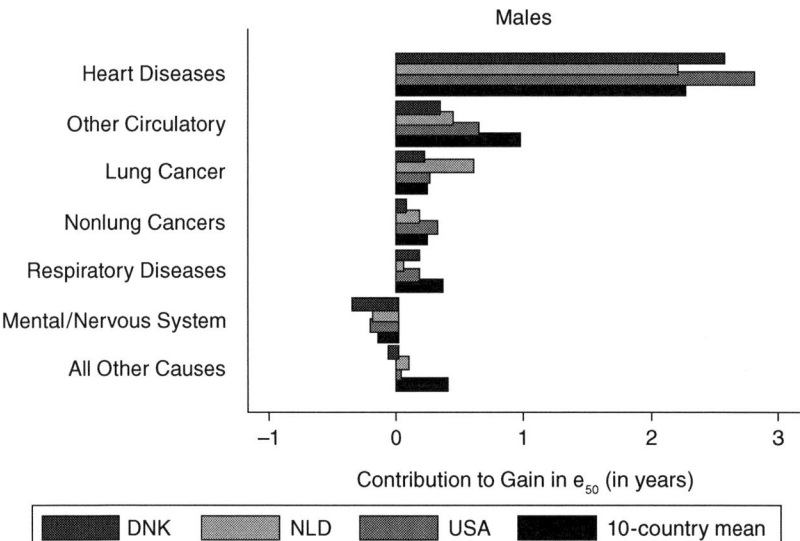

FIGURE 2-9 Contributions by cause of death to gain in e_{50}, 1980-2004.
NOTES: Deaths from ill-defined causes have been redistributed proportionately to all other categories. DNK = Denmark, NLD = the Netherlands, USA = United States.
SOURCES: Calculations by authors based on data from the Human Morality Database and the World Health Organization Mortality Database.

Recent Progress in Denmark and the Netherlands

Danish women resumed progress after the mid-1990s. Between 1980 and 1995, women in the United States made bigger gains in e_{50} than their Danish counterparts (1.1 versus 0.0 year, respectively). In contrast, since 1995 the Danes have fared better (2.1 years versus 1.0 in the United States). The recent progress among women in Denmark is evident for most causes except mental and nervous system diseases. In the 10-year period from 1995 to 2005, Danish women made greater gains than in the previous 15 years for heart diseases, other circulatory diseases, and other cancers and replaced losses with gains for other smoking-related cancers, breast cancer, respiratory diseases, and "all other causes" (see Figure 2-10). Whereas during the earlier period (1980-1995) U.S. women made bigger gains from heart diseases, other circulatory diseases, and breast cancer than their Danish counterparts, in the most recent period (1995-2005), women fared better in Denmark than in the United States against these same causes as well as other cancers and "all other causes."

Starting around 2002, women in the Netherlands also began to make faster gains in e_{50}. Whereas Dutch women did worse than their U.S. counterparts during the period 1980-2002 (1.0 versus 1.5 years gained, respectively), they did somewhat better during the period 2002-2005 (0.8 versus 0.5). Notably, women's e_{50} in the Netherlands increased by almost as much during the 4 years since 2002 as in the 22-year period from 1980 to 2002.

Compared with Denmark, recent gains in the Netherlands are of quite different origin. Since 2002, this country fared no better than the United States for heart diseases (see Figure 2-11). Dutch women also continued to exhibit losses due to lung cancer, other smoking-related cancers, and respiratory diseases, whereas their U.S. counterparts made small gains since 2002. Nonetheless, the Netherlands made bigger gains than the United States against several of the same causes that contributed to Denmark's recent advantage: other circulatory diseases, breast cancer, other cancers, and "all other causes." Unlike Denmark, they also began to convert their earlier losses for mental and nervous system diseases into gains, while the United States continued to make losses.

Compared with the United States, Denmark and the Netherlands appear to be two different cases. Figure 2-12 shows that age-specific contributions to female gains in e_{50} since 1980 were quite different in Denmark compared with the Netherlands and the United States. During the period in which gains in e_{50} were lagging (1980-1995), Denmark exhibited important losses at ages 60-74 while the Netherlands and the United States were still making progress at these ages. Conversely, when Denmark resumed gains in e_{50} after 1995, this progress was largely due to mortality decline at the same adult ages, whereas gains in the Netherlands and United States tended to

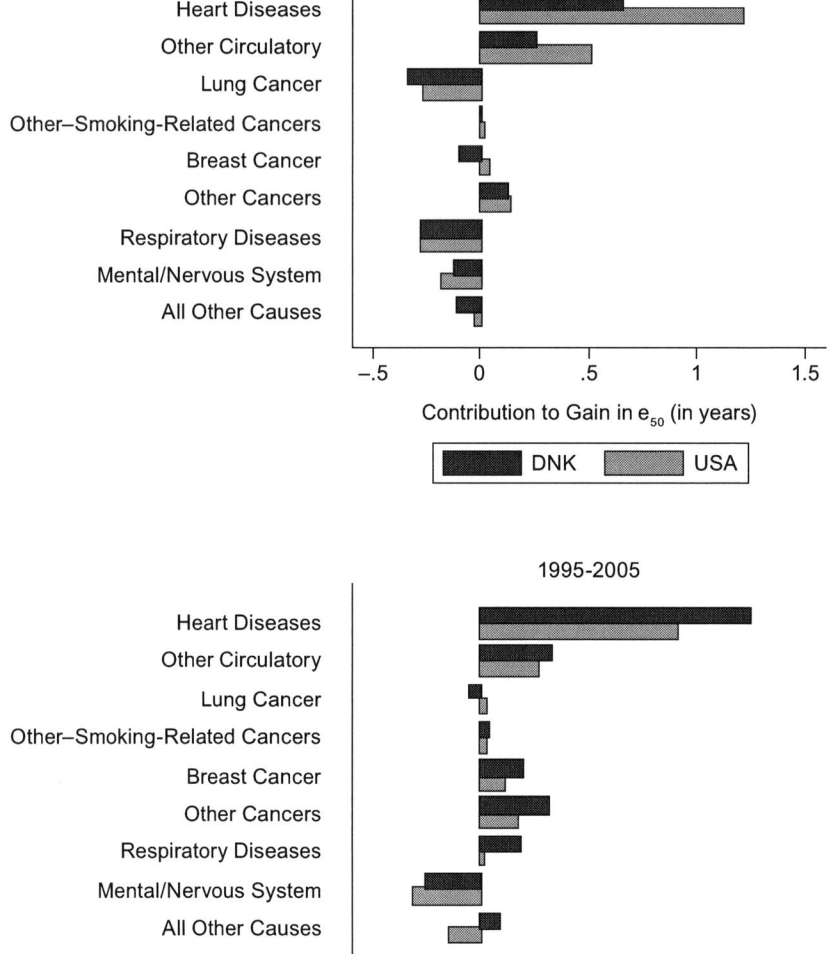

FIGURE 2-10 Cause-of-death contributions to female gains in e_{50} since 1980, Denmark and the United States.
NOTES: Deaths from ill-defined causes have been redistributed proportionately to all other categories. DNK = Denmark, USA = United States.
SOURCE: Calculations by authors based on data from the Human Mortality Database and the World Health Organization Mortality Database.

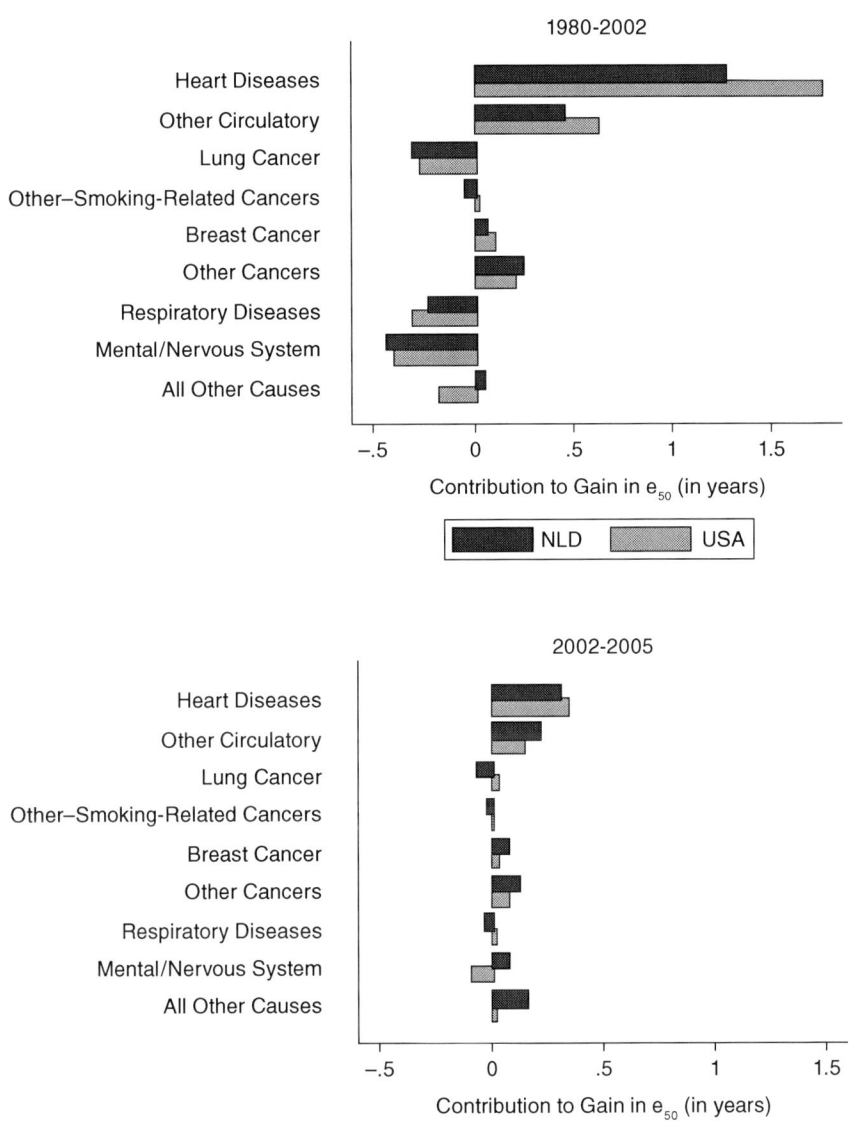

FIGURE 2-11 Cause-of-death contributions to female gains in e_{50} since 1980, the Netherlands and the United States.
NOTES: Deaths from ill-defined causes have been redistributed proportionately to all other categories. NLD = the Netherlands, USA = United States.
SOURCES: Calculations by authors based on data from the Human Mortality Database and the World Health Organization Mortality Database.

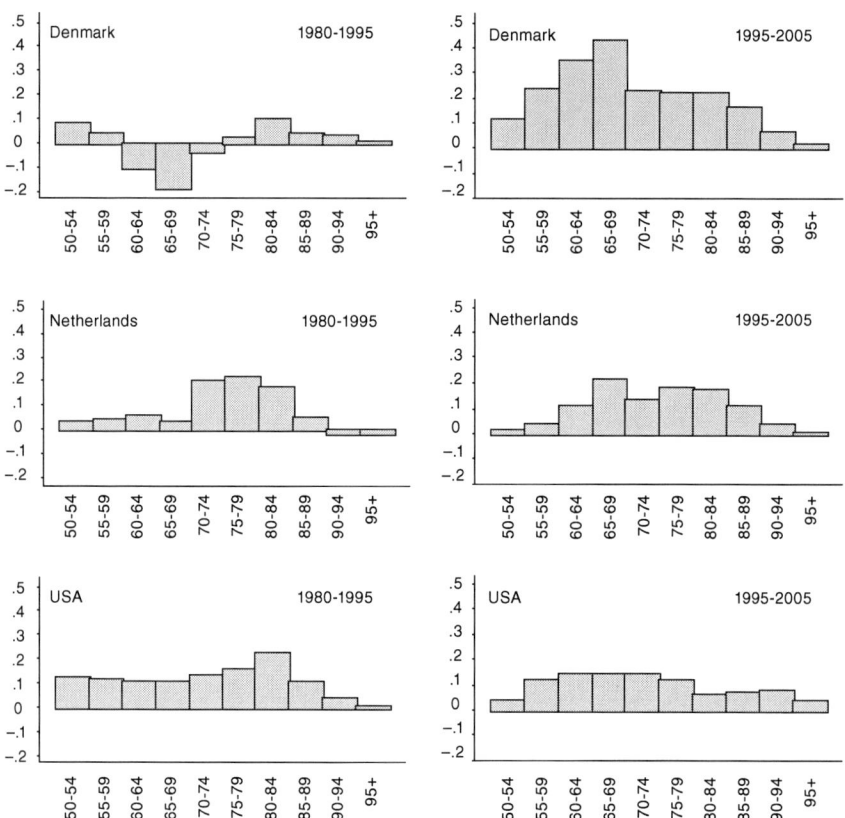

FIGURE 2-12 Age components of female gains in e_{50} since 1980, Denmark, the Netherlands, and the United States.
SOURCES: Calculations by authors based on data from the Human Mortality Database and the World Health Organization Mortality Database.

be distributed more evenly across all older ages. Further analyses among ages 60-74 during the period 1980-1995 (data not shown) indicate that Denmark suffered much bigger losses than the Netherlands and the United States due to smoking-related cancers, breast cancer, respiratory diseases, and digestive diseases. These same causes also appear to be the main source of the reversal since 1995: Denmark succeeded in converting losses into gains at ages 60-74 as mortality from these causes began to decline. Compared with the Netherlands and the United States, Denmark was late to join the cardiovascular revolution and the fight against "man-made diseases"[5]

---

[5] As defined by Omran in his "epidemiologic transition" theory (Omran, 1971).

but is now completing this main step of the health transition (Vallin and Meslé, 2004). The current lagging of the Netherlands and the United States, compared with leaders like France and Japan, could be more related to a third step of the health transition, pertaining to the ability to fight old-age pathologies (Meslé and Vallin, 2006). For that reason, it is interesting to focus on a comparison of the United States with France, Japan, and the Netherlands.

A SPECIAL FOCUS ON RECENT TRENDS IN U.S. FEMALE MORTALITY COMPARED WITH FRANCE, JAPAN, AND THE NETHERLANDS

We further explore the age and cause-specific contributions to changes in life expectancy at old ages among women in four countries: two laggards, the Netherlands and the United States, and two leaders, France and Japan. We concentrate here on ages above 65, which accounted for the vast majority of divergence among women (see Figure 2-4). We also tried to take into account some more detailed causes, such as mental disorders, which were subsumed within a broader category above (mental disorders and nervous system diseases).[6] These more detailed analyses build on previous work focusing on the same four countries between 1984 and 2000 (see Meslé and Vallin, 2006), updated here through 2005.

Figure 2-13 displays the impact on life expectancy at age 65 (e_{65}) of mortality changes for age groups 65-69, . . . 90-94, 95+. The left panel displays gains for the entire period 1984-2005, and the right panel shows two graphs for 1984-2002 and 2002-2005, respectively. From 1984 to 2005, both the Netherlands and the United States gained less than 1.3 years of female life expectancy at age 65, whereas France gained 3.3 years and Japan gained 4.5 years. In every age group, French and Japanese gains are higher than those in the Netherlands and the United States, although they are closer at ages 65-69. At ages 90 and older, the United States fared worse than France and Japan, but the Netherlands did the worst, making no gain at the oldest ages. Interestingly, Japan was the only country that achieved notable gains at the oldest ages (95+).

---

[6]Since ICD-9, Alzheimer's disease (AD) has been included with diseases of the nervous system. For 2002 and 2005, during which all four countries were using the International Classification of Diseases, version 10 (ICD-10), we have included deaths due to AD with mental disorders. However, we do not have sufficiently detailed data to identify AD deaths in 1984, when these countries were using ICD-9. Consequently, some of the apparent increase in mortality due to mental disorders implied by Figures 2-14 and 2-15 may be a statistical artifact resulting from the fact that deaths coded to AD are included with mental disorders in 2002 and 2005 but not in 1984. In 1984, AD deaths remain in the residual category of "other diseases." However, such an artifact cannot impact results much, because at the time AD was rarely registered as a primary cause of death.

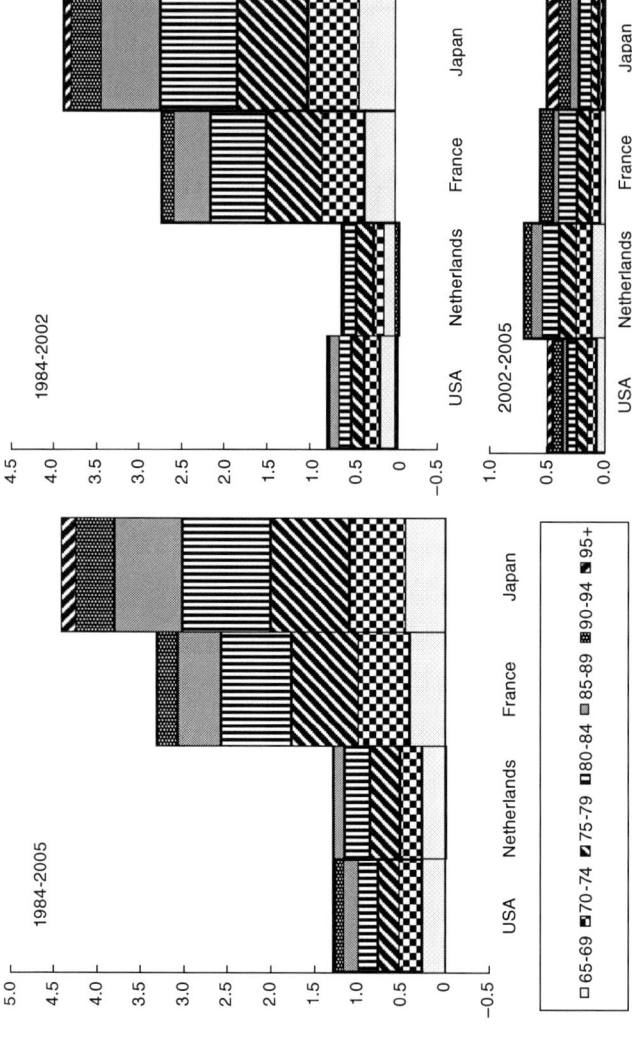

FIGURE 2-13 Age contributions to gains in e_{65} among women in the United States, the Netherlands, France, and Japan in two recent periods, 1984-2002 and 2002-2005.
SOURCES: Calculations by authors based on data from the Human Mortality Database; the World Health Organization Mortality Database; National Center for Health Statistics (1987, Table 8.5); Vallin and Meslé (1988, 1998); Institut National d'Études Démographiques (see http://www-causfra.ined.fr [accessed January 2009]); electronic files from CepiDc INSERM; Statistics and Information Department (1984, Tables 1 and 2); Statistics Netherlands (1984; data provided by Fanny Janssen of the University of Groningen); and Meslé and Vallin (2006).

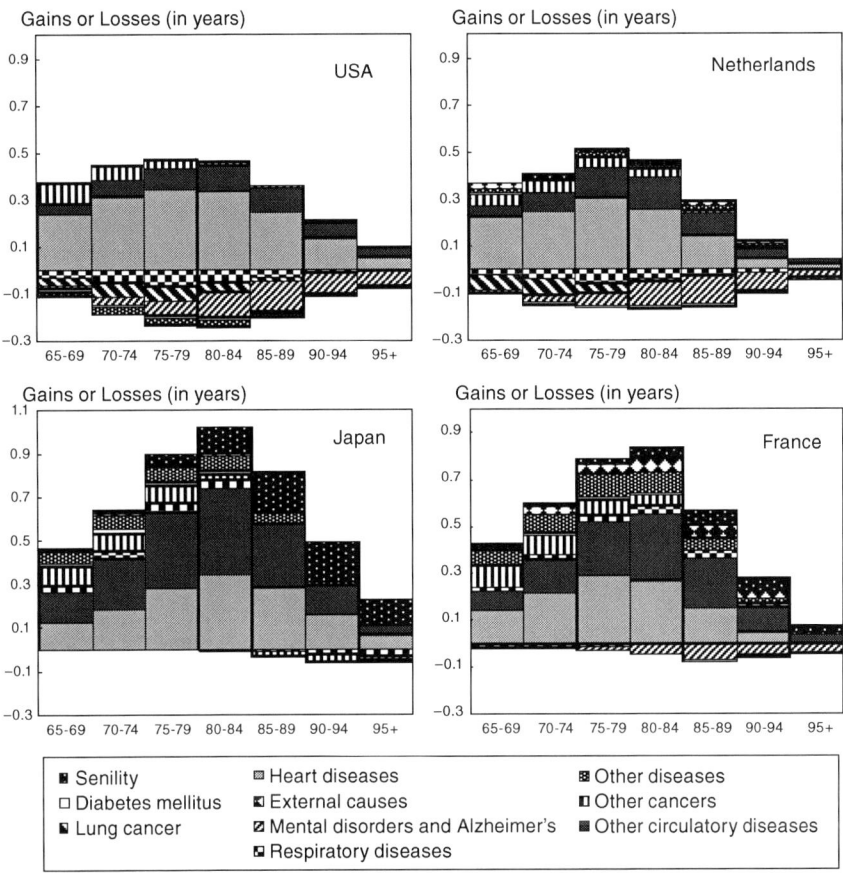

FIGURE 2-14 Age and cause contributions to gains in e_{65} among women in the United States, the Netherlands, France, and Japan, 1984-2005.
NOTES: Deaths due to Alzheimer's disease are included with mental disorders for 2005 but not in 1984. Thus, the losses attributed to this category are probably slightly overstated (see also footnote 7). Senility is separated from other ill-defined causes, which were redistributed proportionately to the other cause groups.
SOURCES: Calculations by authors based on data from the Human Mortality Database; the World Health Organization Mortality Database; National Center for Health Statistics (1987, Table 8.5); Vallin and Meslé (1988, 1998); Institut National d'Études Démographiques (see http://www-causfra.ined.fr [accessed January 2009]); electronic files from CepiDc INSERM; Statistics and Information Department (1984, Tables 1 and 2); Statistics Netherlands (1984; data provided by Fanny Janssen of the University of Groningen); and Meslé and Vallin (2006).

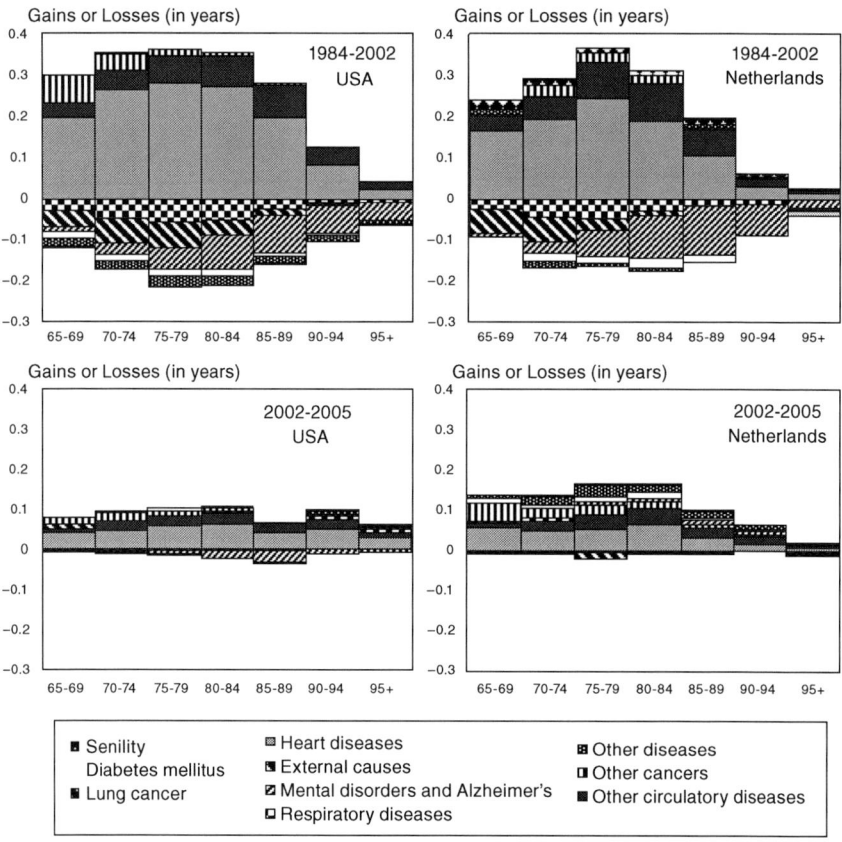

FIGURE 2-15 Age and cause contributions to gains in e_{65} among women in the United States and the Netherlands in two recent periods, 1984-2002 and 2002-2005.

NOTES: Deaths due to Alzheimer's disease are included with mental disorders for 2005 but not in 1984. Thus, the losses attributed to this category are probably slightly overstated (see also footnote 7). Senility is separated from other ill-defined causes, which were redistributed proportionately to the other cause groups.

SOURCES: Calculations by authors based on data from the Human Mortality Database; the World Health Organization Mortality Database; National Center for Health Statistics (1987, Table 8.5); Vallin and Meslé (1988, 1998); Institut National d'Études Démographiques (see http://www-causfra.ined.fr [accessed January 2009]); electronic files from CepiDc INSERM; Statistics and Information Department (1984, Tables 1 and 2); Statistics Netherlands (1984; data provided by Fanny Janssen of the University of Groningen); and Meslé and Vallin (2006).

When dividing the period into two subperiods to take into account the positive changes observed in the Netherlands since 2002, the disadvantaged position of that country for the period 1984-2002 is even more obvious. During that period, Dutch women gained even less than their U.S. counterparts, in particular because of the very tiny gain at ages 85-89 and increased mortality at ages 90-94.

Conversely, from 2002 to 2005, women in the Netherlands made bigger gains in e_{65} than the other three. Japan's only advantage during this short recent period was a larger contribution at age 90+, especially at the oldest ages (95+). Interestingly, the United States also demonstrated a non-negligible impact of mortality decline at ages 95+.

Figure 2-14 displays the respective impact of cause- and age-specific mortality changes over the entire 1984-2005 period in each of the four countries, and Figure 2-15 compares the United States and the Netherlands for the two subperiods. From 1984 to 2005, once again, gains in France and especially Japan are very impressive when compared with both the United States and the Netherlands, where smaller gains are offset by sizeable losses. But the differential impact of causes by age is even more remarkable.

First, whereas in France and Japan, very few age groups exhibit the negative effect of some causes, the impact of which is also very small, the United States and the Netherlands are hit by mortality increases for several causes across all age groups accumulating into substantial losses. The greatest negative impact is due to mental disorders (including AD). At age 85-89, for example, mortality increase for that cause is responsible for about 0.2 years of life expectancy loss at age 65 in both the United States and the Netherlands. Similar losses of 0.1 to 0.2 years are observed for all age groups from 75 to 95, whereas France shows smaller losses and Japan displays no losses from this cause. Total losses due to that cause are half a year in the United States and 0.4 year in the Netherlands, but only 0.2 in France and and even smaller (but positive) in Japan. Admittedly, these intercountry differences may be affected by variations in coding practice.[7]

Respiratory diseases are the second source of losses to e_{65} in the United States and the Netherlands, whereas they contributed some gains in France and Japan. In total, they reduced e_{65} among U.S. and Dutch women by 0.2 year, opposed to an increase of 0.1 in Japan and France.

Almost as important as respiratory diseases, lung cancer is the third source of losses in the United States and the Netherlands (−0.2 year in both

---

[7]As noted earlier, the exclusion of AD deaths in 1984 means that the losses attributed to mental disorders (including AD) are probably overstated. However, if some AD deaths were misclassified as dementia (under mental disorders) in 1984, then it would attenuate this bias. If this type of misclassification was more common in country X than country Y, then the losses due to mental disorders will be overstated, more so for the latter than for the former.

cases), while having virtually no effect in France and Japan. The difference between losses caused by lung cancer and mental disorders observed in the United States and the Netherlands is that the lung cancer impact comes mainly from ages 65-84, whereas that of mental disorders comes mainly from the oldest ages (especially 80+). The negative effects of respiratory diseases are more concentrated in the intermediate ages (70-84).

The second difference between the United States and the Netherlands on one hand, and France and Japan on the other, is that for the former two countries, most gains are due to the decline of heart diseases, while France and Japan enjoyed greater declines in mortality from other diseases of the circulatory system.

Senility also makes an important contribution to gains in e_{65} for France and especially Japan, but not for the United States or the Netherlands because they rarely use this International Classification of Diseases (ICD) code as an underlying cause. Redistributing senility proportionately, as we do for the other ill-defined causes, would mainly increase the positive impact of declines in cardiovascular mortality for France and Japan while being neutral in the two other countries. Yet such redistribution would be inappropriate, because senility is much more related to mental disorders than any other cause (Meslé, 2006). Thus, a more appropriate redistribution of senility would create a positive impact for mental disorders in Japan and change its negative effect into a positive one in France.

Furthermore, France and Japan differ substantially from the Netherlands and the United States in terms of the positive effects of other causes. Compared with the latter two countries, the former benefit from greater reductions in diabetes (especially Japan) and in causes that are here grouped as "other diseases." The latter group contributes an additional 0.4 year of female life expectancy at age 65 in France and more than 0.3 in Japan versus 0.1 in the Netherlands and –0.1 in the United States.

The great similarity observed between the United States and the Netherlands when considering the whole period 1984-2005 must be nuanced by taking into account the very recent change observed in the Netherlands. Figure 2-15 compares two subperiods (1984-2002 and 2002-2005). In spite of the great difference in length between these two periods, the comparison enlightens some features that could be important for the future.

Naturally, the upper part of Figure 2-15 is largely similar to Figure 2-14 for the two countries, but some notable details appear when comparing the two periods. First, the negative effect of lung cancer, quite important in the first period, almost vanished in the second one. From that point of view, the United States did even better than the Netherlands since 2002: lung cancer had a negative effect only in the latter country. Second, the negative effect of diabetes, quite visible in the first period, disappears in the United States and becomes positive in the Netherlands. But the most important fact is that the large negative effect of mental disorders, which was even greater for the Netherlands than the United States during the first period, disappears in the Netherlands during the second period but remains negative in the United States. In general, a greater diversity of causes accounts for Dutch gains since 2002, unlike the relatively monotonous (cardiovascular) source of progress in the United States.

Two main conclusions can be drawn from this special focus on four countries. First, for about 20 years the United States and the Netherlands encountered very similar difficulties in terms of cause patterns and trends in mortality and it would be very useful to know if some common facts in social development and public health were involved, or if the same results occurred from quite different causes. Second, if the Netherlands resumed progress within the past 4 years, it is because they were more successful in fighting diseases like mental disorders, diabetes, and "other diseases." Third, it must be underlined that the United States also achieved some important success in the recent period by eliminating several negative effects (especially from lung cancer, infectious and respiratory diseases, and diabetes), which gives some hope for the future. It remains to be seen whether those former negative effects can be converted into positive effects in the future.

DISCUSSION

In this chapter, we explore which age groups and which causes of death account for the post-1980 slowdown in mortality decline among women in Denmark, the Netherlands, and the United States. The results suggest that compared with the earlier period (1955-1980), these countries made smaller gains at ages 65-79 in particular and slower progress against all causes except heart diseases and nonlung cancers.

Since 1980, women in these three countries made smaller gains in e_{50} than their counterparts in other countries. These differences appear to stem from smaller gains at ages 65 and older, especially at the oldest ones (75+), and weaker progress against other circulatory diseases, respiratory diseases, lung cancer, and the residual category of other remaining causes. In contrast, they generally fared as well as other countries against heart diseases and nonlung cancers.

Interestingly, women in Denmark, the Netherlands, and the United States also made much smaller post-1980 gains in e_{50} than their male compatriots. This female disadvantage results from smaller gains at ages below 80 and less progress against lung cancer, respiratory diseases, heart diseases, and mental disorders, and diseases of the nervous system. Yet within these three countries, women fared as well or better than their male counterparts against other circulatory diseases and nonlung cancers, especially those less affected by smoking.

The common denominator for all of these comparisons is that since 1980 women in Denmark, the Netherlands, and the United States have exhibited bigger increases in mortality due to lung cancer and respiratory diseases compared with the earlier period (1955-1980), compared with their counterparts in other countries, and compared with their male compatriots. While this analysis identifies cause-of-death categories that underlie the mortality trends, we can only speculate about the causal factors that explain these differences. Based on the evidence presented here, the most obvious explanation for the slowing of mortality decline among women in Denmark, the Netherlands, and the United States is smoking, which is strongly correlated with lung cancer and such respiratory diseases as chronic obstructive pulmonary disease. Moreover, the fact that the differences in mortality decline occur not only between countries but also between men and women within the same country suggests that the main explanation pertains to factors that may differ by sex in the same social environment. There are clear sex differences in smoking patterns, with declines in smoking occurring earlier among men than among women (Forey et al., 2007).

However, when using more detailed causes of death among four countries, other important features appear. First, when mental disorders, including Alzheimer's disease, are isolated from other diseases of the nervous system, this category is an important source of contrast between the United States and the Netherlands on one hand and France and Japan on the other. That difference is reinforced when isolating senility. If this specific category is proportionally redistributed among "true" causes of death (as for other ill-defined causes), the greatest part is attributed to cardiovascular causes. Actually, we would argue that a greater proportion should be attributed to mental disorders (Meslé, 2006). Because reductions in senility are a bigger contributor to gains in France and Japan compared with the United States and the Netherlands, we may underestimate the true contrast between these countries in terms of mental disorders.

A secondary goal we posed at the outset was to investigate why women in Denmark and more recently the Netherlands have resumed progress while U.S. women have not. In fact, Denmark and the Netherlands are quite different cases in terms of timing and cause-of-death patterns. The stagnation of Danish life expectancy started much earlier and also ended earlier (1995 instead of 2002). And in terms of causes of death, after 1960, Denmark was more comparable to Eastern European countries than to Western ones in showing difficulty in overcoming the "age of degenerative diseases and man-made diseases" described by Omran (1971). This country was late entering the "cardiovascular revolution" (Vallin and Meslé, 2001, 2004). Actually, Denmark fully entered this step of the health transition in 1995. Its trajectory is hardly comparable to that of the United States, which entered it as soon as the late 1960s, like most Western countries.

The comparison between the Netherlands and the United States is much more informative, since the two countries followed quite similar cause-of-death trends and patterns until the early 2000s. Yet we must rely on a very short period to appreciate the causes of the recent Dutch reversal. Nevertheless, some features appear that may have consequences for the future. Indeed, the United States also made some progress in very recent years for lung cancer and diabetes. In fact, it did even better than the Netherlands in terms of lung cancer. The somewhat greater success of the Netherlands in terms of overall gains in female life expectancy at old ages mainly relies on two facts: (1) changes in mortality from mental disorders turned from important losses into significant gains and (2) it made greater gains than the United States against some other causes of death, including diabetes.

Admittedly, this study is not without limitations. Although mortality data tend to be more reliable than other kinds of data (e.g., estimates of morbidity based on clinical diagnoses, self-reports of health status), there can still be data quality problems, such as incomplete coverage and age misreporting. In particular, previous studies suggest problems of age exaggeration in the historical data for the United States (Coale and Kisker, 1986, 1990; Elo and Preston, 1994; Preston, Elo, and Stewart, 1999). Thus, estimates of life expectancy at the oldest ages may have been overestimated in previous years, and the apparent slowing of mortality decline among women in the United States could actually be a statistical artifact resulting from improvements in data quality. Yet it seems unlikely that such a problem would affect women but not men; moreover, it would not explain the similar slowing of mortality decline among women in Denmark and the Netherlands, where data quality is very high (Meslé and Vallin, 2006). The Social Security Administration (SSA) in the United States provides alternative estimates of mortality and life expectancy; for ages 65 and older, it uses estimates based on Medicare data. Its estimates of mortality at the oldest ages (90+) tend to be higher than those given in the HMD (U.S. Social Security Administration, 2009). Nonetheless, the SSA estimates for e_{50} in 1955, 1980, and 2004 would suggest that the slowing of gains in e_{50} among U.S. women were even worse than the HMD data would suggest, especially for the period 1980-2004.

The comparability of cause-of-death data may also be comprised by variation in coding practice across time and place. We noted such a problem for AD (see the Annex). By combining mental disorders with diseases of the nervous system, we eliminated most of the discontinuities at changes in the ICD. Nonetheless, it is unclear whether the increase in mortality from this group of causes observed during 1980-2004 among virtually all countries is real or whether it is simply an artifact of changes in coding practice over time (Meslé and Vallin, 2006). A more precise comparison was made by focusing on four countries (France, Japan, the Netherlands, the United States) in which we could isolate mental disorders (including Alzheimer's disease for the most recent period covered by ICD-10). Nonetheless, some difficulty remains regarding how to handle senility. If we accept the idea that this ICD code should be disproportionately attributed to "mental disorders," it could widen the gap in mental disorders among these four countries (i.e., France and Japan would have greater gains against these causes). We think that proportional redistribution of senility underestimates the role played by mental disorders, but we do not know by how much. Furthermore, given evidence of shifts in coding for respiratory diseases, it is possible that we have overestimated the contribution of this category to post-1980 gains in Canada, France, and the United Kingdom (see the Annex). Nonetheless, we observed notable gains from respiratory diseases among women in several other countries that contrast with the losses found among women in Denmark, the Netherlands, and the United States.

In sum, the evidence presented here is consistent with the hypothesis that smoking was an important factor accounting for the slowing of mortality decline among women in these three countries. If so, when smoking ceases to rise, then the rate of mortality decline may return to normal; if smoking declines, then it may begin to catch up. Yet we see little evidence that recent progress among women in Denmark and the Netherlands is due to declines in smoking. Still, the lag between smoking behavior and its health consequences means the full benefits of a decline in smoking will not be realized until several decades later. Moreover, countries in which smoking continues to increase among women may in future years reveal the negative effects and perhaps a slowing of mortality decline. Nonetheless, smoking is probably not the only cause of divergence between the United States or the Netherlands and the other countries. More detailed analyses suggest that mental disorders could also be playing a role. Since 2002, e_{50} among Dutch women resumed a steady increase, in part because they succeeded in replacing losses with gains in the field of mental disorders and other smaller causes of death.

ACKNOWLEDGMENTS

This project received financial support from the National Institute on Aging (grant R01 AG11552) and from Institut National d'Études Démographiques (INED research project no. P-05-3-7). We thank Sam Preston, Eileen Crimmins, and Johan Mackenbach for their comments and suggestions regarding this paper.

REFERENCES

Anderson, R.N., Miniño, A.M., Hoyert, D.L., and Rosenberg, H.M. (2001). *Comparability of Cause of Death Between ICD-9 and ICD-10: Preliminary Estimates*. (National Vital Statistics Reports, vol. 49, no. 2.) Hyattsville, MD: National Center for Health Statistics.

Armstrong, D.L., Wing, S.B., and Tyroler, H.A. (1995). United States mortality from ill-defined causes, 1968-1988: Potential effects on heart disease mortality trends. *International Journal of Epidemiology*, 24(3), 522-527.

Coale, A.J., and Kisker, E.E. (1986). Mortality crossovers: Reality or bad data? *Population Studies*, 49, 389-401.

Coale, A.J., and Kisker, E.E. (1990). Defects in data on old-age mortality in the United States. *Asian and Pacific Population Forum*, 4(1), 1-31.

Elo, I.T., and Preston, S.H. (1994). Estimating African-American mortality from inaccurate data. *Demography*, 31(3), 427-458.

Forey, B., Hamling, J., Hamling, J., and Lee, P. (2007). *International Smoking Statistics, Web Edition: A Collection of Worldwide Historical Data. Comparisons Between Countries*. Sutton, England: P. N. Lee Statistics and Computing Ltd.

Human Mortality Database. (2009). *University of California, Berkeley (USA), and Max Planck Institute for Demographic Research (Germany)*. Available http://www.mortality.org [accessed November 2009].

Janssen, F., and Kunst, A.E. (2004). ICD coding changes and discontinuities in trends in cause-specific mortality in six European countries, 1950-99. *Bulletin of the World Health Organization*, 82(12), 904-913.

Mathers, C.D., Fat, D.M., Inoue, M., Rao, C., and Lopez, A.D. (2005). Counting the dead and what they died from: An assessment of the global status of cause of death data. *Bulletin of the World Health Organization*, 83(3), 171-177.

Meslé, F. (2006). Causes of death among the oldest-old: Validity and comparability. In J. Robine, E.M. Crimmins, S. Horiuchi, and Y. Zheng (Eds.), *Human Longevity, Individual Life Duration, and the Growth of the Oldest-Old Population* (pp. 191-214). Dordrecht, The Netherlands: Springer.

Meslé, F., and Vallin, J. (2006). Diverging trends in female old-age mortality: The United States and the Netherlands versus France and Japan. *Population and Development Review*, 31(1), 123-145.

National Center for Health Statistics. (1987). *Vital Statistics of the United States 1984*. (Volume II, Mortality, Part B.) Hyattsville, MD: U.S. Department of Health and Human Services, Public Health Service.

Office of Population Censuses and Surveys. (1995). *Mortality Statistics: Causes 1993/1994*. London, England: Author.

Omran, A.R. (1971). The epidemiological transition: A theory of the epidemiology of population change. *Milbank Memorial Fund Quarterly*, 49(4), 509-538.

Pollard, J.H. (1988). On the decomposition of changes in expectation of life and differentials in life expectancy. *Demography*, 25(2), 265-276.

Preston, S.H., Elo, I.T., and Stewart, Q. (1999). Effects of age misreporting on mortality estimates at older ages. *Population Studies*, 53(2), 165-177.

Royal College of Physicians of London. (2000). *Nicotine Addiction in Britain*. London, England: Author.

Statistics and Information Department. (1984). *Vital Statistics 1984 Japan*. (Volume 3.) Tokyo, Japan: Ministry of Health and Welfare.

Statistics Canada. (2005). *Comparability of ICD-10 and ICD-9 for Mortality Statistics in Canada*. (Catalogue No. 84-548-XIE, Bridge-Coding Studies.) Ottawa: Minister of Industry.

Statistics Netherland. (1984). *Deaths by Cause of Death* [in Dutch]. Voorburg/Heerlen: Author.

U.S. Department of Health and Human Services. (1989). *Reducing the Health Consequences of Smoking: 25 Years of Progress. A Report of the Surgeon General.* (DHHS Publication CDC 89-8411.) Rockville, MD: Centers for Disease Control and Prevention, Center for Chronic Disease Prevention and Health Promotion, Office on Smoking and Health.

U.S. Social Security Administration. (2009). *United States Life Table Functions and Actuarial Functions at 2.9 Percent Interest Based on the Alternative 2 Mortality Probabilities Used in the 2008 Trustees Report.* Unpublished manuscript.

Vallin, J., and Meslé, F. (1988). *Les Causes de Décès en France de 1925 à 1978.* Paris: Institut National d'Études Démographiques.

Vallin, J., and Meslé, F. (1998). Comment suivre l'évolution de la mortalité par cause malgré les discontinuities de la statistique. Le cas de la France de 1925 à 1993. In G. Pavillon (Ed.), *Enjeux des Classifications Internationales en Santé* (pp. 113-156). Paris: Éditions INSERM.

Vallin, J., and Meslé, F. (2001). Trends in mortality in Europe since 1950: Age-, sex- and cause-specific mortality. In J. Vallin, F. Meslé, and T. Valkonen (Eds.), *Trends in Mortality and Differential Mortality* (pp. 131-186). Strasbourg, France: Council of Europe.

Vallin, J., and Meslé, F. (2004). Convergences and divergences in mortality. A new approach to health transition. *Demographic Research, Special Collection,* 2(Article 2), 12-44.

World Bank. (1976). *World Tables 1976.* Washington, DC: Author.

World Bank. (2008). *2008 World Development Indicators.* Washington, DC: Author.

World Health Organization. (2009). *Detailed Data Files of the WHO Mortality Database.* Available http://www.who.int/whosis/mort/download/en/index.htm [accessed December 2009].

ANNEX 2A

Detailed Age Group Contributions to Gains in e_{50}

The decomposition by age group uses death rates from the HMD (2009). We use the Pollard (1988) method to decompose the gains in e_{50} into the contributions by age (see Tables 2A-1 and 2A-2).

Variation in Coding Practice Across Time and Place

Coding to Ill-Defined and Other Nonspecific Causes

One indicator that is often used as a measure of the overall reliability and accuracy of cause-specific mortality data is the proportion of death coded to ill-defined categories (Armstrong, Wing, and Tyroler, 1995). As shown in Table 2A-3, this proportion varies considerably across the 10 study countries. Among deaths at ages 50 and older in 1955, the percentage of ill-defined ranged from 19 percent in France and Spain and 16 percent in Japan to less than 2 percent in Australia, Canada, Denmark, and the United States. In most countries, the category termed "senility" comprises the majority of these ill-defined causes, but it varies across countries. In Italy, Japan, and the United Kingdom, more than 85 percent of ill-defined deaths at ages 50 and older in 1955 were coded to senility, whereas the corresponding percentages were 27-48 percent in France, the Netherlands, Spain, and the United States.

Over time, the percentage of ill-defined declined in most countries; by 2004, ill-defined had fallen to 3 percent in Japan and Spain and 6 percent in France. In half of these countries (Australia, Canada, Italy, Japan, and the Netherlands), most of this decline resulted from decreased use of the code for senility. The most extreme example is Japan, for which senility coding declined from 13.5 percent in 1955 to 2.5 percent in 2004. Denmark was the only study country for which ill-defined coding actually increased since 1955; all of the increase occurred in other ill-defined causes.

In addition to the ill-defined codes included in the ICD chapter entitled "Symptoms, Signs, and Ill-defined Conditions," there are nonspecific codes included in other ICD chapters. Called "garbage codes," these include cardiovascular categories lacking diagnostic meaning (e.g., "cardiac arrest," "heart failure"), cancers coded to secondary or unspecified sites, and injuries with undetermined intent (Mathers et al., 2005). In 2004, garbage coding comprised an even larger proportion of deaths than ill-defined causes. For example, in the Netherlands, nearly one-tenth of all deaths were coded to these other nonspecific codes, mostly cardiovascular (Table 2A-3). Overall, nonspecific causes—including both ill-defined and garbage codes—are currently used most commonly in France (15 percent), the Netherlands (14

TABLE 2A-1 Age Group Contributions to Gains in e_{50}, 1955-1980

	AUS	CAN	DNK	ESP	FRA	GBR	ITA
Females							
Ages 50-64	0.9	0.9	0.3	1.3	1.2	0.4	0.9
50-54	0.2	0.2	0.0	0.3	0.3	0.1	0.2
55-59	0.3	0.3	0.1	0.4	0.4	0.1	0.3
60-64	0.4	0.4	0.2	0.6	0.5	0.2	0.4
Ages 65-79	1.7	1.7	1.5	2.2	2.0	1.2	1.6
65-69	0.5	0.5	0.4	0.7	0.6	0.3	0.5
70-74	0.6	0.6	0.5	0.8	0.7	0.4	0.5
75-79	0.6	0.7	0.6	0.7	0.7	0.5	0.6
Ages 80+	0.7	0.9	0.7	0.6	0.8	0.6	0.5
80-84	0.4	0.4	0.4	0.4	0.5	0.4	0.3
85-89	0.2	0.3	0.2	0.2	0.2	0.2	0.1
90+	0.1	0.1	0.1	0.0	0.1	0.1	0.0
Total gain in e_{50}	3.3	3.5	2.4	4.0	4.0	2.2	2.9
Males							
Ages 50-64	0.9	0.7	−0.4	1.0	1.0	0.7	0.2
50-54	0.2	0.2	−0.1	0.3	0.2	0.2	0.1
55-59	0.3	0.2	−0.1	0.3	0.4	0.2	0.1
60-64	0.3	0.3	−0.2	0.4	0.4	0.3	0.1
Ages 65-79	0.9	0.6	−0.4	1.2	1.0	0.6	0.0
65-69	0.4	0.2	−0.1	0.4	0.3	0.3	0.0
70-74	0.3	0.2	−0.2	0.4	0.3	0.2	0.0
75-79	0.2	0.2	−0.1	0.4	0.3	0.2	0.1
Ages 80+	0.2	0.2	0.1	0.3	0.3	0.2	0.1
80-84	0.1	0.1	0.1	0.2	0.2	0.1	0.1
85-89	0.1	0.1	0.0	0.1	0.1	0.1	0.0
90+	0.0	0.0	0.0	0.0	0.0	0.0	0.0
Total gain in e_{50}	1.9	1.5	−0.7	2.5	2.2	1.5	0.3

NOTE: AUS = Australia, CAN = Canada, DNK = Denmark, ESP = Spain, FRA = France, GBR = United Kingdom, ITA = Italy, JPN = Japan, NLD = the Netherlands, USA = United States.
[a]Based on the simple mean across countries.
[b]Data for various countries are aggregated before calculating death rates; thus, the results represent a weighted mean.
SOURCES: Calculations by authors based on data from the Human Mortality Database and the World Health Organization Mortality Database.

percent), Denmark (13 percent), and Spain (11 percent) and least often in Australia (5 percent) and Canada (6 percent).

Although high levels of garbage coding may reflect inappropriate use of these codes (Mathers et al., 2005), they have less effect on our results than coding to ill-defined causes. For the decomposition analyses, garbage

DIVERGING TRENDS IN LIFE EXPECTANCY AT AGE 50

					Excluding DNK, NLD, and USA	
JPN	NLD	USA	Mean[a]	Composite[b]	Mean[a]	Composite[b]
2.0	0.7	0.8	0.9	1.0	1.1	1.2
0.6	0.2	0.2	0.2	0.3	0.3	0.3
0.7	0.2	0.3	0.3	0.3	0.3	0.4
0.8	0.3	0.3	0.4	0.4	0.5	0.5
2.5	1.9	1.5	1.8	1.8	1.8	1.9
0.9	0.5	0.4	0.6	0.5	0.6	0.6
0.9	0.7	0.5	0.6	0.6	0.6	0.7
0.7	0.7	0.6	0.6	0.6	0.6	0.6
0.6	1.0	0.7	0.7	0.7	0.7	0.6
0.4	0.5	0.4	0.4	0.4	0.4	0.4
0.2	0.3	0.2	0.2	0.2	0.2	0.2
0.0	0.1	0.1	0.1	0.1	0.1	0.1
5.1	3.6	3.0	3.4	3.5	3.6	3.7
2.0	−0.1	1.0	0.7	1.0	0.9	1.1
0.5	0.0	0.3	0.2	0.3	0.2	0.3
0.7	0.0	0.3	0.2	0.3	0.3	0.4
0.8	−0.1	0.3	0.2	0.4	0.4	0.4
1.9	−0.3	0.6	0.6	0.8	0.9	1.0
0.8	−0.2	0.3	0.2	0.3	0.3	0.4
0.7	−0.2	0.2	0.2	0.3	0.3	0.3
0.4	0.0	0.2	0.2	0.2	0.2	0.3
0.3	0.2	0.2	0.2	0.2	0.2	0.2
0.2	0.1	0.1	0.1	0.1	0.1	0.1
0.1	0.1	0.1	0.1	0.1	0.1	0.1
0.0	0.0	0.0	0.0	0.0	0.0	0.0
4.2	−0.2	1.8	1.5	2.0	2.0	2.3

codes are grouped with their respective chapters (e.g., the category for heart diseases includes such nonspecific codes as "cardiac arrest" and "heart failure"). In contrast, if deaths due to heart disease were inappropriately coded to ill-defined causes, then our results would understate the true level of heart disease.

TABLE 2A-2 Age Group Contributions to Gains in e_{50}, 1980-2004

	AUS	CAN	DNK	ESP	FRA	GBR	ITA
Females							
Ages 50-64	1.1	0.8	0.7	0.8	0.7	1.1	0.9
50-54	0.3	0.2	0.2	0.2	0.2	0.3	0.2
55-59	0.4	0.3	0.2	0.2	0.2	0.4	0.3
60-64	0.4	0.3	0.3	0.4	0.3	0.5	0.4
Ages 65-79	1.9	1.3	0.4	2.0	1.9	1.6	2.3
65-69	0.5	0.4	0.1	0.5	0.4	0.5	0.6
70-74	0.7	0.4	0.1	0.7	0.6	0.6	0.8
75-79	0.7	0.5	0.2	0.8	0.8	0.6	0.9
Ages 80+	1.1	0.7	0.5	1.2	1.7	0.9	1.7
80-84	0.6	0.4	0.3	0.7	0.8	0.5	0.8
85-89	0.4	0.2	0.2	0.4	0.6	0.3	0.6
90+	0.1	0.1	0.1	0.1	0.3	0.1	0.3
Total gain in e_{50}	4.1	2.7	1.6	4.0	4.3	3.6	5.0
Males							
Ages 50-64	2.3	1.8	1.2	1.0	1.6	2.0	2.1
50-54	0.6	0.5	0.2	0.2	0.5	0.4	0.6
55-59	0.8	0.6	0.4	0.3	0.5	0.7	0.7
60-64	0.9	0.7	0.6	0.4	0.6	0.8	0.8
Ages 65-79	2.9	2.1	1.4	1.6	2.2	2.5	2.5
65-69	1.1	0.8	0.6	0.5	0.8	0.9	0.9
70-74	1.0	0.7	0.5	0.6	0.8	0.9	0.9
75-79	0.8	0.6	0.4	0.5	0.7	0.7	0.7
Ages 80+	0.8	0.6	0.2	0.6	0.9	0.7	0.9
80-84	0.5	0.4	0.2	0.4	0.5	0.4	0.5
85-89	0.2	0.2	0.1	0.2	0.3	0.2	0.3
90+	0.1	0.0	0.0	0.1	0.1	0.1	0.1
Total gain in e_{50}	5.9	4.4	2.9	3.2	4.7	5.2	5.5

NOTE: AUS = Australia, CAN = Canada, DNK = Denmark, ESP = Spain, FRA = France, GBR = United Kingdom, ITA = Italy, JPN = Japan, NLD = the Netherlands, USA = United States.

[a]Based on the simple mean across countries.

[b]Data for various countries are aggregated before calculating death rates; thus, the results represent a weighted mean.

SOURCES: Calculations by authors based on data from the Human Mortality Database and the World Health Organization Mortality Database.

Discontinuities at the Time of Changes in the Classification System

Changes in the system of classification can create discontinuities in historical trends, both at the time of change from one ICD version to the next, but also within an ICD version, because of changes in the implementation of coding rules. Given that different countries adopt a new ICD version at varying times, these transitions also contribute to variation across countries.

DIVERGING TRENDS IN LIFE EXPECTANCY AT AGE 50

JPN	NLD	USA	Mean[a]	Composite[b]	Excluding DNK, NLD, and USA Mean[a]	Composite[b]
0.8	0.3	0.6	0.8	0.8	0.9	0.9
0.2	0.0	0.2	0.2	0.2	0.2	0.2
0.2	0.1	0.2	0.3	0.3	0.3	0.3
0.4	0.2	0.2	0.3	0.4	0.4	0.4
2.6	0.9	0.8	1.6	1.7	1.9	2.2
0.6	0.2	0.3	0.4	0.4	0.5	0.6
0.9	0.3	0.3	0.6	0.6	0.7	0.7
1.1	0.4	0.3	0.7	0.7	0.9	0.9
2.7	0.5	0.6	1.2	1.3	1.4	1.7
1.2	0.3	0.3	0.6	0.6	0.8	0.8
0.9	0.2	0.2	0.4	0.4	0.6	0.6
0.7	0.0	0.1	0.2	0.2	0.3	0.3
6.1	1.6	2.1	3.7	3.7	4.3	4.8
0.9	1.4	1.5	1.6	1.5	1.7	1.6
0.3	0.3	0.4	0.4	0.4	0.4	0.4
0.3	0.4	0.5	0.5	0.5	0.6	0.5
0.4	0.6	0.6	0.7	0.6	0.7	0.6
2.1	1.8	1.8	2.1	2.2	2.3	2.3
0.6	0.7	0.7	0.7	0.8	0.8	0.8
0.7	0.6	0.7	0.7	0.8	0.8	0.8
0.8	0.5	0.5	0.6	0.6	0.7	0.7
1.1	0.2	0.6	0.7	0.8	0.8	0.9
0.6	0.2	0.4	0.4	0.4	0.5	0.5
0.4	0.0	0.2	0.2	0.2	0.3	0.3
0.2	0.0	0.1	0.1	0.1	0.1	0.1
4.1	3.3	3.9	4.4	4.4	4.7	4.8

Some countries have conducted comparability (i.e., "bridge-coding") studies to assess the impact of ICD revisions. Specifically, deaths for a given year are dual-coded using successive revisions of the ICD and a comparability ratio is calculated based on the number of deaths classified to a specific cause using the new ICD divided by the corresponding number using the old ICD. Even for the most recent revision, bridge-coding studies

TABLE 2A-3 Nonspecific Coding Among Deaths at Age 50 and Older by Country, 1955-2004*

	AUS	CAN	DNK	ESP	FRA	GBR	ITA	JPN	NLD	USA
% Ill-defined[a,b]										
1955	1.7	1.5	1.2	18.9	19.0	2.1	8.4	15.7	5.2	1.1
1980	0.2	0.9	3.7	3.7	5.8	0.2	2.8	5.3	4.2	1.1
2004*	0.4	0.9	4.7	2.8	6.1	2.1	1.7	3.1	4.4	1.0
% Senility[a]										
1955	1.4	0.8	0.9	7.6	8.9	2.0	7.4	13.5	2.5	0.3
1980	0.1	0.1	0.3	2.3	2.1	0.2	2.5	5.2	0.9	0.1
2004*	0.1	0.2	0.7	0.8	1.1	1.9	1.0	2.5	1.1	0.2
% Other ill-defined[b]										
1955	0.3	0.7	0.3	11.3	10.1	0.1	1.0	2.1	2.7	0.8
1980	0.1	0.7	3.5	1.4	3.7	0.0	0.3	0.1	3.4	1.0
2004*	0.4	0.7	3.9	1.9	5.0	0.2	0.7	0.6	3.3	0.8
% Other nonspecific, 2004*	4.7	5.5	8.2	8.6	8.8	5.0	8.1	6.7	9.9	5.8
Cardiovascular[c]	2.6	3.3	5.9	6.9	6.1	2.3	6.7	6.2	8.0	4.3
Cancers[d]	2.2	2.1	2.1	1.7	2.7	2.5	1.4	0.4	1.9	1.4
Injuries[e]	0.0	0.1	0.1	0.0	0.0	0.1	0.0	0.1	0.0	0.1
% All nonspecific, 2004*	5.2	6.4	12.8	11.4	15.0	7.0	9.8	9.9	14.2	6.8

NOTE: AUS = Australia, CAN = Canada, DNK = Denmark, ESP = Spain, FRA = France, GBR = United Kingdom, ITA = Italy, JPN = Japan, NLD = the Netherlands, USA = United States.
*Based on data from 2003 for Italy.
[a]Includes ICD-7/ICD-8 code 794, ICD-9 code 797, and ICD-10 code R54.
[b]Includes all other causes included in the ICD chapter entitled "symptoms, signs, and ill-defined conditions."
[c]Includes ICD-10 codes I46, I47.2, I49.0, I50, I51.4-I51.6, I51.9, and I70.9.
[d]Includes ICD-10 codes Y10-Y34 and Y87.2.
[e]Includes ICD-10 codes C76, C80, and C97.
SOURCE: Calculations by authors based on data from the World Health Organization Mortality Database.

are available only for a select number of countries (e.g., Canada, England and Wales, France, Italy, Sweden, the United States). For earlier revisions, such comparability studies are rarely available (exceptions are the United States, England and Wales).

The most recent revision (to ICD-10) created more substantial changes than past revisions because of a large increase in the number of codes (from approximately 5,000 to 8,000), changes in coding rules, and conceptual revisions (Anderson et al., 2001; Mathers et al., 2005). For example, one cause that created a big discontinuity was Alzheimer's disease (AD). Bridge-coding studies from both the United States and Canada suggested that deaths coded to this cause increased by more than 50 percent as a result of the change to ICD-10 (Anderson et al., 2001; Statistics Canada, 2005). Prior to ICD-9, AD was not coded separately; it was probably included with senile or presenile dementia in the chapter for mental disorders. Starting with ICD-9, diseases of the nervous system include a code for AD (331.0), but the huge increase in AD with the change to ICD-10 resulted mostly from deaths coded as presenile dementia (290.1) in ICD-9 (Anderson et al., 2001). Given the big changes in coding practice for this disease, we have grouped mental disorders with diseases of the nervous system in order to better capture AD and minimize discontinuities.

Among the 10 study countries, Denmark was the first to adopt ICD-10 (1994; it skipped over ICD-9 entirely), whereas Italy was the last (2003). In 1955, all 10 countries were using ICD-7. By 1980, Denmark was still using ICD-8 but the others had adopted ICD-9. In 2004, all study countries were using ICD-10.

Looking at the country-level trends for the cause of death groups examined in this chapter (see Table 2A-4 for a detailed list by ICD codes), there are a few apparent discontinuities at the transitions from one ICD version to the next. For example, in Spain at the transition from ICD-7 to ICD-8 in 1968, there is a big jump in heart disease as a proportion of all deaths at ages 50 and older mirrored by a decrease in the proportion due to ill-defined causes (see Figure 2A-1). Yet even after redistributing ill-defined causes proportionately to the other categories, a substantial disruption remains in the trend for heart disease. Thus, for Spain during the period 1955-1980, we may underestimate the contribution of heart disease to gains in e_{50}.

In Japan, there was a drop in heart disease mortality at the change to ICD-10 (in 1995); it is mirrored by an increase in other circulatory diseases (see Figure 2A-2). These discontinuities suggest that the change to ICD-10 may have caused coding shift from heart disease to other circulatory diseases in Japan. Thus, for Japan during the period 1980-2004, we may overestimate the contribution of heart disease to gains in e_{50} and understate the role of other circulatory diseases.

For respiratory diseases, many countries exhibit an increase in mortality rates at the transition to ICD-8. Canada, France, and the United Kingdom also show a sudden drop in respiratory diseases at the change to ICD-10. The most extreme of these discontinuities occurs in the United Kingdom (see Figure 2A-3). The jump in respiratory diseases at ICD-8 could be partly because we were not able to include hay fever, asthma, and pneumonia of the newborn for the period covered by ICD-7; they are instead grouped with the residual category "all else" (see Table 2A-2). Consequently, for the period 1955-1980, the gains in e_{50} attributable to respiratory diseases may be downwardly biased for many countries. At the transition to ICD-10, the drop in respiratory diseases in the United Kingdom is reflected by an increase

TABLE 2A-4 Cause-of-Death Groupings for ICD-7 Through ICD-10

Cause Groupings	ICD-7	ICD-8	ICD-9	ICD-10
1) Heart diseases	400-447	390-429	390-429	I00-I51
2) Other circulatory diseases	330-334, 450-468	430-458	430-459	I60-I99, G45.8, G45.9
3) Lung cancer	162, 163	162	162	C33, C34
4) Other smoking-related cancers[a]				
a) Cancer of the esophagus	150	150	150	C15
b) Cancer of the lip/oral cavity/pharynx	140-148	140-149	140-149	C00-C14
c) Cancer of the larynx	161	161	161	C32
d) Cancer of the pancreas	157	157	157	C25
e) Cancer of the bladder	188	188	188	C67
f) Cancer of the kidney(s)	180	189	189	C64-C66, C68
5a) Breast cancer (for women)	170	174	174, 175	C50
5b) Prostate cancer (for men)	177	185	185	C61
6) All other cancers	151-156, 158-160, 164-165, 171-176, 178, 179, 190-239	151-156, 158-160, 163, 170-173, 180-184, 186, 187, 190-239	151-156, 158-160, 163-165, 170-173, 179-184, 186, 187, 190-239	C16-C24, C26, C30-C31, C37-C49, C51-C60, C62, C63, C69-C97, D00-D48
7) Respiratory diseases[b]	470-527	460-519	460-519	J00-J98, U04
8) Mental disorders; diseases of the nervous system and sense organs[c]	300-326, 340-398	290-389	290-389	F01-F99, G00-G45.4, G45-H93
a) Mental disorders	300-326	290-315	290-319	F01-F99
b) Alzheimer's disease	[c]	[c]	[c]	G30
c) Other diseases of the nervous system	340-398	320-389	320-389	G00-G26, G31-G45.4, G47-H93
9) Ill-defined causes	780-795	780-796	780-799	R00-R99
a) Senility	794	794	797	R54
b) Other ill-defined	780-793, 795	780-793, 795-796	780-796, 798-799	R00-R53, R55-R99
10) Other remaining causes				
a) External causes	E800-E999	E800-E999	E800-E999	V01-Y89
b) Infectious diseases	001-138, 600, 690-698	000-136, 590, 680-686	001-139, 279.5, 279.6[d], 590, 680-686	A00-B99, N10-N12, N13.6, N15, L00-L08

c) Diabetes mellitus	260	250	E10-E14
d) Skin and musculoskeletal diseases	700-749	690-739	L10-M99
e) Digestive diseases	530-587	520-579	K00-K92
f) Genitourinary diseases	590-594	580-589, 591-629	N00-N07, N13.0-N13.5, N13.7-N14, N17-N98
g) All else	240-254, 270-299, 640-689, 751-776	240-246, 251-289, 630-678, 740-779	240-246, 251-279.4, 279.8, 279.9, 280-289, 630-676, 740-779	E00-E07, E15-E88, D50-D89, O00-Q99

[a] Includes cancers for which at least 25 percent of deaths (among men or women) are attributable to smoking according to the CPS-II study (U.S. Department of Health and Human Services, 1989, Table 2-11). Although we refer to this grouping as "other smoking-related cancers," we recognize that it is an oversimplification: smoking is likely to account for a substantial fraction of these deaths, but this category includes many deaths that are not due to smoking, while excluding deaths from other causes that are due to smoking.

[b] For ICD-7, this category excludes hay fever (240), asthma (241), and pneumonia of newborns (763) because the WHO data are not sufficiently detailed to identify these particular causes. In 2003, among all deaths at ages 50+ in this category for the 10 study countries, 38.1 percent resulted from COPD (ICD-10: J40-J44, J47), 6.2 percent from pneumonia (J12-J18), 37.6 percent from lung disease due to external agents (J60-J70), 1.8 percent from asthma, 0.8 percent from influenza, and 15.5 percent from other respiratory diseases.

[c] Alzheimer's disease was not coded separately under ICD-7 or ICD-8 (it was probably coded as senile or presenile dementia under mental disorders). In ICD-9, a code for Alzheimer's (331.0) was included with diseases of the nervous system, but we do not have data at the 4-digit level required to identify these deaths. In 2003, among all deaths at ages 50+ in this category for the 10 study countries, 65.4 percent resulted from dementia and Alzheimer's (ICD-10: F01, F03, G30), 11.9 percent from Parkinson's (G20), 0.3 percent from Huntington's (G10), and 22.4 percent from other mental disorders and diseases of the nervous system.

[d] In order to be comparable with ICD-10 coding of HIV/AIDS (B20-B24), we have included ICD-9 codes 279.5 (human immunodeficiency virus disease) and 279.6 (AIDS-related complex) with other infectious diseases.

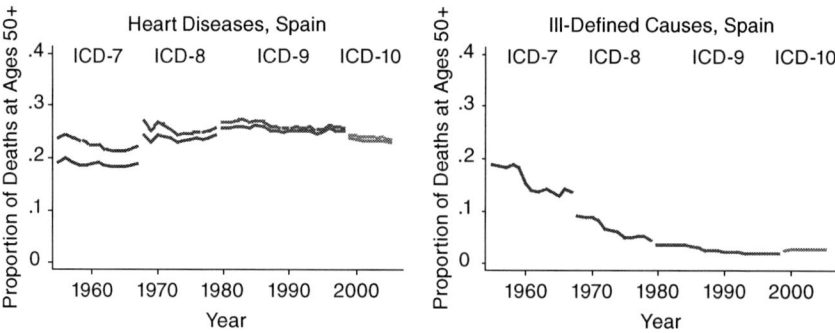

FIGURE 2A-1 Proportion of deaths due to heart disease and ill-defined causes, Spain.
NOTES: Solid line = unadjusted proportion; dashed line = adjusted proportion after redistributing ill-defined causes.
SOURCE: Calculations by authors based on data from the World Health Organization Mortality Database.

in mental disorders and diseases of the nervous system (Figure 2A-3). We see a similar pattern for Canada and France (not shown). Thus, for the period 1980-2004, we may overestimate the decline in respiratory diseases among these three countries. Within ICD-9, the United Kingdom also exhibits a curious drop in respiratory diseases in 1984 and a later increase in 1993, which is mirrored by a "hump" in mental disorders and diseases of the nervous system. A similar (albeit somewhat smaller) hump is apparent in other remaining causes (not shown). During the period 1984-1992, England and

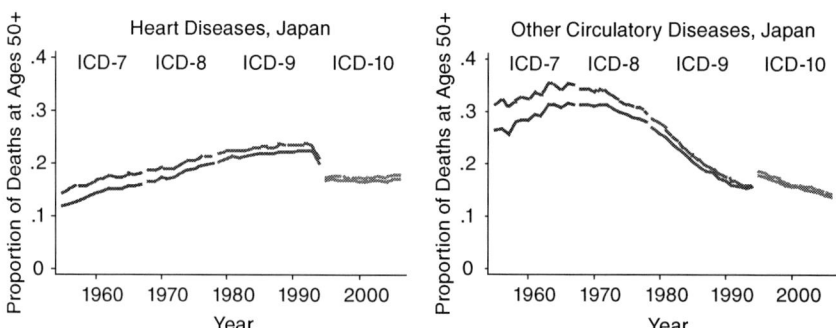

FIGURE 2A-2 Proportion of deaths due to heart and other circulatory diseases, Japan.
NOTES: Solid line = unadjusted proportion; dashed line = adjusted proportion after redistributing ill-defined causes.
SOURCE: Calculations by authors based on data from the World Health Organization Mortality Database.

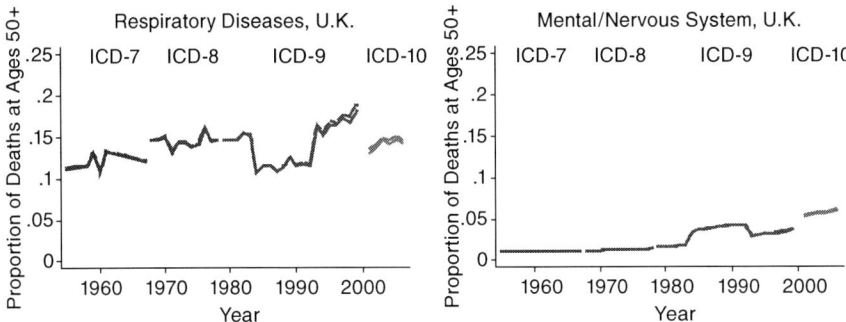

FIGURE 2A-3 Proportion of deaths due to respiratory diseases and mental/nervous system, United Kingdom.
NOTES: Solid line = unadjusted proportion; dashed line = adjusted proportion after redistributing ill-defined causes.
SOURCE: Calculations by authors based on data from the World Health Organization Mortality Database.

Wales broadened coding rule 3, and as a result contributing causes of death were more frequently coded as the underlying cause of death (Janssen and Kunst, 2004; Office of Population Censuses and Surveys, 1995).

Detailed Cause of Death Contributions to Gains in e_{50}

For the decomposition by cause of death, we extracted death counts by sex, age group, and cause of death from the WHO Mortality Database (World Health Organization, 2009). Data were available through 2003 for Italy and through 2004 for all other countries. In most cases, the WHO data are given by the following age groups: 0, 1-4, 5-9, . . . 80-84, 85+. For the most recent year, more detailed data at the oldest ages (85-89, 90-94, 95+) are available for all countries except Canada. All-cause death rates and exposure estimates come from the HMD (2009). To obtain cause-specific death rates, we apply the distribution of death counts by cause based on the WHO data to the all-cause death rates from the HMD. In cases in which the WHO data are available only to ages 85+, we apply the distribution by cause for deaths at age 85+ to the all-cause death rates at ages 85-89, 90-94, and 95+. We use the Pollard (1988) method to decompose the gains in e_{50} into the contributions by cause of death. The contribution of ill-defined causes is shown separately here (see Tables 2A-5 and 2A-6), but for Figures 2-6 to 2-11 (in the main text) we have redistributed ill-defined deaths proportionately to all other cause groups before decomposing the gains in e_{50} by cause group.

TABLE 2A-5 Cause-of-Death Contributions to Gains in e_{50}, 1955-1980

	AUS	CAN	DNK	ESP	FRA
Females					
Cardiovascular diseases	2.4	2.8	2.0	1.0	1.5
Heart diseases	1.4	1.7	0.9	0.5	0.7
Cerebrovascular & other circulatory diseases	1.1	1.1	1.1	0.5	0.8
Cancers	0.0	0.1	0.1	0.0	0.3
Lung cancer	−0.1	−0.2	−0.2	0.0	0.0
Other smoking-related cancers	−0.1	0.0	−0.1	0.0	−0.1
Breast cancer	0.0	−0.1	0.0	−0.1	−0.1
All other cancers	0.2	0.3	0.4	0.2	0.4
Respiratory diseases	0.1	0.0	−0.2	0.5	0.4
Mental disorders/nervous system/sense organs	0.0	0.0	0.0	0.1	0.2
Ill-defined causes	0.2	0.1	−0.2	1.8	1.6
Other remaining causes	0.6	0.5	0.6	0.6	0.1
External causes	0.1	0.1	0.1	0.0	−0.1
Infectious diseases	0.1	0.1	0.2	0.2	0.1
Diabetes mellitus	0.1	0.1	0.0	−0.1	0.0
Digestive diseases	0.1	0.0	0.3	0.2	0.1
Genitourinary diseases	0.1	0.2	0.1	0.2	0.0
All else	0.1	0.1	0.0	0.1	−0.1
Total gain in e_{50}	3.3	3.5	2.4	4.0	4.0
Males					
Cardiovascular diseases	1.5	1.7	0.0	0.3	0.9
Heart diseases	1.1	1.2	−0.4	−0.1	0.4
Cerebrovascular and other circulatory diseases	0.5	0.5	0.4	0.5	0.6
Cancers	−0.5	−0.5	−0.4	−0.5	−0.7
Lung cancer	−0.4	−0.5	−0.5	−0.3	−0.4
Other smoking-related cancers	−0.1	0.0	−0.2	−0.2	−0.3
Prostate cancer	0.0	0.0	−0.1	−0.1	0.0
Other cancers	0.0	0.1	0.3	0.0	0.0
Respiratory diseases	0.0	−0.2	−0.4	0.3	0.2
Mental disorders/nervous system/sense organs	0.0	0.0	0.0	0.1	0.2
Ill-defined causes	0.1	0.0	−0.3	1.5	1.1
Other remaining causes	0.8	0.5	0.5	0.8	0.5
External causes	0.2	0.1	0.1	0.0	0.1
Infectious diseases	0.2	0.1	0.1	0.4	0.4
Diabetes mellitus	0.0	0.0	0.0	−0.1	0.0
Digestive diseases	0.1	0.0	0.1	0.1	0.0
Genitourinary diseases	0.2	0.2	0.3	0.2	0.1
All else	0.1	0.1	0.0	0.2	0.0
Total gain in e_{50}	1.9	1.5	−0.7	2.5	2.2

NOTE: AUS = Australia, CAN = Canada, DNK = Denmark, ESP = Spain, FRA = France, GBR = United Kingdom, ITA = Italy, JPN = Japan, NLD = the Netherlands, USA = United States.
  [a]Based on the simple mean across countries.
  [b]Data for various countries are aggregated before calculating death rates; thus, the results represent a weighted mean.
SOURCES: Calculations by authors based on data from the Human Mortality Database and the World Health Organization Mortality Database.

							Excluding DNK, NLD, and USA	
GBR	ITA	JPN	NLD	USA	Mean[a]	Composite[b]	Mean[a]	Composite[b]
1.9	1.7	1.4	2.2	2.7	2.0	2.1	1.8	1.7
1.1	1.0	0.0	0.9	1.6	1.0	1.1	0.9	0.8
0.8	0.7	1.4	1.2	1.1	1.0	1.0	0.9	0.9
−0.2	0.0	0.1	0.3	0.0	0.1	0.1	0.0	0.1
−0.2	−0.1	−0.1	−0.1	−0.3	−0.1	−0.2	−0.1	−0.1
0.0	−0.1	−0.1	−0.1	0.0	0.0	0.0	0.0	0.0
−0.1	−0.1	0.0	−0.1	0.0	−0.1	0.0	−0.1	−0.1
0.2	0.2	0.3	0.5	0.3	0.3	0.3	0.3	0.3
−0.1	0.3	0.1	0.3	−0.1	0.1	0.1	0.2	0.2
0.0	0.1	0.1	0.1	−0.1	0.1	0.0	0.1	0.1
0.2	0.6	1.7	0.2	0.0	0.6	0.7	0.9	1.0
0.3	0.2	1.7	0.5	0.4	0.6	0.5	0.6	0.6
0.1	−0.1	0.0	0.0	0.2	0.0	0.1	0.0	0.0
0.1	0.1	0.4	0.1	0.1	0.1	0.1	0.2	0.2
0.0	−0.1	−0.1	0.2	0.1	0.0	0.0	0.0	0.0
0.0	0.1	0.8	0.1	0.1	0.2	0.2	0.2	0.2
0.0	0.1	0.3	0.1	0.1	0.1	0.1	0.1	0.1
0.1	0.1	0.2	0.1	0.0	0.1	0.1	0.1	0.1
2.2	2.9	5.1	3.6	3.0	3.4	3.5	3.6	3.7
0.6	0.3	1.3	0.0	1.9	0.9	1.3	0.9	0.9
0.2	−0.1	0.0	−0.5	1.3	0.3	0.7	0.4	0.3
0.4	0.4	1.3	0.5	0.7	0.6	0.6	0.6	0.6
−0.1	−0.9	−0.3	−0.8	−0.4	−0.5	−0.4	−0.5	−0.4
−0.2	−0.6	−0.3	−0.7	−0.5	−0.4	−0.4	−0.4	−0.3
0.0	−0.2	−0.1	−0.2	0.0	−0.1	−0.1	−0.1	−0.1
0.0	0.0	0.0	0.0	0.0	0.0	0.0	0.0	0.0
0.1	0.0	0.1	0.1	0.1	0.1	0.1	0.0	0.1
0.3	0.0	0.0	0.0	−0.3	0.0	0.0	0.1	0.1
0.0	0.1	0.1	0.1	−0.1	0.0	0.0	0.1	0.1
0.1	0.4	1.2	0.1	0.0	0.4	0.4	0.6	0.7
0.6	0.4	1.9	0.5	0.5	0.7	0.7	0.8	0.8
0.1	0.0	0.1	0.1	0.2	0.1	0.1	0.1	0.1
0.2	0.3	0.6	0.1	0.2	0.3	0.3	0.3	0.4
0.0	−0.1	0.0	0.0	0.0	0.0	0.0	0.0	0.0
0.1	−0.1	0.7	0.1	0.1	0.1	0.1	0.1	0.2
0.2	0.1	0.2	0.2	0.1	0.2	0.2	0.2	0.2
0.1	0.1	0.3	0.1	0.0	0.1	0.1	0.1	0.1
1.5	0.3	4.2	−0.2	1.8	1.5	2.0	2.0	2.2

TABLE 2A-6 Cause of Death Contributions to Gains in e_{50}, 1980-2004*

	AUS	CAN	DNK	ESP	FRA
Females					
Cardiovascular diseases	3.9	3.1	2.1	3.2	2.6
Heart diseases	2.5	2.2	1.7	1.2	1.3
Cerebrovascular & other circulatory diseases	1.5	0.9	0.5	2.0	1.3
Cancers	0.2	0.0	0.0	0.2	0.4
Lung cancer	−0.1	−0.4	−0.4	0.0	−0.1
Other smoking-related cancers	0.0	0.0	0.0	0.0	0.0
Breast cancer	0.1	0.1	0.0	0.0	0.0
Other cancers	0.2	0.2	0.4	0.3	0.5
Respiratory diseases	0.0	−0.1	−0.2	0.3	0.2
Mental disorders/nervous system/sense organs	−0.2	−0.4	−0.4	−0.4	−0.1
Ill-defined causes	0.0	0.0	0.0	0.3	0.3
Other remaining causes	0.2	0.1	−0.1	0.4	1.0
External causes	0.1	0.1	0.2	0.1	0.3
Infectious diseases	0.0	−0.1	0.0	0.0	0.0
Diabetes mellitus	0.0	0.0	−0.1	0.2	0.0
Digestive diseases	0.1	0.1	−0.1	0.2	0.4
Genitourinary diseases	0.0	0.0	0.0	0.0	0.1
All else	0.0	0.0	−0.1	−0.1	0.1
Total gain in e_{50}	**4.1**	**2.7**	**1.6**	**4.0**	**4.3**
Males					
Cardiovascular diseases	4.5	3.6	2.8	2.6	2.3
Heart diseases	3.4	2.9	2.5	1.3	1.3
Cerebrovascular & other circulatory diseases	1.1	0.8	0.3	1.4	1.1
Cancers	0.6	0.5	0.3	−0.3	0.7
Lung cancer	0.4	0.3	0.2	−0.2	0.0
Other smoking-related cancers	0.1	0.1	0.0	−0.1	0.4
Prostate cancer	0.0	0.0	0.0	0.0	0.1
Other cancers	0.1	0.1	0.1	0.0	0.2
Respiratory diseases	0.5	0.3	0.2	0.3	0.4
Mental disorders/nervous system/sense organs	−0.1	−0.2	−0.3	−0.2	0.0
Ill-defined causes	0.0	0.0	0.1	0.2	0.2
Other remaining causes	0.4	0.2	−0.1	0.6	1.1
External causes	0.2	0.2	0.2	0.1	0.4
Infectious diseases	0.0	−0.1	0.0	0.0	0.0
Diabetes mellitus	0.0	−0.1	−0.1	0.0	0.0
Digestive diseases	0.2	0.2	−0.1	0.4	0.6
Genitourinary diseases	0.1	0.0	0.0	0.1	0.1
All else	0.0	0.0	−0.1	0.0	0.1
Total gain in e_{50}	**5.9**	**4.4**	**2.9**	**3.2**	**4.7**

NOTE: AUS = Australia, CAN = Canada, DNK = Denmark, ESP = Spain, FRA = France, GBR = United Kingdom, ITA = Italy, JPN = Japan, NLD = the Netherlands, USA = United States.
*Based on data from 2003 for Italy.
[a]Based on the simple mean across countries.
[b]Data for various countries are aggregated before calculating death rates; thus, the results represent a weighted mean.
SOURCES: Calculations by authors based on data from the Human Mortality Database and the World Health Organization Mortality Database.

	GBR	ITA	JPN	NLD	USA	Mean[a]	Composite[b]	Excluding DNK, NLD, and USA	
								Mean[a]	Composite[b]
	3.0	3.1	4.1	2.0	2.8	3.0	3.1	3.3	3.4
	2.0	1.8	1.7	1.5	2.0	1.8	1.9	1.8	1.8
	1.0	1.3	2.4	0.6	0.7	1.2	1.2	1.5	1.6
	0.3	0.2	0.4	0.0	0.1	0.2	0.3	0.2	0.4
	−0.1	−0.1	0.0	−0.3	−0.3	−0.2	−0.1	−0.1	−0.1
	0.0	0.0	0.0	−0.1	0.0	0.0	0.0	0.0	0.0
	0.2	0.0	−0.1	0.1	0.1	0.1	0.1	0.0	0.1
	0.2	0.3	0.5	0.3	0.3	0.3	0.3	0.3	0.4
	0.5	0.3	0.2	−0.2	−0.3	0.1	0.1	0.2	0.3
	−0.2	−0.2	0.0	−0.4	−0.4	−0.3	−0.3	−0.2	−0.1
	−0.1	0.2	0.8	0.1	0.0	0.2	0.1	0.2	0.2
	0.1	0.5	0.7	0.1	−0.1	0.3	0.3	0.4	0.5
	0.1	0.2	0.1	0.2	0.0	0.1	0.1	0.2	0.2
	0.0	0.0	0.0	0.0	−0.1	0.0	−0.1	0.0	0.0
	0.0	0.2	0.1	−0.1	−0.1	0.0	0.0	0.1	0.1
	−0.1	0.3	0.3	0.0	0.1	0.1	0.2	0.2	0.2
	0.0	0.0	0.1	0.0	−0.1	0.0	0.0	0.0	0.0
	0.0	−0.1	0.1	0.0		0.0	0.0	0.0	0.0
	3.6	4.1	6.1	1.6	2.1	3.4	3.6	4.1	4.7
	3.7	2.9	3.0	2.5	3.4	3.1	3.2	3.2	3.1
	2.9	1.8	1.2	2.1	2.8	2.2	2.3	2.1	1.9
	0.8	1.1	1.8	0.4	0.6	0.9	1.0	1.1	1.2
	0.7	0.5	0.2	0.7	0.5	0.4	0.5	0.4	0.4
	0.6	0.2	−0.1	0.6	0.3	0.2	0.2	0.2	0.2
	0.0	0.2	−0.1	0.0	0.1	0.1	0.1	0.1	0.1
	0.0	0.0	−0.1	0.0	0.1	0.0	0.0	0.0	0.0
	0.1	0.1	0.4	0.2	0.2	0.1	0.2	0.1	0.2
	0.9	0.5	0.1	0.0	0.2	0.3	0.3	0.4	0.4
	−0.1	−0.1	0.0	−0.2	−0.2	−0.1	−0.1	−0.1	−0.1
	0.0	0.1	0.3	0.2	0.1	0.1	0.1	0.1	0.1
	0.1	0.9	0.5	0.1	0.0	0.4	0.4	0.5	0.6
	0.1	0.2	0.0	0.1	0.1	0.2	0.1	0.2	0.1
	0.0	0.0	0.1	0.0	−0.1	0.0	0.0	0.0	0.0
	0.0	0.1	0.0	−0.1	−0.1	0.0	0.0	0.0	0.0
	−0.1	0.6	0.4	0.0	0.2	0.2	0.3	0.3	0.4
	0.1	0.1	0.1	0.1	0.0	0.0	0.0	0.1	0.1
	0.0	−0.1	0.0	0.0	0.0	0.0	0.0	0.0	0.0
	5.2	4.8	4.1	3.3	4.0	4.3	4.4	4.6	4.7

TABLE 2A-7 Age Group Contributions to Gap in e_{50} in 2004

	AUS	CAN	DNK	ESP	FRA	GBR	ITA
Females							
Ages 50-64	0.9	0.6	0.0	1.1	0.8	0.4	1.0
50-54	0.3	0.2	0.0	0.3	0.1	0.1	0.2
55-59	0.3	0.2	0.0	0.4	0.3	0.1	0.3
60-64	0.4	0.2	0.0	0.5	0.4	0.2	0.4
Ages 65-79	1.1	0.7	−0.6	1.4	1.6	0.1	1.3
65-69	0.4	0.3	−0.1	0.5	0.5	0.1	0.5
70-74	0.4	0.3	−0.3	0.5	0.6	0.1	0.5
75-79	0.3	0.2	−0.2	0.4	0.5	−0.1	0.4
Ages 80+	0.1	0.1	−0.7	−0.2	0.4	−0.5	0.1
80-84	0.2	0.2	−0.2	0.1	0.3	−0.1	0.2
85-89	0.0	0.0	−0.2	−0.1	0.1	−0.2	0.0
90+	−0.1	−0.1	−0.2	−0.2	0.0	−0.2	−0.1
Total gap in e_{50}	2.2	1.4	−1.2	2.3	2.8	0.1	2.4
Males							
Ages 50-64	1.3	0.8	0.1	0.5	0.2	0.6	1.0
50-54	0.4	0.3	0.1	0.2	0.0	0.2	0.4
55-59	0.4	0.3	0.0	0.1	0.0	0.2	0.3
60-64	0.4	0.3	0.0	0.2	0.2	0.2	0.3
Ages 65-79	0.9	0.5	−0.7	0.3	0.5	0.0	0.5
65-69	0.4	0.2	−0.1	0.2	0.2	0.1	0.3
70-74	0.3	0.2	−0.3	0.1	0.2	0.0	0.2
75-79	0.2	0.1	−0.3	0.0	0.1	−0.1	0.1
Ages 80+	−0.1	−0.1	−0.6	−0.2	−0.1	−0.4	−0.2
80-84	0.1	0.0	−0.3	−0.1	0.1	−0.2	0.0
85-89	−0.1	−0.1	−0.2	−0.1	−0.1	−0.1	−0.1
90+	−0.1	−0.1	−0.1	−0.1	−0.1	−0.1	−0.1
Total gap in e_{50}	2.0	1.3	−1.2	0.6	0.7	0.3	1.3

NOTE: AUS = Australia, CAN = Canada, DNK = Denmark, ESP = Spain, FRA = France, GBR = United Kingdom, ITA = Italy, JPN = Japan, NLD = the Netherlands.

[a]Based on the simple mean across countries.

[b]Data for various countries are aggregated before calculating death rates; thus, the results represent a weighted mean.

SOURCES: Calculations by authors based on data from the Human Mortality Database and the World Health Organization Mortality Database.

Current Gap in e_{50}: The United States Versus Other High-Income Countries

For the tables in this Annex, the gap in e_{50} is defined as: $e_{50}^{CountryX} - e_{50}^{USA}$. For example, among women, the gap of 4.3 for Japan indicates that, on average, women in Japan can expect to live 4.3 years longer after age 50 than their U.S. counterparts (see Table 2A-7).

JPN	NLD	Mean[a]	Composite[b]	Excluding DNK and NLD	
				Mean[a]	Composite[b]
1.1	0.4	0.7	0.9	0.8	0.9
0.3	0.1	0.2	0.2	0.2	0.2
0.4	0.1	0.2	0.3	0.3	0.3
0.5	0.2	0.3	0.4	0.4	0.4
2.0	0.5	0.9	0.9	1.2	1.4
0.6	0.2	0.3	0.3	0.5	0.5
0.7	0.2	0.3	0.3	0.5	0.5
0.7	0.1	0.2	0.3	0.4	0.4
1.1	−0.6	0.0	0.2	0.2	0.3
0.6	−0.1	0.1	0.2	0.2	0.3
0.3	−0.2	0.0	0.0	0.1	0.1
0.3	−0.2	−0.1	0.0	0.0	0.0
4.3	0.3	1.6	1.9	2.2	2.6
0.9	0.7	0.7	0.7	0.8	0.8
0.3	0.3	0.2	0.3	0.3	0.3
0.3	0.2	0.2	0.2	0.2	0.2
0.3	0.2	0.2	0.3	0.3	0.3
0.9	−0.2	0.3	0.5	0.5	0.6
0.4	0.1	0.2	0.3	0.3	0.3
0.3	−0.1	0.1	0.2	0.2	0.2
0.2	−0.2	0.0	0.1	0.1	0.1
0.1	−0.6	−0.2	−0.1	−0.1	−0.1
0.1	−0.3	−0.1	0.0	0.0	0.0
0.0	−0.2	−0.1	−0.1	−0.1	−0.1
0.0	−0.1	−0.1	−0.1	−0.1	−0.1
1.9	−0.1	0.8	1.1	1.2	1.2

TABLE 2A-8 Cause-of-Death Contributions to Gap in e_{50} in 2004*

	AUS	CAN	DNK	ESP	FRA
Females					
Cardiovascular diseases	0.7	0.9	0.1	0.8	1.6
Heart diseases	0.9	0.8	0.5	0.9	1.4
Cerebrovascular & other circulatory diseases	−0.1	0.1	−0.4	−0.1	0.2
Cancers	0.3	−0.2	−0.9	0.8	0.5
Lung cancer	0.4	0.0	−0.1	0.6	0.6
Other smoking-related cancers	0.0	0.0	−0.2	0.1	0.0
Breast cancer	0.0	0.0	−0.2	0.1	−0.1
Other cancers	−0.1	−0.1	−0.4	0.0	−0.1
Respiratory diseases	0.3	0.3	−0.2	0.4	0.7
Mental disorders/nervous system/sense organs	0.2	0.0	0.0	0.1	0.1
Ill-defined causes	0.1	0.0	−0.4	−0.1	−0.4
Other remaining causes	0.6	0.3	0.0	0.4	0.4
External causes	0.1	0.0	0.0	0.1	−0.1
Infectious diseases	0.1	0.1	0.1	0.1	0.1
Diabetes mellitus	0.1	0.1	0.1	0.1	0.2
Digestive diseases	0.1	0.0	−0.2	0.0	0.0
Genitourinary diseases	0.1	0.1	0.1	0.1	0.2
All else	0.0	0.0	0.0	0.1	0.0
Total gap in e_{50}	2.2	1.4	−1.3	2.3	2.8
Males					
Cardiovascular diseases	0.9	0.8	0.0	0.9	1.2
Heart diseases	1.0	0.8	0.5	1.1	1.3
Cerebrovascular & other circulatory diseases	−0.1	0.0	−0.5	−0.2	0.0
Cancers	0.0	−0.1	−0.7	−0.5	−0.7
Lung cancer	0.3	0.1	0.0	0.0	0.0
Other smoking-related cancers	0.0	0.0	−0.2	−0.2	−0.2
Prostate cancer	−0.1	0.0	−0.2	0.0	−0.1
Other cancers	−0.2	−0.2	−0.3	−0.3	−0.5
Respiratory diseases	0.3	0.2	0.0	−0.1	0.4
Mental disorders/nervous system/sense organs	0.2	0.0	−0.2	0.1	0.0
Ill-defined causes	0.0	0.0	−0.4	−0.1	−0.4
Other remaining causes	0.6	0.4	0.1	0.3	0.2
External causes	0.2	0.1	0.1	0.1	−0.1
Infectious diseases	0.2	0.1	0.1	0.1	0.1
Diabetes mellitus	0.1	0.0	0.0	0.2	0.2
Digestive diseases	0.1	0.0	−0.2	−0.2	−0.1
Genitourinary diseases	0.1	0.1	0.0	0.1	0.1
All else	0.0	0.0	0.0	0.1	0.0
Total gap in e_{50}	2.1	1.3	−1.2	0.6	0.7

NOTE: AUS = Australia, CAN = Canada, DNK = Denmark, ESP = Spain, FRA = France, GBR = United Kingdom, ITA = Italy, JPN = Japan, NLD = the Netherlands.

*Based on data from 2003 for Italy.

[a]Based on the simple mean across countries.

[b]Data for various countries are aggregated before calculating death rates; thus, the results represent a weighted mean.

SOURCES: Calculations by authors based on data from the Human Mortality Database and the World Health Organization Mortality Database.

						Excluding DNK and NLD	
GBR	ITA	JPN	NLD	Mean[a]	Composite[b]	Mean[a]	Composite[b]
0.1	0.1	1.8	0.4	0.7	1.0	0.9	1.0
0.6	0.4	1.9	0.6	0.9	1.1	1.0	1.1
−0.5	−0.3	−0.1	−0.2	−0.2	−0.1	−0.1	−0.1
−0.2	0.3	0.8	−0.3	0.1	0.4	0.3	0.4
0.2	0.5	0.6	0.2	0.3	0.4	0.4	0.5
−0.1	0.0	0.1	−0.1	0.0	0.0	0.0	0.0
−0.1	0.0	0.3	−0.1	0.0	0.1	0.0	0.1
−0.2	−0.3	−0.1	−0.3	−0.2	−0.1	−0.1	−0.1
−0.2	0.6	0.3	0.2	0.3	0.3	0.3	0.3
0.1	0.3	0.8	−0.1	0.2	0.3	0.2	0.3
−0.1	0.0	−0.2	−0.3	−0.2	−0.1	−0.1	−0.1
0.4	0.4	0.8	0.3	0.4	0.5	0.5	0.5
0.1	0.0	0.0	0.0	0.0	0.0	0.0	0.0
0.1	0.2	0.1	0.1	0.1	0.1	0.1	0.1
0.2	0.0	0.3	0.1	0.1	0.2	0.1	0.2
−0.2	0.0	0.1	−0.1	0.0	0.0	0.0	0.0
0.1	0.1	0.1	0.1	0.1	0.1	0.1	0.1
0.1	0.1	0.2	0.1	0.0	0.1	0.1	0.1
0.1	1.6	4.3	0.3	1.5	2.4	2.1	2.5
−0.1	0.3	1.5	0.3	0.7	0.9	0.8	0.9
0.4	0.6	1.9	0.6	0.9	1.1	1.0	1.2
−0.4	−0.4	−0.4	−0.3	−0.2	−0.3	−0.2	−0.3
−0.2	−0.6	−0.3	−0.6	−0.4	−0.4	−0.3	−0.4
0.2	0.0	0.3	−0.1	0.1	0.1	0.1	0.1
−0.1	−0.1	0.0	−0.1	−0.1	−0.1	−0.1	−0.1
−0.1	0.0	0.1	−0.1	0.0	0.0	0.0	0.0
−0.2	−0.5	−0.6	−0.2	−0.3	−0.4	−0.4	−0.4
−0.2	0.3	−0.2	0.0	0.1	0.0	0.1	0.0
0.1	0.2	0.4	0.0	0.1	0.2	0.1	0.2
0.0	0.0	−0.1	−0.3	−0.1	−0.1	−0.1	−0.1
0.7	0.5	0.4	0.5	0.4	0.4	0.4	0.4
0.2	0.1	−0.1	0.2	0.1	0.0	0.1	0.0
0.2	0.2	0.1	0.1	0.1	0.1	0.1	0.1
0.2	0.1	0.2	0.1	0.1	0.2	0.1	0.2
−0.1	0.0	0.0	0.0	0.0	0.0	0.0	0.0
0.1	0.1	0.1	0.1	0.1	0.1	0.1	0.1
0.1	0.1	0.1	0.1	0.0	0.1	0.0	0.1
0.3	0.6	1.9	−0.1	0.7	1.0	1.1	1.1

3

Are International Differences in Health Similar to International Differences in Life Expectancy?

Eileen M. Crimmins, Krista Garcia, and Jung Ki Kim

The question addressed in this chapter is whether people in countries with relatively low life expectancy after age 50 have worse health than those in countries with longer life expectancy. We begin with a short discussion of the theoretical relationships between mortality and population health and the potential complexity of the link between measures of health and mortality. We then examine how indicators of health vary across countries and how closely differences in a set of health indicators correspond to differences in mortality across 10 countries. We note at the outset that most of the data we examine reflect analysis of cross-sectional differences in health; without comparable longitudinal data, there is little we can say about how the differences arose. The countries compared include Australia, Canada, Denmark, England, France, Italy, Japan, the Netherlands, Spain, and the United States.

MEASURES OF POPULATION HEALTH

A number of people have addressed the question of whether populations that live longer are or should be "healthier." Answers range from yes, because there is a "compression of morbidity" (Fries, 1980), to no, as there is a "failure of success" (Gruenberg, 1977), to no change, as there is dynamic equilibrium (Manton, 1982). It was probably true that improved health and increased life expectancy went together in the past, when mortality was highly related to death from infectious disease. It is not necessarily true when mortality is largely the result of chronic conditions that exist over long periods of the life span and are treated but not cured. Successful treatment can leave more people with a condition surviving in the population. If more people survive with more health problems, it becomes difficult to know when one country is "healthier" than another.

At the moment, most of the data available for cross-national comparisons indicate the prevalence of health problems in the population. The prevalence of a health problem at a given time depends on how many people have experienced the onset of the problem or condition and how long they survived with the problem. The onset rate or incidence of a problem depends on risk for the condition in the exposed population, whereas the survival rate can depend on whether the case is treatable and, if treated, whether death or the progression of severity of disease is delayed. Populations can be in better health because the incidence of a disease is lower, but they could also have a lower prevalence of poor health if those with diseases did not survive as long. For instance, if life expectancy among the diseased and disabled increases, population health as measured by disability could deteriorate. Two countries with the same level of disease incidence but different approaches to treatment could have differences in population health; where disease is aggressively treated and death prevented, the level of disease prevalence as well as life expectancy could be higher. So the health status of a population depends on a set of processes of onset and survival that cannot be inferred from one or more snapshots of the prevalence of health problems in the population.

There can also be variation in the presence of diseases and conditions across countries and across time for a number of reasons. Diagnostic definitions can differ across countries and change over time. For instance, the blood pressure cutoff value indicating hypertension has gotten lower over time, so that diagnosis occurs at an earlier stage of severity in more recent years. Countries may adopt changes in definitions at different times, leading to variability of the definition of conditions at one time. Another example is differences in the diagnostic criteria for diabetes (DECODE Study Group, 1998; Wareham and O'Rahilly, 1998). Differences in national emphasis on screening for conditions can also affect variability in knowledge of the existence of diseases and reported prevalence. This is true for cancer, hypertension, high cholesterol, and diabetes (Ashworth, Medina, and Morgan, 2008; Gregg et al., 2004; Wareham and O'Rahilly, 1998). It is also possible that recognition of disease varies over time and across countries. For instance, Alzheimer's disease (AD) is now a recognized cause of both morbidity and mortality but was virtually unknown and unrecognized in the 1950s. The timing of accepting AD as a cause of mortality and morbidity can differ across countries. It is also possible that there are national or cultural differences in the way doctors disclose conditions to patients (Asai, 1995).

There are multiple dimensions of health to be considered in evaluating national differences in health. Health change with age in populations begins with the onset of risk factors, progresses to diseases and impairments, and then to functioning loss and to the inability to perform expected tasks or disability, frailty, and death (Crimmins, Kim, and Vasunilashorn, 2010). This can be termed the "morbidity process." No one individual needs to experience problems reflecting all of these dimensions, as some people die very suddenly with no warning that their health has begun to deteriorate. In addition, for individuals the process is not always unidirectional, but back and forth movement is possible (Crimmins, Hayward, and Saito, 1994). These dimensions of population health relate to mortality differently. For instance, many important causes of disability are not highly related to mortality, for instance, arthritis. In contrast, cancer is highly related to mortality but not disability. Heart disease tends to be a major cause of both mortality and disability. In this analysis, we examine self-reported indicators of functioning, disability, and disease presence and cancer incidence from registries. We also examine both self-reports and measured prevalence of high cholesterol and high blood pressure, along with body mass index based primarily on self-reports.

DATA

Where possible, our analysis uses information on health for the population ages 50 and older, or 65 and older, in the 10 countries. However, in some cases, we expand or limit the age range because of data unavailability. Most of the countries have conducted national surveys of their older populations, which provide individual-level data on a number of health indicators, risk factors, and drug usage. Many of the self-reported indicators of health status come from a family of surveys designed to be comparable: (1) the Health and Retirement Study (HRS) for 2004 for the United States (Health and Retirement Study, 2006); (2) the Surveys of Health, Ageing and Retirement in Europe (SHARE) for 2004 for Denmark, France, Italy, the Netherlands, and Spain (Börsh-Supan and Jurges, 2005; Börsch-Supan et al., 2005); and (3) the English Longitudinal Study of Ageing (ELSA) for England collected in 2002 (Marmot et al., 2007). Sometimes we employ information for England and Wales or the United Kingdom when we use other sources. All of these surveys use similar formats for their questionnaires and survey national samples of people ages 50+. The Nihon University Japanese Longitudinal Study on Aging (Nihon University Japanese Longitudinal Study on Aging, 2009) provides a representative sample of those ages 65+ for Japan, with most of the data used in this analysis from the 2003 wave. For Canada, much of the self-reported information comes from the 2003 Canadian Community Health Survey (CCHS), and for Australia, the source is often the National Health Survey 2004-2005.

Our comparison of national cancer rates is not based on self-reports from surveys but is taken from the GLOBOCAN 2002 database from the

Descriptive Epidemiology Group of the International Agency for Research on Cancer (IARC), part of the World Health Organization (WHO). Cancer registries reflecting national populations or samples from selected regions of countries are the basis for these data (Ferlay et al., 2004).

Our data on measured biological risk draw on resources from the WHO Global Infobase (World Health Organization, 2009), Organisation for Economic Co-operation and Development (OECD) (2008), the U.S. National Health and Nutrition Examination Survey (NHANES) (2001-2006), ELSA (2004) for England, and the Japanese Health and Nutrition Survey Report (2004) (Ministry of Health, Labour and Welfare of Japan, 2006). For Australia, data came from a report based on the Australian Diabetes, Obesity and Lifestyle Study (AusDiab) conducted in 1999-2000 (Dunstan et al., 2001). We link our health measures to estimates of life expectancy at age 50 and differences in life expectancy relative to those in the United States due to specified causes from Glei, Meslé, and Vallin (Chapter 2, in this volume) and to life expectancy at ages 50 and 65 in 2004 from the Human Mortality Database.

After examining country differences in the prevalence of health conditions and risk factors, we use the microdata in a pooled equation for surveys designed to be comparable to examine country differences among individuals in health outcomes with controls for age, diseases, and health behaviors.

CROSS-NATIONAL DIFFERENCES IN POPULATION HEALTH

We begin our examination of health differences at the end of the morbidity process with indicators of loss of functioning and disability. We then examine diseases that are important causes of mortality. Finally, we turn to selected risk factors and bioindicators related to the diseases we have examined.

Disability and Functioning Loss

Many studies of health trends in older populations have focused on trends in disability and functioning loss. Trends in the United States have shown that there has been some improvement in functioning and reduction in disability over the past 25 years (Freedman et al., 2004). The improvement in less severe disability began earlier, and improvement in the most severe category of disability began later and has probably been the smallest. It should be noted that some recent studies have found that improvement in disability may no longer be occurring among the U.S. young-old population (Seeman et al., 2010). Time trends in disability have varied in the other countries we are comparing to the United States (Aijanseppa et al.,

2005). A study comparing trends in severe disability in 12 OECD countries for people ages 65+ (Lafortune, Balestat, and the Disability Study Expert Group Members, 2007) found clear evidence of a decline in disability in Denmark, Italy, the Netherlands, and the United States; an increase in disability in Japan; and no clear direction of change in France or the United Kingdom. Not all studies of trends agree; Schoeni et al. (2006) find some recent improvement in disability in Japan.

We examine two indicators of problems with functioning and disability self-reported in surveys collected in the first half of the decade: (1) having difficulty performing at least 1 of 10 functioning tasks known as Nagi functions and (2) having difficulty performing at least 1 of 6 activities of daily living (ADLs). Difficulties with functioning problems should reflect problems with strength, balance, mobility, and dexterity, and they are an indicator of less severe functioning loss. ADL difficulty reflects difficulty in performing tasks related to self-maintenance and more severe disability. Although some measures of disability can be influenced by the challenge of the environment, as well as the intrinsic health of the person, these measures should primarily reflect perceptions of intrinsic ability.

An examination of the prevalence of functioning problems in the 50+ populations across countries in the early 2000s indicates that people in the United States report more functioning problems than any of the other countries (see Table 3-1). People in Denmark and the Netherlands report the fewest functioning problems. For men, the prevalence of functioning problems in these two countries is about half of the U.S. level; for women, it is about two-thirds of the U.S. level. When the sample is limited to persons ages 65+, the differences between the United States and other countries are not as great. From this, one can infer that U.S. functioning ability is worse relative to that in other countries in the 50-64 range than at older ages. Among women ages 65+, levels of functioning problems in France, Italy, England, and Spain are close to those among U.S. women; U.S. men exceed men in all countries in functioning problems. The country with the lowest level of reported functioning problems at ages 65+ is Japan, for which data were not available in the 50-64 age range. Among the older age group, Denmark and the Netherlands have relatively good functioning.

Americans age 50 and over report more ADL difficulty than anyone except the British. In the older age range, ADL difficulties are fairly similar among Denmark, France, Italy, Spain, and the United States. Again, ADL functioning problems are greater among the English. Only in Japan and the Netherlands is the level of ADL disability notably lower. Differences between the United States and other countries in ADL difficulties also appear to be greater in the younger part of the age range than after age 65.

TABLE 3-1 Functioning Difficulty, Difficulty with Activities of Daily Living (ADLs), and Ratios to U.S. Level, by Gender and Country

	Ages 50+				Ages 65+			
	Men		Women		Men		Women	
Country	%	Ratio/U.S.	%	Ratio/U.S.	%	Ratio/U.S.	%	Ratio/U.S.
Functioning Difficulty								
United States	61.5	1.00	74.0	1.00	67.6	1.00	78.6	1.00
Denmark	34.2	0.56	50.3	0.68	48.5	0.72	63.5	0.81
France	38.3	0.62	59.0	0.80	53.9	0.80	74.4	0.95
Italy	43.8	0.71	60.2	0.81	56.7	0.84	72.1	0.92
Netherlands	31.7	0.52	51.5	0.70	43.4	0.64	62.8	0.80
Spain	43.1	0.70	64.9	0.88	57.8	0.86	77.5	0.99
England	49.2	0.80	64.0	0.86	61.3	0.91	75.3	0.96
Japan	NA	NA	NA	NA	31.4	0.46	46.0	0.59
ADL Difficulty								
United States	13.9	1.00	18.0	1.00	16.1	1.00	21.4	1.00
Denmark	9.9	0.71	11.0	0.61	15.4	0.96	16.7	0.78
France	12.8	0.92	12.5	0.69	19.3	1.20	19.7	0.92
Italy	10.1	0.73	13.9	0.77	15.5	0.96	21.7	1.01
Netherlands	6.4	0.46	10.7	0.59	9.0	0.56	16.7	0.78
Spain	10.2	0.73	15.1	0.84	14.7	0.91	22.5	1.05
England	19.5	1.40	21.8	1.21	25.3	1.57	30.2	1.41
Japan	NA	NA	NA	NA	11.2	0.70	15.0	0.70

NOTES: ADL = activities of daily living. NA = not available. Functioning tasks (10): walking blocks (100 meters, 100 yards); sitting 2 hrs; getting up from a chair; climbing one flight of stairs; climbing several flights of stairs; stooping, crouching, kneeling; reaching over head; pushing/pulling large objects; lifting or carrying 10 lbs (5 kilos); picking up a coin. ADL tasks (6): walking across room, dressing, bathing, eating, getting in or out of bed, using the toilet. In Japan, the functioning tasks do not include picking up a coin or pushing and pulling large objects, but they do include shaking hands and grasping with fingers. Survey question for the English Longitudinal Study of Ageing (ELSA) and the Surveys of Health, Ageing and Retirement in Europe (SHARE): "Please tell me if you have any difficulty with these because of a physical, mental, emotional or memory problem." For the Health and Retirement Study (HRS): "Because of a health or memory problem do you have any difficulty with. . . ." For the Nihon University Japanese Longitudinal Study on Aging (NUJLSOA): "Do you find it difficult to ___ due to your health or physical state?"

SOURCES: Data from HRS (2004) for the United States; from ELSA (2002) for England; from SHARE (2004) for Denmark, France, Italy, the Netherlands, and Spain; and from NUJLSOA (2003) for Japan.

The relationship between national level of life expectancy at age 50 or 65 and the percentage of the population with functioning problems or ADL disability is not very strong. An example of the relationship between national levels of ADL disability and life expectancy at age 65 is shown in Figure 3-1, which displays a statistically insignificant relationship between lower life expectancy and worse ADL functioning.

Differences in Disease Prevalence

We examine cross-national differences in self-reports of three diseases from national surveys: heart disease, stroke, and diabetes (see Table 3-2). Heart disease accounts for more than half of the female gap in life expectancy at age 50 between the United States and nine other countries studied here (0.8 years out of 1.4) and the difference in the gap in life expectancy due to heart disease is greater than the overall male gap (0.8 out of 0.6) (Chapter 2, in this volume, see Table 2A-8). We also examine differences in stroke prevalence, as the U.S. ranking for cerebrovascular death rates relative to other countries has fallen recently, although Americans still have lower death rates than in the average of the nine countries (Chapter 2, in this volume, Table 2A-8). Diabetes deaths contribute to lower life expectancy in the United States compared with the average of the other nine countries of 0.1 year for both men and women at age 50 (Chapter 2, in this volume, see Table 2A-8).

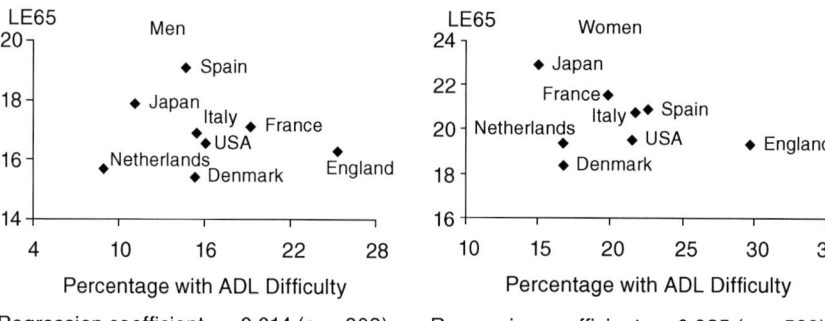

FIGURE 3-1 National percentage of activities of daily living (ADL) difficulty at ages 65+ and life expectancy at age 65 (LE65).
SOURCES: Data on ADL difficulty from Table 3-1; data on life expectancy for 2004 from the Human Mortality Database (see http://www.mortality.org [accessed March 2009]). Life expectancy data extracted from country-specific life tables from the HMD.

TABLE 3-2 Prevalence of Self-Reported Disease in the 50+ and 65+ Populations

	Ages 50+				Ages 65+			
	Men		Women		Men		Women	
Country	%	Ratio/ U.S.	%	Ratio/ U.S.	%	Ratio/ U.S.	%	Ratio/ U.S.
(a) Heart Disease								
United States	28.4	1.00	22.1	1.00	36.4	1.00	28.0	1.00
Denmark	9.9	0.35	7.8	0.35	15.9	0.44	13.0	0.46
France	18.5	0.65	10.8	0.49	28.8	0.79	16.3	0.58
Italy	12.4	0.44	10.1	0.46	18.7	0.51	14.3	0.51
Netherlands	13.6	0.48	8.8	0.40	21.7	0.60	12.9	0.46
Spain	11.3	0.40	11	0.50	15.1	0.41	15.5	0.55
England	23.0	0.81	19.0	0.86	32.2	0.88	26.4	0.94
Japan	NA	NA	NA	NA	14.4	0.40	12.2	0.44
Canada	13.8	0.49	10.7	0.48	21.8	0.60	18.1	0.65
(b) Stroke								
United States	7.3	1.00	6.4	1.00	9.4	1.00	8.6	1.00
Denmark	6.0	0.82	4.9	0.77	9.9	1.05	7.3	0.85
France	3.5	0.48	3.8	0.59	5.5	0.59	5.8	0.67
Italy	3.7	0.51	2.7	0.42	5.8	0.62	4.0	0.47
Netherlands	4.4	0.60	4.8	0.75	7.1	0.76	7.8	0.91
Spain	2.4	0.33	1.9	0.30	2.9	0.31	2.8	0.33
England	4.9	0.67	4.0	0.63	8.2	0.87	6.4	0.74
Japan	NA	NA	NA	NA	9.3	0.99	6.0	0.70
Canada	2.8	0.38	2.4	0.38	5.2	0.55	3.9	0.45
(c) Diabetes								
United States	19.5	1.00	16.5	1.00	21.4	1.00	17.6	1.00
Denmark	8.2	0.42	6.8	0.41	11.1	0.52	8.7	0.49
France	10.9	0.56	8.6	0.52	13.0	0.61	10.8	0.61
Italy	12.8	0.66	11.4	0.69	17.6	0.82	15.7	0.89
Netherlands	7.8	0.40	9.2	0.56	10.6	0.50	12.2	0.69
Spain	15.3	0.78	13.9	0.84	20.4	0.95	17.1	0.97
England	8.6	0.44	6.2	0.38	11.2	0.52	8.0	0.45
Japan	NA	NA	NA	NA	10.1	0.47	7.5	0.43
Canada	11.9	0.61	9.1	0.55	15.6	0.73	11.9	0.68
Australia					16.2	0.76	11.5	0.65

NOTE: ADL = activities of daily living. NA = not available.
SOURCE: Data on self-reported diseases from HRS (2004) for the United States; from ELSA (2002) for England; from SHARE (2004) for Denmark, France, Italy, the Netherlands, and Spain; for NUJLSOA (2003) for Japan; from CCHS (2003) for Canada; and from the Australian Bureau of Statistics (2006a) [http://www.abs.gov.au/ausstats, accessed December 5, 2009] and NHS (2004-2005) for Australia.

Heart Disease

Americans ages 65+ report more heart disease than persons in any of the other countries. The prevalence is only slightly lower in England than in the United States. Denmark and Japan have prevalence values of only about half of the U.S. values (see Table 3-2[a]).[1] Each country's age-sex group ratio to the U.S. value is higher among the 50+ population than among the 65+ population, indicating larger differences at younger ages. National heart disease prevalence is not closely related to national life expectancy (see Figure 3-2[a]).

A number of studies in the United States have reported increases over time in the prevalence of heart disease in the population (Crimmins and Saito, 2001; Cutler and Richardson, 1997), although a recent study reports that this increase may have ended after 1997 (Freedman et al., 2007). An increase in the proportion of the population with heart disease is perhaps not surprising in light of the fact that declining death rates from heart disease have been such a strong contributor to mortality trends (Jemal et al., 2005). Even in the short period from 2000 to 2006, U.S. cases of atrial fibrillation increased by 30 percent and heart failure cases increased by 8 percent among Medicare beneficiaries (Chronic Condition Data Warehouse, 2009).[2]

Stroke

At ages 50+, Americans report the highest prevalence of stroke. For women, the Netherlands and Denmark have prevalences that are about three-fourths of the U.S. level. For the 65+ population, the prevalence of self-reported stroke is highest among Danish men. U.S. and Japanese men have levels very similar to those of the Danes, followed closely by English men (see Table 3-2[b]).[3] This high level of stroke among Japanese men is not surprising, as high levels of stroke with low levels of heart disease have long characterized the Japanese (Reed, 1990). For women, the highest levels

---

[1]The Organisation for Economic Co-operation and Development reports the number of hospital discharges per 100,000 population for acute myocardial infarction (AMI) and cerebrovascular disease. While these are not age-specific rates, they provide some comparison of the self-reports to other sources. The rate of hospital discharge for AMI is highest in Denmark and second in the United States (Organisation for Economic Co-operation and Development, 2008).

[2]A recent paper based on the Framingham Study provides some explanation for the finding that heart attack rates have been relatively constant over recent decades (Parikh et al., 2009). Over the last four decades, improved methods of diagnosis of AMI have led to an increase in the number of cases; if diagnosis had remained the same as in the 1960s and 1970s, the rates of AMI would have declined.

[3]Hospital discharge rates for cerebrovascular conditions are only weakly related to the level of self-reported stroke. Discharge rates are high among the Japanese and Danes but also among Italians, who self-report low stroke prevalence (Organisation for Economic Co-operation and Development, 2008).

INTERNATIONAL DIFFERENCES IN HEALTH AND LIFE EXPECTANCY 77

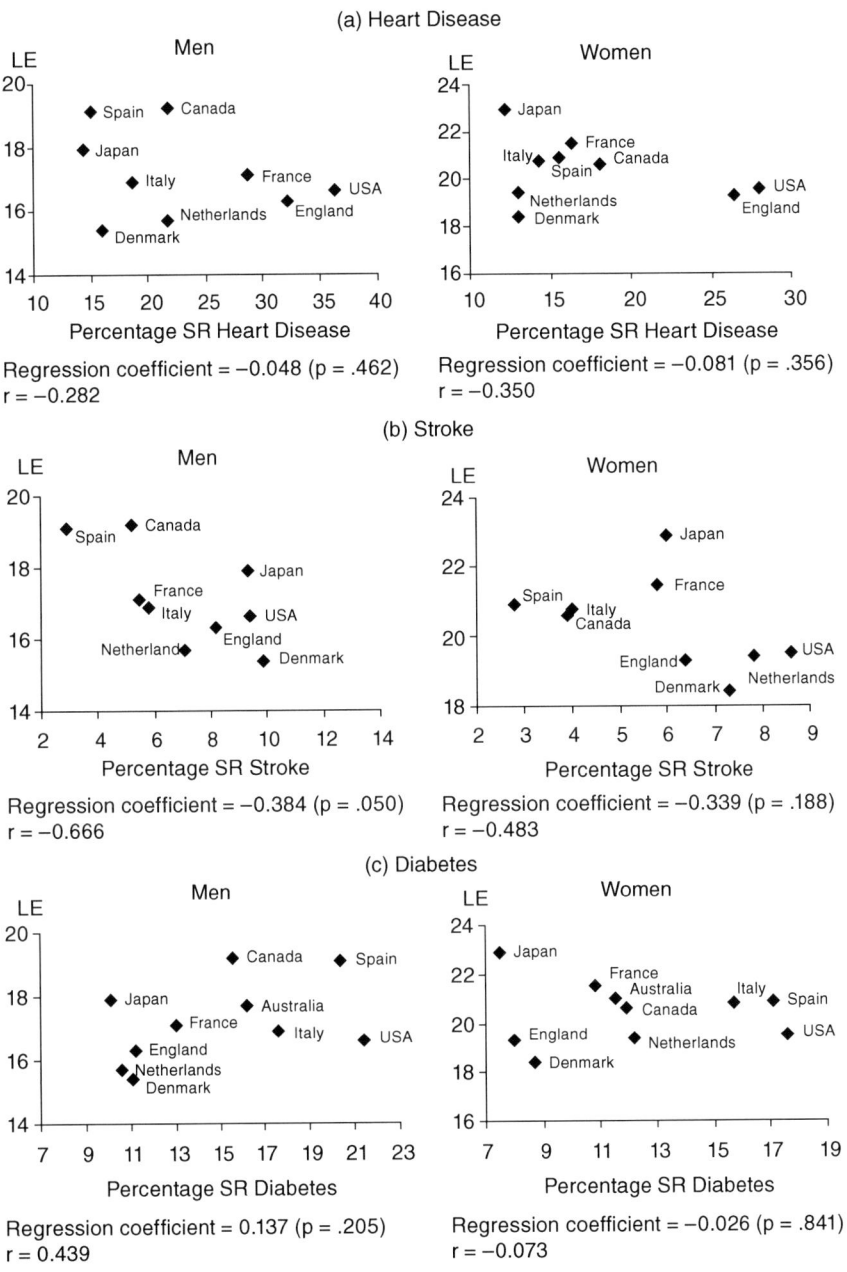

FIGURE 3-2 National percentage self-reporting (SR) disease (65+) and life expectancy (LE) at age 65.
SOURCES: Data on disease from Table 3-2; data on life expectancy for 2004 from the Human Mortality Database (HMD) (see http://www.mortality.org [accessed March 2, 2009]). Life-expectancy data extracted from country-specific life tables from HMD.

of stroke are reported among Americans; Japanese women have lower levels of stroke than Americans, Danes, the Dutch, and the English. This finding that Japanese women now have a lower prevalence of stroke than Americans fits with the observation that, in recent years, mortality related to stroke among Japanese women has been lower than that for U.S. women (Crimmins et al., 2008).

National levels of mortality and stroke prevalence have a stronger association than that observed for heart disease. For women, it is the countries with adverse mortality trends— Denmark, the Netherlands, and the United States—that have relatively high levels of female stroke prevalence (see Figure 3-2[b]).

Diabetes

For those ages 50 and older, diabetes prevalence is reported to be the highest in the United States. For men, only Italy, France, and Spain have levels that exceed half of the U.S. value. Among women, Denmark and England have levels of diabetes only about 40 percent of that in the United States. At ages 65+, the United States has the highest level, followed closely by that of Spain and Italy (see Table 3-2[c]). In Denmark, England, and Japan, self-reported diabetes prevalence at ages 65+ is only about half of that of the United States (Table 3-2[c]).[4] Again, the differences between the United States and other countries appear to be greater in the younger part of the age range examined, as the ratios to the U.S. values are higher at older ages in every case. The link between national levels of self-reported diabetes and mortality is not significant (see Figure 3-2[c]).

In sum, self-reports of disease presence tend to place people in the United States in the high-prevalence group for each of these diseases. Although other countries tend to be high in only one of the three diseases, the United States tends to have high levels in all three. The differences between the United States and other countries in the prevalence of all three diseases are greater among those ages 50-64 than over age 65.

Figure 3-3 shows the level of the three diseases self-reported in each country as related to country-level life expectancy differences from U.S. life expectancy due to heart disease (for heart disease), cerebrovascular disease (for stroke), and diabetes (for diabetes) from Glei, Meslé, and Vallin. (Chapter 2, in this volume). Neither heart disease nor stroke is significantly

---

[4]We also examined diabetes prevalence for the age-standardized population ages 20-79 from OECD reports, which are based on a combination of measured biological markers and self-reports—and therefore are not truly comparable across countries. This is also true because the age groups for which data are available are quite different. The OECD prevalence of diabetes for ages 20-79 is highest in the United States (Organisation for Economic Co-operation and Development, 2008).

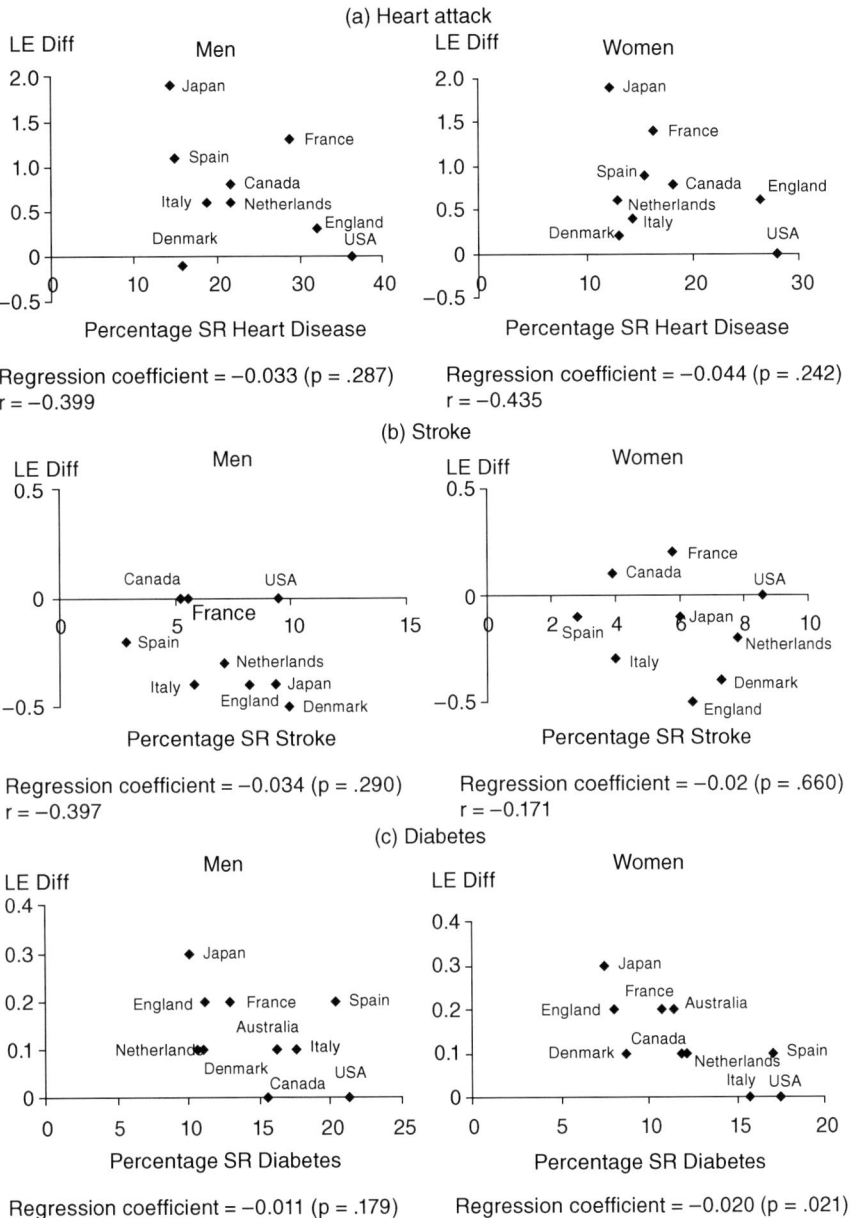

FIGURE 3-3 National percentage self-reporting (SR) disease (65+) and difference from U.S. life expectancy (LE) at age 50 from heart disease, stroke, and diabetes. SOURCES: Data on disease from Table 3-2; data on life expectancy from Glei et al. (Chapter 2, in this volume, Table 2A-8). Life-expectancy data extracted from country-specific life tables from HMD.

related to the national life expectancy differentials, but the level of diabetes and life expectancy lost due to diabetes are significantly related for women, indicating some link between the level of disease and differences in life expectancy.

Cancer

Overall, cancer death rates for men in the United States are shown to be lower than those for the other countries we are considering (contribution to the life expectancy gap between the United States and the other nine countries is –0.4 years); however, for women, lung cancer is a cause of lower life expectancy in the United States (contribution to the gap of lung cancer is 0.3) (Chapter 2, in this volume). We examine differences in incidence of all cancers except nonmelanoma skin cancer but also for four specific cancers: prostate cancer for men, breast cancer for women, lung cancer, and colorectal cancer. The recorded incidence or onset rate of prostate, breast, and colorectal cancers will be affected by policies toward screening, which vary markedly across countries (Banta and Oortwiin, 2001; Hakama et al., 2008; Preston and Ho, Chapter 9, in this volume; Quinn, 2003). Countries with intensive screening are likely to find more cancers. This will include early cancers and cancers that might never produce any symptoms or lead to death. Identifying and treating cancers early should reduce mortality. We also examine mortality rates from cancer to assess incidence relative to mortality (see Figure 3-4).

The United States has the highest recorded incidence of all cancers for both men and women. However, all-cancer mortality rates are moderate for men in the United States; national all-cancer mortality rates for U.S. women could be characterized as among the higher but not the highest levels. The incidence of both prostate and breast cancers are highest in the United States. Mortality from these cancers is not particularly high in the United States. Prostate cancer mortality is higher in Denmark and the Netherlands; breast cancer mortality is higher in Denmark, the Netherlands, and the United Kingdom. Incidence and mortality from both of these cancers are particularly low in Japan.

For both men and women, lung cancer incidence is highest in the United States. Lung cancer mortality is highest among men in the Netherlands; among women, rates are highest among the Danes, and almost as high in the United States and Canada. The difference between the incidence rate and the mortality rate is greatest in the United States. The incidence of colorectal cancer is highest among Japanese men, and it is high among Australians of both genders. Colorectal cancer mortality rates vary little across countries, with the exception that Denmark appears to have higher mortality from colorectal cancer than other countries.

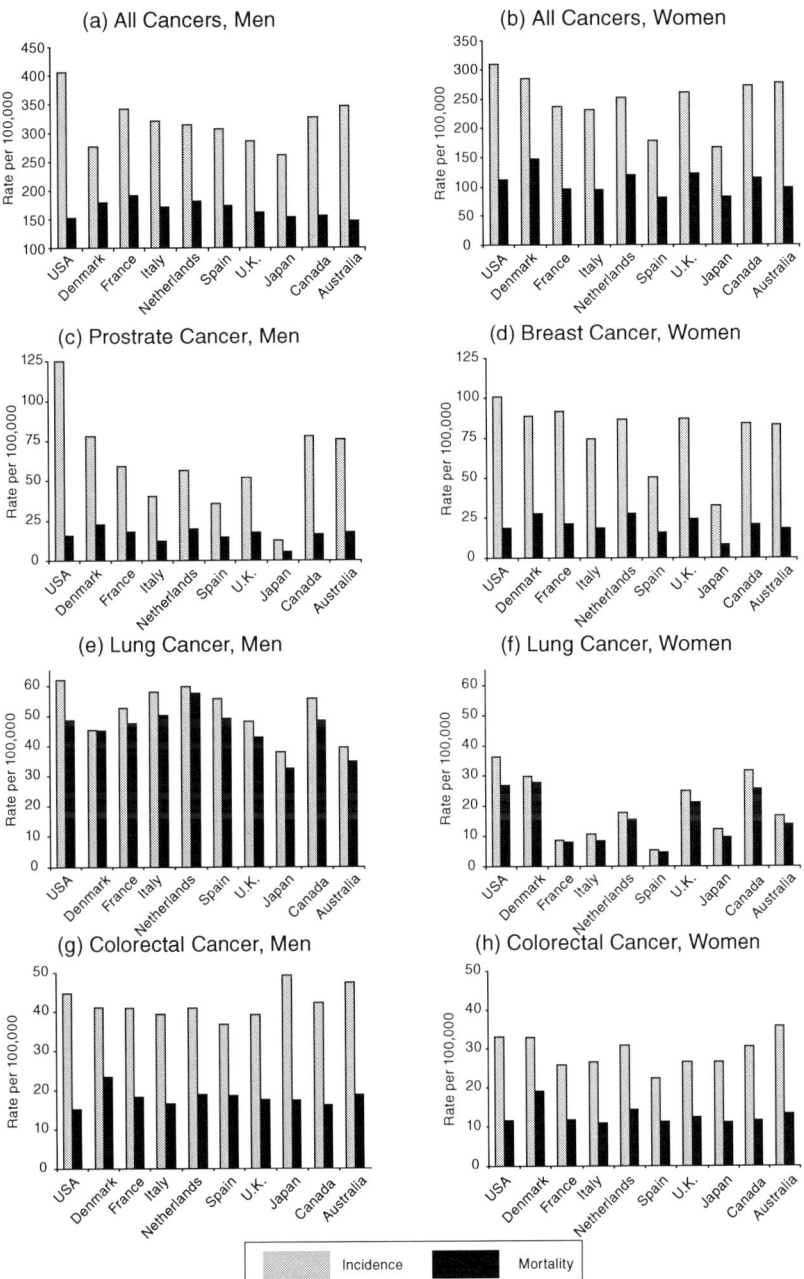

FIGURE 3-4 Age-standardized cancer incidence and mortality rates, 2002. All cancers excluding nonmelanoma skin cancer.
SOURCE: GLOBOCAN 2002 database (Ferlay et al., 2004; see http://www-dep.iarc.fr [accessed June 2010]). Data from summary tables created in online database.

The high incidence of breast and prostate cancers in the United States could reflect high levels of screening (Preston and Ho, Chapter 9, in this volume). This is not true for lung cancer. In contrast to the cardiovascular diseases and diabetes discussed above, the United States does not have particularly high mortality from cancer except for lung cancer for women.

Differences in Risk Factors

Recent research has reported higher levels of some biological risk factors among Americans compared with English and Japanese persons of the same age (Banks et al., 2006; Crimmins et al., 2008). We examine national differences in the prevalence of three indicators of physiological dysregulation that are risk factors for mortality, cardiovascular disease, and diabetes: high cholesterol, high blood pressure, and obesity. Each of these can be either self-reported or measured in populations; we report both types of data. In comparing countries, measured risk avoids some of the problems of self-report that could reflect cultural differences in knowledge about health; however, measured values are much less available. It is also true that measured levels of cholesterol and blood pressure are affected by the use of medications, which is rapidly changing in most countries, making it difficult to compare data collected in different years.

Cholesterol

First, we examine self-reports of having ever been told one has high cholesterol. Self-reported high cholesterol is very high in the United States, 2-3 times higher than in other countries examined (see Table 3-3). About half of the U.S. population ages 50+ reported being told they had high cholesterol (48.2 percent for men; 49.0 percent for women); values are similar at ages 65+ (49.3 percent for men and 42.7 percent for women).

Measured high cholesterol is available for older age groups for a smaller number of countries in the early 2000s. The prevalence of people with high measured cholesterol is low in the United States relative to that in other countries (see Table 3-3). Among those ages 50-64, the percentage with raised measured cholesterol is highest among persons in England. In this age group, U.S. women have the lowest levels of raised measured cholesterol; the percentage of U.S. men with measured high cholesterol is higher than that of the Japanese but lower than in all other countries. Among those ages 65+, Americans and Japanese have relatively low values compared with other countries.

National levels of measured high cholesterol are shown relative to levels of life expectancy in Figure 3-5. In this small group of countries, there is no statistical association between a country's level of raised cholesterol and life expectancy in either the 50-64 or 65+ age group.

TABLE 3-3 Self-Reported Prevalence of High Cholesterol, Measured Level of High Cholesterol, and Ratios to U.S. Level

Country	Men %	Ratio/ U.S.	Women %	Ratio/ U.S.	Men %	Ratio/ U.S.	Women %	Ratio/ U.S.
	Self-Reported High Cholesterol							
	Ages 50+				Ages 65+			
United States	48.2	1.00	49.0	1.00	49.3	1.00	42.7	1.00
Denmark	17.1	0.35	13.6	0.28	21.2	0.43	15.4	0.36
France	23.7	0.49	22.5	0.46	23.7	0.48	26.3	0.62
Italy	18.5	0.38	20.5	0.42	19.8	0.40	20.5	0.48
Netherlands	16.3	0.34	13.4	0.27	15.3	0.31	14.9	0.35
Spain	22.5	0.47	24.9	0.51	21.3	0.43	28.2	0.66
Australia	23.8	0.49	21.6	0.44	16.3	0.33	16.6	0.89
	Measured Prevalence of High Cholesterol (≥240mg/dL)[a]							
	Ages 50-64				Ages 65+			
United States	19.7	1.00	26.7	1.00	10.1	1.00	23.2	1.00
Netherlands	23.8	1.21	28.3	1.06	15.5	1.53	32.2	1.39
Spain	24.3	1.23	32.8	1.23				
England	38.7	1.96	51.2	1.92	24.2	2.40	48.0	2.07
Japan	14.4	0.73	28.6	1.07	10.7	1.06	15.7	0.68
Canada	27.8	1.41	28.6	1.07	25.0	2.48	44.0	1.90

[a]Many values estimated for age groups from the original data. The definition of measured high cholesterol in the Netherlands (≥250mg/dL); England ages 52-64; Canada ages 65-74. Data collection year for measured high cholesterol: United States (2001-2006), the Netherlands (2001), Spain-subnational (1992), England (2004), Japan (2004), and Canada (1990).
SOURCE: Data on self-reported high cholesterol: from NHANES (2001-2006) for the United States; from SHARE (2004) for Denmark, France, Italy, the Netherlands, and Spain; and from AIHW (2006) and NHS (2004-2005) for Australia. Data on measured high cholesterol: from NHANES (2001-2006) for the United States; from ELSA (2004) for England; from the Ministry of Health, Labour and Welfare of Japan (2006) and NHNS (2004) for Japan; and from the WHO Global InfoBase for the Netherlands, Spain, and Canada.

High cholesterol can be fairly effectively controlled by lipid-lowering drugs, so high national use of drugs will reduce the number of persons with high measured cholesterol. The high use of lipid-lowering drugs in the United States is the explanation for why ever having a diagnosis of high cholesterol is relatively high but the prevalence of measured high cholesterol is relatively low. While we do not have data for all of the countries, we have self-reports of the use of lipid-lowering drugs around the same time period in eight countries. The United States has the highest use of lipid-lowering drugs; only Canada and France come close to it in the level of drug use for high cholesterol (see Table 3-4). The United States has been recognized

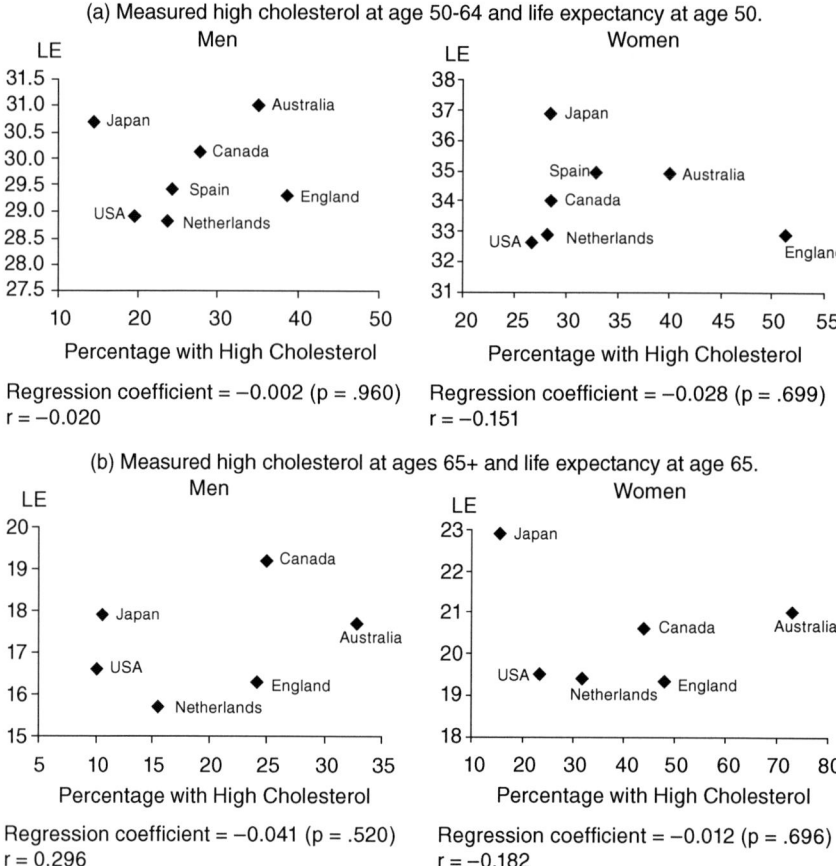

FIGURE 3-5 Measured high cholesterol (≥240mg/dL) and life expectancy (LE). SOURCES: Data on measured high cholesterol from Table 3-3; data on life expectancy for 2004 from the Human Mortality Database (see http://www.mortality.org [accessed March 2009]). Life-expectancy data extracted from country-specific life tables from HMD.

as a country that aggressively treats with pharmaceuticals, but a number of European countries have markedly increased the use of lipid-lowering drugs in this decade. In only three years, from 2000 to 2003, the number of daily doses per person almost tripled in England, more than doubled in Italy, and increased by more than 50 percent in France and the Netherlands (Mantel-Teeuwisse et al., 2002; Walley et al., 2005). Usage also continues to increase in the United States (Crimmins et al., 2010).

TABLE 3-4 Percentage of the Population Taking Lipid-Lowering Drugs

	Ages 50+		Ages 65+	
Country	Men	Women	Men	Women
United States	26.8	24.1	33.1	31.3
Denmark	12.9	9.4	19.9	11.3
France	23.3	21.6	25.3	26.9
Italy	12.2	12.9	14.9	14.3
Netherlands	15.0	12.3	18.4	15.5
Spain	15.4	16.1	16.5	19.6
Japan	8.3	15.1	11.3	20.6
Canada	24.5	20.3	30.7	28.9
Australia	16.3	16.5	16.6	20.9

SOURCES: Data from NHANES (2001-2006) for United States; from SHARE (2004) for Denmark, France, Italy, the Netherlands, and Spain; from Ministry of Health, Labour and Welfare of Japan (2006) and NHNS (2004) for Japan; from CCHS (2003) for Canada; and from Dunstan et al. (2001) and AusDiab (1999-2000) for Australia.

High Blood Pressure

The United States has been described in the past as having levels of measured blood pressure lower than a number of European countries (Wolf-Maier et al., 2003). Based on an analysis of people ages 35-64 and using data from the late 1990s and early 2000s, measured blood pressure was shown to be lower in the United States and Canada and higher in European countries including Italy, England, and Spain. The treatment of hypertension in the United States was also more prevalent, which led to the conclusion that hypertensive treatment was more aggressive there (Wang, Alexander, and Stafford, 2007).

We examine available data on more recent national differences in the prevalence of self-reports of having been told one has hypertension, measured hypertension, and measured hypertension or using antihypertensive medications in Table 3-5. On one hand, self-reports of having been diagnosed with hypertension from survey data are highest for Americans. For those ages 50+, the range across countries of the ratio of national levels to the U.S. level is .43 to .70. At age 65, the range is .48 to .79.

On the other hand, the United States has relatively low levels of measured hypertension. Only English and Australian women ages 50+ and English women ages 65+ have lower levels of measured hypertension than Americans. In France, ratios indicate levels 1.48 to 2.35 times higher than those of Americans. The Japanese also have higher levels of measured hypertension, particularly men.

Some countries report hypertension by combining measured high blood pressure with reported use of drugs to control hypertension. If we consider

TABLE 3-5 Prevalence of High Blood Pressure and Ratio to U.S. Level

Country	Men %	Ratio/ U.S.	Women %	Ratio/ U.S.	Men %	Ratio/ U.S.	Women %	Ratio/ U.S.
	Self-Reported Hypertension							
	Ages 50+				Ages 65+			
United States	53.6	1.00	55.1	1.00	57.2	1.00	62.7	1.00
Denmark	30.4	0.57	28.1	0.51	41.8	0.73	32.6	0.52
France	25.5	0.48	31.7	0.58	31.4	0.55	39.3	0.63
Italy	35.8	0.67	38.1	0.69	43.8	0.77	46.4	0.74
Netherlands	22.8	0.43	27.8	0.50	27.4	0.48	32.7	0.52
Spain	27.0	0.50	37.6	0.68	34.3	0.60	49.5	0.79
England	36.0	0.67	38.7	0.70	41.7	0.73	47.0	0.75
Japan	NA	NA	NA	NA	30.5	0.53	34.3	0.55
Canada	29.5	0.55	35.2	0.64	37.3	0.65	47.1	0.75
Australia	24.4	0.46	29.2	0.53	36.7	0.64	41.8	0.67
	Measured High Blood Pressure (≥140/90mmHg)							
	Ages 50-64				Ages 65+			
United States	28.1	1.00	36.6	1.00	34.3	1.00	49.5	1.00
France	60.6	2.16	65.2	1.78	80.5	2.35	73.1	1.48
England	33.4	1.19	27.9	0.76	44.6	1.30	46.3	0.94
Japan	52.5	1.87	41.2	1.13	66.7	1.94	62.7	1.27
Australia	39.0	1.39	33.4	0.91	72.2	2.10	71.8	1.45
	Measured High (≥140/90mmHg) or Using Medication							
	Ages 50-64				Ages 65+			
United States	50.6	1.00	57.9	1.00	61.9	1.00	73.2	1.00
Netherlands	53.0	1.05	47.0	0.81	76.0	1.23	71.0	0.97
Spain	52.3	1.03	53.9	0.93	60.3	0.97	65.2	0.89
England (2003)	53.1	1.05	44.7	0.77	66.6	1.08	72.1	0.98
Japan	48.8	0.96	39.7	0.69	68.7	1.11	68.7	0.94
Canada					61.1	0.99	43.5	0.59
Australia	46.7	0.92	42.7	0.74	71.8	1.16	70.5	0.96

NOTES: For measured data, estimates made for specified age groups for Australia, France, and Japan.

SOURCES: Data on self-reported hypertension from HRS (2004) for United States; from SHARE (2004) for Denmark, France, Italy, the Netherlands, and Spain; from ELSA (2002) for England; from NUJLSOA (2003) for Japan; from CCHS (2003) for Canada; from AIHW (2006) and NHS (2004-2005) for Australia (50+); and from Australian Bureau of Statistics (2006a) [http://www.abs.gov.au/ausstats, accessed December 5, 2009] and NHS (2004-2005) for Australia (65+). Data on measured hypertension from NHANES (2001-2006) for the United States; from ELSA (2004) for England; and from the WHO Global Infobase for France (1996), Japan (2000), and Australia (1999-2000). Data on measured and measured plus medication from NHANES (2001-2006) for the United States; from the WHO Global Infobase for the Netherlands (2001), Spain (1990), England (2003), Canada limited to Ontario (1990), and Japan (2000); and from Dunstan et al. (2001) and AusDiab (1999-2000) for Australia.

the proportions who either have measured hypertension, or are using medication, American women have the highest level of hypertension, and the difference is greater in the 50-64 age range.[5] For men ages 50-64, there is almost no variability in the proportion with measured hypertension or who use medication across countries; ages 65+, U.S. men appear to have a relatively low level and men in the Netherlands appear to have the highest level. National levels of the percentage with measured high blood pressure and hypertension levels defined as including antihypertensive use are shown relative to life expectancy in Figure 3-6. The relationship is not significant.

Trends in the use of antihypertensives have been similar to those for lipid-lowering drugs, although the uptake of these drugs initially occurred a decade or so earlier. Self-reports of the use of antihypertensives are available for all 10 countries (see Table 3-6). Use of antihypertensives is highest in the United States, although it has increased recently in Europe (Ashworth, Medina, and Morgan, 2008; Primatesta, Brookes, and Poulter, 2001). Italy is the country with the next highest usage, and the ratio of Italian use to American use is .72 and .77 for men and women ages 50+, and .86 and .85 for men and women ages 65+. Overall, the Netherlands appears to be the country with the lowest use of antihypertensives. All of this makes it somewhat hard to determine the relative risk across countries due to elevated blood pressure. Quite clearly, the United States has the most diagnosed high blood pressure but also the fewest people with measured high levels because of the aggressive use of drugs.

Weight

Weight has been increasing throughout the developed world in recent decades, and the increase in the United States has been larger and at earlier ages (Andreyeva, Michaud, and van Soest, 2007; Bleich et al., 2008; Rabin, Boehmer, and Brownson, 2007). Recent rates of increase in obesity have been fastest in the United States, England, and Australia. Data in Table 3-7 are developed from self-reports of height and weight in most countries and measured in others. Self-reports from HRS and SHARE are corrected for tendencies to misreport height and weight (Michaud, van Soest, and Andreyeva, 2007). This is not true for Canada, Australia, or older (65+) Japanese. Body mass index, which is based on measured height and weight, is included for England, the United States, and Japanese ages 50+.

At ages 50+, the level of obesity is highest in the United States. Only English men and Spanish women have levels of obesity even close to those in the United States (ratios of .88 and .89, respectively). Among the Japanese,

---

[5]The value for Canada here is based only on Ontario, so it may not be representative of the entire country.

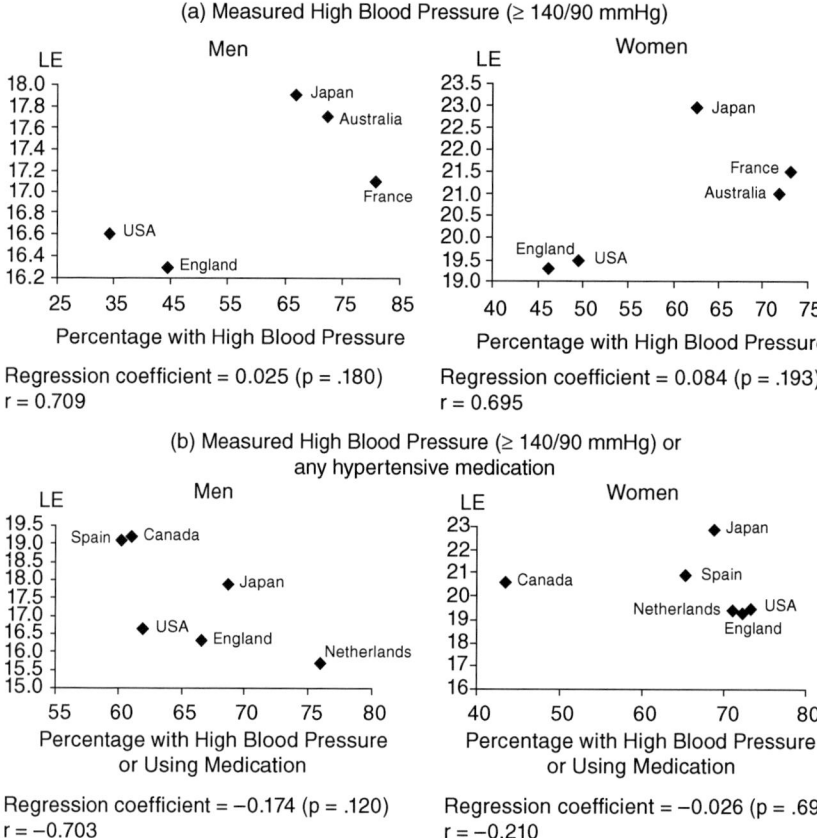

FIGURE 3-6 Measured high blood pressure and life expectancy (LE) at age 65.
SOURCES: Data on high blood pressure from Table 3-5; data on life expectancy for 2004 from the Human Mortality Database (see http://www.mortality.org [accessed March 2, 2009]). Life-expectancy data extracted from country-specific life tables from HMD.

obesity is almost nonexistent (ratios to the United States at 50+ of .10 for men and .08 for women). At ages 65+, obesity in English men and women and Spanish women actually exceeds that in the United States. Again, obesity at this age is extremely low in Japan.

The national prevalence of obesity is graphed against life expectancy at age 50 in Figure 3-7; again, there is no significant relationship, although the association appears stronger among women than men.

TABLE 3-6 Use of Antihypertensive Drugs

	Ages 50+				Ages 65+			
	Men		Women		Men		Women	
Country	%	Ratio/U.S.	%	Ratio/U.S.	%	Ratio/U.S.	%	Ratio/U.S.
United States	47.2	1.00	50.4	1.00	52.1	1.00	58.3	1.00
Denmark	28.3	0.60	25.8	0.51	44.0	0.84	33.1	0.57
France	29.4	0.62	34.6	0.69	39.3	0.75	45.2	0.78
Italy	34.1	0.72	38.8	0.77	45.0	0.86	49.4	0.85
Netherlands	22.4	0.47	27.7	0.55	31.7	0.61	38.2	0.66
Spain	24.6	0.52	36.9	0.73	32.5	0.62	51.3	0.88
England	27.7	0.59	29.8	0.59	35.4	0.68	39.9	0.68
Japan[a]	28.0	0.59	31.0	0.62	38.6	0.74	44.5	0.76
Canada	27.0	0.57	30.7	0.61	39.3	0.75	46.1	0.79
Australia[a]	28.0	0.59	36.2	0.72	34.1	0.65	45.1	0.77

[a]Estimates made for specified age groups.
SOURCES: Data from HRS (2004) for the United States; from SHARE (2004) for Denmark, France, Italy, the Netherlands, and Spain; from ELSA (2002) for England; from CCHS (2003) for Canada (using medication in past month); from the Ministry of Health, Labour and Welfare of Japan (2006) and NHNS (2004) for Japan; and from Dunstan et al. (2001) and AusDiab (1999-2000) for Australia.

MICRO-LEVEL ANALYSIS OF DISEASE PRESENCE, FUNCTIONING LOSS, AND DISABILITY

Taking advantage of the harmonization of the HRS, SHARE, and ELSA data, we can also examine results from individual-level regressions indicating the effect of being a resident of each country while controlling for age and two individual health behaviors: smoking and weight. This analysis does not include data from Australia, Canada, or Japan. Without controls for the behaviors, the odds ratios from logit models for self-reported presence of disease provide an indication of country-level differences assuming the same age distribution. These results should largely reproduce the descriptive results above. With controls for health behaviors, the odds ratios provide an indication of country-level differences in the health indicators, assuming the levels of past and current smoking and weight are similar. Country effects are shown relative to the United States, the omitted category.

The relative level of heart disease is lower in every country than in the United States, with the odds ratios ranging from .31 to .72 (see Table 3-8). There is very little change when health behaviors are controlled, although being obese and having been a smoker are linked to more heart disease. The effect of being obese on heart disease presence is to increase by 50 to 60 percent the relative likelihood of heart disease compared with those who

TABLE 3-7 Prevalence of Obesity and Ratio to U.S. Level

Country	Ages 50+				Ages 65+			
	Men		Women		Men		Women	
	%	Ratio/ U.S.	%	Ratio/ U.S.	%	Ratio/ U.S.	%	Ratio/ U.S.
United States (HRS 2004, self-reported)	30.7	1.00	37.9	1.00	21.2	1.00	21.8	1.00
Denmark	17.5	0.57	18.2	0.48	12.3	0.58	12.4	0.57
France	16.2	0.53	20.3	0.54	13.8	0.65	15.2	0.70
Italy	15.6	0.51	23.4	0.62	14.7	0.69	17.4	0.80
Netherlands	15.3	0.50	23.2	0.61	11.5	0.54	15.9	0.73
Spain	20.8	0.68	33.6	0.89	19.8	0.93	26.3	1.21
England	27.0	0.88	30.7	0.81	24.1	1.14	29.6	1.36
Japan	3.0	0.10	3.0	0.08	1.1	0.04	2.5	0.11
Canada	18.1	0.59	17.7	0.47	14.2	0.67	15.1	0.69
Australia	19.2	0.63	19.9	0.53	13.9	0.66	14.7	0.67
United States (NHANES 2001-2006, measured)	32.9	1.07	35.5	0.94	27.8	1.31	30.8	1.41

NOTES: Obesity is defined as a body mass index (BMI) ≥ 30. Self-reported data from SHARE (50+) for Denmark, France, Italy, the Netherlands, and Spain have been corrected for misreporting by Michaud et al. (2007). Measured data used for England (52+). For Japan estimates were made for BMI≥30 for the 50+ population because only overweight (BMI ≥ 25) is reported; for the 65+ population, estimates were computed from self-reports in the NUJLSOA (2003). For Canada and Australia, BMI was calculated from self-reported height and weight. Estimates were made for specified age groups for Australia. Data collection year: for the United States, self-report (2004), measured (2001-2006); for Denmark (2004), France (2004), Italy (2004), the Netherlands (2004), Spain (2004), England (2004), Japan 50+ (2004), 65+ (2003), Canada (2003), Australia (2004-2005).

SOURCES: Data on obesity (50+) from Michaud et al. (2007, Table 1) for the United States, Denmark, France, Italy, the Netherlands, and Spain; from ELSA (2004) for England; from the Ministry of Health, Labour and Welfare of Japan (2006) and NHNS (2004) for Japan; from Statistics Canada (see http://www.statcan.gc.ca [accessed July 7, 2009]) and CCHS (2003) for Canada; from the Australian Bureau of Statistics (2006b) (see http://www.abs.gov.au/ausstats [accessed December 5, 2009]) and NHS (2004-2005) for Australia; from NHANES (2001-2006) for the United States (measured). Data on obesity (65+) from HRS (2004) for United States; from SHARE (2004) for Denmark, France, Italy, the Netherlands, and Spain; from ELSA (2004) for England; from NUJLSOA (2003) for Japan; from CCHS (2003) for Canada; and from the Australian Bureau of Statistics (2006b) (see http://www.abs.gov.au/ausstats [accessed December 5, 2009]) and NHS (2004-2005) for Australia.

are not obese. Having been a smoker increases the relative likelihood of heart disease by more than 30 percent.

Relative to the United States, male stroke prevalence is significantly lower in each of these countries except Denmark (OR .33 to .73). This is true with or without controls for health behaviors. Women in the United States, Denmark, and the Netherlands have similar levels of stroke; in other

INTERNATIONAL DIFFERENCES IN HEALTH AND LIFE EXPECTANCY

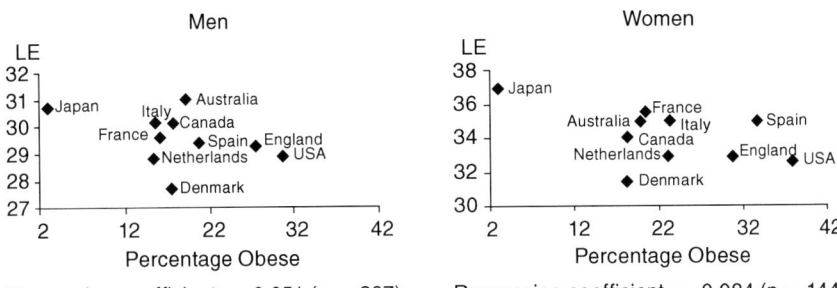

FIGURE 3-7 National percentage obese and national life expectancy at age 50. SOURCE: Data on obesity from Table 3-7; data on life expectancy for 2004 from the Human Mortality Database (see http://www.mortality.org [accessed March 2009]). Life-expectancy data extracted from country-specific life tables from HMD.

countries, the levels are lower than those in the United States. Having been a smoker for both sexes, currently smoking for men, and being obese for women are strongly associated with having had a stroke.

Every country has significantly lower levels of diabetes than the United States for both men and women, with or without the controls for weight. The odds ratios for other countries on diabetes range from .29 to .82 and are not changed much by controls for weight and smoking, although being overweight or obese is strongly associated with being diabetic. Overweight is linked to odds ratios indicating a doubling of the relative likelihood of having diabetes, whereas being obese multiplies the odds ratios by 3.54 times for men and 5.2 times for women.

The effects of country of interview on functioning and ADLs disability with and without controls for the health behaviors and for the presence of the three diseases (heart disease, diabetes, and stroke) that are potential causes of disability and functioning loss are shown in Table 3-9. When controlled for all these variables, these odds ratios for countries represent the level of functioning and ADL problems in each country relative to the United States if the prevalence of these diseases and the health behaviors were the same across countries.

Both men and women in the United States have more functioning problems. Without controls, the odds ratios for functioning problems for other countries range from .36 to .73. With controls, the odds ratios generally become higher or closer to the United States, indicating that some of the explanations of the difference in functioning problems are the higher level of disease and obesity among Americans. Each disease as well as higher weight and smoking raises the likelihood of functioning problems.

TABLE 3-8 Odds Ratios from Logistic Regressions of Country, Age, and Health Behaviors on Self-Reported Prevalence of Heart Disease, Stroke, and Diabetes

	Heart Disease				Stroke				Diabetes			
	Men		Women		Men		Women		Men		Women	
	M1	M2	M1	M2	M1	M2	M1	M2	M1	M2	M1	M2
Age	1.06*	1.06*	1.05*	1.06*	1.05*	1.06*	1.06*	1.07*	1.02*	1.03*	1.02*	1.03*
United States (ref)												
Denmark	0.34*	0.35*	0.31*	0.33*	1.01	0.97	0.84	0.82	0.41*	0.48*	0.38*	0.49*
France	0.68*	0.72*	0.44*	0.50*	0.55*	0.57*	0.62*	0.72*	0.54*	0.63*	0.50*	0.60*
Italy	0.40*	0.43*	0.42*	0.46*	0.58*	0.58*	0.44*	0.49*	0.65*	0.73*	0.66*	0.75*
Netherlands	0.48*	0.50*	0.36*	0.38*	0.73*	0.70*	0.84	0.87	0.38*	0.45*	0.51*	0.60*
Spain	0.36*	0.38*	0.43*	0.47*	0.33*	0.32*	0.31*	0.36*	0.75*	0.80*	0.82*	0.78*
England	0.64*	0.63*	0.72*	0.68*	0.41*	0.40*	0.44*	0.41*	0.38*	0.36*	0.29*	0.25*
Overweight		1.08		1.08		1.02		1.05		1.79*		2.02*
Obese		1.47*		1.61*		1.12		1.32*		3.54*		5.20*
Current smoker		0.90		0.98		1.34*		1.21		0.98		0.96
Ever smoker		1.36*		1.31*		1.47*		1.42*		1.24*		1.00
N	15,211		19,493		15,216		19,498		15,212		19,495	

*p < 0.05.
SOURCE: Data from HRS, SHARE, ELSA Countries, 50+ Sample, 2004.

TABLE 3-9 Odds Ratios from Logistic Regressions of Country, Age, and Health Behaviors on Self-Reported Prevalence of Functioning and ADL Difficulty

	Functioning Difficulty				ADL Difficulty			
	Men		Women		Men		Women	
	M1	M2	M1	M2	M1	M2	M1	M2
Age	1.06*	1.06*	1.05*	1.06*	1.05*	1.05*	1.06*	1.06*
United States (ref)								
Denmark	0.39*	0.46*	0.39*	0.49*	0.82	1.00	0.60*	0.77*
France	0.45*	0.53*	0.56*	0.74*	1.09	1.39*	0.70*	0.93
Italy	0.56*	0.69*	0.57*	0.72*	0.80*	1.02	0.80*	1.03
Netherlands	0.36*	0.41*	0.42*	0.50*	0.52*	0.64*	0.62*	0.77*
Spain	0.53*	0.60*	0.66*	0.76*	0.73*	0.91	0.78*	0.93
England	0.69*	0.75*	0.73*	0.73*	1.50*	1.83*	1.31*	1.49*
Heart disease		2.13*		2.42*		1.68*		1.87*
Stroke		2.55*		2.51*		3.45*		3.11*
Diabetes		1.68*		1.46*		1.62*		1.81*
Overweight		1.22*		1.58*		1.00		1.19*
Obese		2.43*		3.89*		1.93*		2.47*
Current smoker		1.33*		1.30*		1.35*		1.42*
Ever smoked		1.43*		1.10*		1.28*		1.05
N	15,204		19,478		15,203		19,484	

*$p < 0.05$.
SOURCE: Data from HRS, SHARE, ELSA Countries, 50+ Sample, 2004.

Differences in ADL functioning between men in the United States and those in other countries are not so consistent as those found above for funtioning difficulty. Without controls, there is no difference in ADL functioning among men in Denmark, France, and the United States. English men have more ADL problems than Americans. Men in the United States have worse ADL functioning than men in Italy, Spain, and the Netherlands. If all the countries had the same presence of the three diseases, smoking, and obesity, U.S. men would only have more ADL functioning problems than men in the Netherlands. U.S. women have worse ADL functioning than those in all other countries except England. If the prevalence of the included diseases and the health behaviors were the same across countries, U.S. women would only fare worse than Dutch and Danish women. These results seem to indicate that the relatively poor ranking of Americans in terms of ADL functioning is largely due to the presence of more diseases, more overweight, and higher smoking levels.

DISCUSSION

Reviewing this complex set of health differences, two conclusions stand out. For many indicators of health, the United States ranks as the country with the highest prevalence of problems. This includes functioning, heart disease, stroke at some ages, diabetes, and obesity. The other generalization is that Japan is often the country ranking as best in a number of health indicators. This includes functioning and ADL disability levels, prevalence of heart disease, diabetes, and obesity, and incidence of some cancers. Many other countries rank poorly in some health indicators but do not rank poorly in others, so it is hard to determine a clear ranking for other countries. Denmark and the Netherlands stand out as having relatively high levels of stroke and mortality from some cancers, yet these countries appear to have relatively good levels of physical functioning. The poor position of the United States and the good position of Japan provide some support for a link between levels of life expectancy and levels of population health, but the overall association is weak for many of the indicators.

Banks and colleagues (2006) have pointed out that Americans in their 50s and 60s had more diseases and worse levels of a number of biomarkers than the English. Crimmins and colleagues (Crimmins et al., 2008; Reynolds et al., 2008) have noted that levels of functioning problems and disability, diseases, and a number of biomarkers are worse among Americans than the Japanese. Poor relative health appears to characterize comparisons of Americans with multiple additional countries. The diseases with higher prevalence among Americans are conditions that are related to health behaviors and lifestyle factors.

For a number of indicators, the relatively poor position of the United States was more exaggerated among people ages 50-64 than in the group ages 65+. This included functioning and ADL disability, heart disease, stroke, and obesity. Although we do not have the ability to examine the effects of mortality and disease onset with these data, these findings could be compatible with earlier onset of disease among Americans.

Obesity is a potential explanation of some of the poor health indicators in the United States, as it is related to each of the diseases we examined, and the diseases are, in turn, related to more functioning problems. Our micro-level analysis indicated the substantial effect of obesity on the presence of each of these diseases, functioning loss, and disability; however, our analysis controlling for overweight and obesity indicates that Americans would report more heart disease, stroke, diabetes, and functioning problems even if they had the same levels of overweight, obesity, and smoking patterns as in the SHARE countries and England. In further analysis, we replicated the regressions in Tables 3-8 and 3-9 after eliminating all obese persons, and the results are hardly changed: nonobese Americans are still likely to have more diseases and worse functioning problems. Both obese and the nonobese Americans have more diseases and disabilities than persons in other countries.

Our disease-specific analyses do not indicate the level of concentration of health problems in individuals. It is possible that the concentration of health problems in individuals differs across countries and is one explanation of why mortality is not strongly related to the prevalence of individual health problems. One hypothesis for why some countries do poorly is that health problems are concentrated in a smaller group in the population. For the countries for which we have individual data, we examined the occurrence of comorbidity of heart disease, stroke, and diabetes. We found dramatically higher levels of comorbidity in the United States than in other countries, indicating a larger portion of the population with multiple serious health risks in the United States (see Table 3-10). The proportion of people with more than one of the three conditions—heart disease, stroke, and diabetes—is generally at least twice as high in the United States as in the other countries. Further analysis should include better information on

TABLE 3-10 Percentage Self-Reporting More Than One of the Three Conditions—Heart Disease, Stroke, and Diabetes

	Men	Women
Among 50+		
United States (HRS 2004, SR)	10.7	8.7
Denmark (SHARE wave 1)	2.4	2.2
France	3.8	3.2
Italy	3.1	3.5
Netherlands	3.6	2.9
Spain	4.5	3.0
England (ELSA wave 2)	4.2	3.3
Japan	NA	NA
Canada	4.2	3.1
Among 65+		
United States (HRS 2004, SR)	13.7	11.1
Denmark	4.4	3.7
France	5.6	4.7
Italy	5.0	4.8
Netherlands	5.9	4.8
Spain	7.0	4.1
England (ELSA wave 2)	6.4	4.7
Japan	4.5	2.4
Canada	6.9	5.2

NOTE: NA = not available.
SOURCES: Data from HRS (2004) for the United States; from SHARE (2004) for Denmark, France, Italy, the Netherlands, and Spain; from ELSA (2004) for England; from NUJLSOA (2003) for Japan; and from CCHS (2003) for Canada.

the concentration of risks and comorbid conditions among individuals. This chapter has not examined social differences in health risks across countries, but they are known to be relatively large in the United States (Avendano et al., 2009; Avendano et al., Chapter 11, in this volume). Both social disadvantages and health disadvantages may be more concentrated in the United States, while health disadvantage may be distributed more equally across the population in other countries.

Our data also have some implications for assessing performance of the U.S. health care system relative to those in other countries. The United States does relatively well at diagnosing and treating hypertension and high cholesterol. Risk is reduced well below what it would be without the widespread use of drug treatment. It is hard to say how countries rank in the relative risk from hypertension and high cholesterol given that the United States has the highest diagnosed levels of these risks but almost the lowest measured levels of current risk, indicating high levels of control. This provides an indication of the role of the U.S. health care system in reducing the risk associated with hypertension and high cholesterol. However, the significantly worse health in the United States for people ages 50-64 occurs in an age group whose health care insurance availability is lower than at older ages.

Cancer death rates, except for lung cancer among women, are relatively low in the United States (see also Preston and Ho, Chapter 9, in this volume). Cancer screening appears to identify a relatively high number of cases in the United States and to result in a lower rate of mortality among incident cases. This could reflect good treatment or the fact that extensive screening identifies cases that have a lower chance of dying. Again, it becomes somewhat difficult to determine relative cancer risk across countries, as our observations are so affected by screening. This high identification of screenable cancers is another indication of the positive role of the U.S. health care system.

Can we rely on the results of our analyses of diseases and functioning problems based on self-reports? Research has shown relatively high agreement between the self-report and medical record report for some conditions: diabetes, stroke, and myocardial infarction (Bush et al., 1989; Goldman et al., 2003; Okura et al., 2004). Because our analysis relied on self-reports of diagnosed heart disease, not limited to myocardial infarction, it is possible that national differences in the prevalence of heart disease are affected by reporting and diagnostic differences. The level of agreement between self-report and medical records for hypertension is generally thought to be lower than that for some other conditions, and this may be the case for the European countries included in SHARE in our analysis. Functioning difficulties and disability are generally self-reported in surveys, not based on a doctor's diagnosis.

Two recent analyses of how Americans and the Dutch report disability have come to different conclusions about relative reporting tendencies. Comparing responses to vignettes indicates that, with a given description of a disability, Americans are less likely than the Dutch to see a person as disabled (Kapteyn, Smith, and van Soest, 2007); however, another comparison of American and Dutch self-reports of disability to measured disabilities shows Dutch individuals have greater limitation when they report themselves disabled (Melzer et al., 2004). It is hard to know how to assess the overall effect of national differences in reporting or diagnostic tendencies; however, most of the differences we observe are quite large, and they are relatively consistent across many conditions. It is hard to believe that all differences arise from differential reporting. Additional sources of differential reporting include cultural context, sociodemographic characteristics, and environmental circumstances (Bago d'Uva, O'Donnell, and van Doorslaer, 2008; Bago d'Uva et al., 2008; Iburg et al., 2001; Melzer et al., 2004).

Finally, to return to our initial discussion about population health, with prevalence data it is difficult to determine the process that resulted in the observed differences. It is obvious that current health status, including mortality, reflects past heath, health behaviors, and health care use. Thus, in order to understand the process leading to mortality, we need information on earlier health behaviors, incidence of, and survival from certain conditions. However, most of our data indicate current prevalence, cancer being the exception. While our results show higher levels of some conditions and risk factors in the United States, longitudinal data are required for a better understanding of the roles of incidence, treatment, and survival in creating current health, including mortality. As we mentioned earlier, increasing survival among people with diseases and functioning problems can lead to a higher prevalence of health problems in the population. Finally, our cross-sectional data are limited in making any connection between earlier risk factors, lifelong health behaviors, and lifetime circumstances that could affect later health.

ACKNOWLEDGMENTS

Support was provided by the U.S. National Institutes of Health (P30 AG17265) and the University of Southern California Humanities and Social Sciences Fund. This chapter uses data from the early release of SHARE 2004. SHARE data collection was primarily funded through the European Commission through the 5th framework program (Project QLK6-CT-2001-0060 in the thematic program "Quality of Life"). Additional funding came from the U.S. National Institute on Aging (U01 AG09740-13S2, P01 AG005842, P01 AG08291, P30 AG12816, Y1-AG-4553-01, and OGHA 04-064). Data collection in Austria, Belgium, and Switzerland was nationally funded. The collection of the Health and Retirement Study was supported by the U.S.

National Institute on Aging (U01 AG009740) and is conducted by the University of Michigan. ELSA was developed by a team of researchers based at the National Centre for Social Research, University College London, and the Institute for Fiscal Studies. The data were collected by the National Centre for Social Research and made available through the UK Data Archive. The funding is provided by the U.S. National Institute on Aging and a consortium of United Kingdom government departments coordinated by the Office for National Statistics. This analysis is based on Statistics Canada's Canadian Community Health Survey, Cycle 2.1 (2003), Public Use Microdata File, which contains anonymized data. All computations on these microdata were prepared by University of Southern California, and the responsibility for the use and interpretation of these data is entirely that of the authors. The developers and funders of the data sets do not bear any responsibility for the analyses or interpretations presented here.

REFERENCES

Aijanseppa, S., Notkola, I.L., Tijhuis, M., van Stavern, W., Kromhout, D., and Nissinen, A. (2005). Physical functioning in elderly Europeans: 10-year changes in the north and south: The HALE project. *Journal of Epidemiology and Community Health, 59*(5), 413-419.

Andreyeva, T., Michaud, P.C., and van Soest, A. (2007). Obesity and health in Europeans aged 50 years and older. *Public Health, 121,* 497-509.

Asai, A. (1995). Should physicians tell patients the truth? *Western Journal of Medicine, 163*(1), 6-39.

Ashworth, M., Medina, J., and Morgan, M. (2008). Effect of social deprivation on blood pressure monitoring and control in England. *British Medical Journal, 337,* a2030.

Australian Bureau of Statistics. (2006a). *Health of Older People in Australia: A Snapshot, 2004-2005.* No. 4833.0.55.001. Canberra: Australian Bureau of Statistics. Available http://www.abs.gov.au/ausstats [accessed December 2009].

Australian Bureau of Statistics. (2006b). *National Health Survey: Summary of Results, Australia 2004-2005.* No. 4364.0. Canberra: Australian Bureau of Statistics. Available http://www.abs.gov.au/ausstats [accessed December 2009].

Australian Institute of Health and Welfare. (2006). *Chronic Diseases and Associated Risk Factors in Australia, 2006.* No. PHE 81. Canberra: Author.

Avendano, M., Glymour, M., Banks, J., and Mackenbach, J.P. (2009). Health disadvantage in U.S. adults aged 50-74 years: A comparison of the health of rich and poor Americans with that of Europeans. *American Journal of Public Health, 99,* 540-548.

Bago d'Uva, T., O'Donnell, O., and Van Doorslaer, E. (2008). Differential health reporting by education level and its impact on the measurement of health inequalities among older Europeans. *International Journal of Epidemiology, 37,* 1375-1383.

Bago d'Uva, T., Van Doorslaer, E., Lindeboom, M., and O'Donnell, O. (2008). Does reporting heterogeneity bias the measurement of health disparities? *Health Economics, 17,* 351-375.

Banks, J., Marmot, M., Oldfield, Z., and Smith, J.P. (2006). Disease and disadvantage in the United States and in England. *Journal of the American Medical Association, 295,* 2037-2045.

Banta, H.D., and Oortwiin, W. (2001). Health technology assessment and screening in the Netherlands: Case studies of mammography in breast cancer, PSA screening in prostate cancer, and ultrasound in normal pregnancy. *International Journal of Technology Assessment in Health Care, 17*(3), 369-379.

Bleich, S., Cutler, D., Murray, C., and Adams, A. (2008). Why is the developed world obese? *Annual Review of Public Health, 29*, 273-295.

Börsch-Supan, A., and Jürges, H. (Eds.). (2005). *The Survey of Health, Ageing and Retirement in Europe: Methodology.* Mannheim, Germany: Mannheim Research Institute for the Economics of Ageing.

Börsch-Supan, A., Brugiavini, A., Jürges, H., Makenbach, J., Siegrist, J., and Weber, G. (Eds.). (2005). *Health, Ageing, and Retirement in Europe: First Results from the Survey of Health, Ageing, and Retirement in Europe.* Mannheim, Germany: Mannheim Research Institute for the Economics of Ageing.

Bush, T., Miller, S., Golden, A., and Hale, W. (1989). Self-report and medical record report agreement of selected medical conditions in the elderly. *American Journal of Public Health, 79*, 1554-1556.

Chronic Condition Data Warehouse. (2009). *Medicare Beneficiary Prevalence for Chronic Conditions for 2000-2007* (Table B.2). Available http://ccwdata.org/downloads/data_tables/CCW_Web_Site_Table_B.2.pdf [accessed June 2009].

Crimmins, E.M., and Saito, Y. (2001). Trends in healthy life expectancy in the United States, 1970-1990: Gender, racial, and educational differences. *Social Science and Medicine, 52*, 1629-1641.

Crimmins, E., Hayward, M., and Saito, Y. (1994). Changing mortality and morbidity rates and the health status and life expectancy of the older U.S. population. *Demography, 31*, 159-175.

Crimmins, E.M., Kim, J.K., Vasunilashorn, S., Hagedorn, A., and Saito, Y. (2008). A comparison of biological risk factors in two populations: The United States and Japan. *Population and Development Review, 34*, 457-482.

Crimmins, E.M., Kim, J.K., and Vasunilashorn, S. (2010). Biodemography: New approaches to understanding trends and differences in population health and mortality. Submitted to *Demography*.

Cutler, D.M., and Richardson, E. (1997). Measuring the health of the U.S. population. In M. Baily, P. Reiss, and C. Winston (Eds.), *Brookings Papers on Economic Activity: Microeconomics* (pp. 214-282). Washington, DC: Brookings Institution.

DECODE Study Group, on behalf of the European Diabetes Epidemiology Study Group. (1998). Will new diagnostic criteria for diabetes mellitus change phenotype of patients with diabetes? Reanalysis of European epidemiological data. *British Medical Journal, 317*, 371-375.

Dunstan, D., Zimmet, P., Welborn, T., Sicree, R., Armstrong, T., Atkins, R., Cameron, A., Shaw, J., and Chadban, S. (2001). *Diabetes and Associated Disorders in Australia—2000: The Australian Diabetes, Obesity and Lifestyle Study (AusDiab).* Available http://www.diabetes.com.au/pdf/AusDiab_Report.pdf [accessed December 2009].

Ferlay, J., Bray, F., Pisani, P., and Parkin, D.M. (2004). *GLOBOCAN 2002: Cancer Incidence, Mortality and Prevalence Worldwide.* IARC CancerBase No. 5. version 2.0. Lyon, France: IARC Press.

Freedman, V.A., Crimmins, E., Schoeni, R.F., Spillman, B.C., Aykan, H., Kramarow, E., Land, K., Lubitz, J., Manton, K., Martin, L.G., Shinberg, D., and Waidmann, T. (2004). Resolving inconsistencies in old-age disability trends: Report from a technical working group. *Demography, 41*, 417-441.

Freedman, V.A., Schoeni, R.F., Martin, L.G., and Cornman, J.C. (2007). Chronic conditions and the decline in late life disability. *Demography, 44*(3), 450-477.

Fries, J.F. (1980). Aging, natural death, and the compression of morbidity. *New England Journal of Medicine, 303,* 130-135.

Goldman, N., Lin, I., Weinstein, M., and Lin,Y. (2003). Evaluating the quality of self-reports of hypertension and diabetes. *Journal of Clinical Epidemiology, 56,* 148-154.

Gregg, E.W., Cadwell, B.L., Cheng, Y.J., Cowie, C.C., Williams, D.E., Geiss, L., Engelgau, M.M., and Vinicor, F. (2004). Trends in the prevalence and ratio of diagnosed to undiagnosed diabetes according to obesity levels in the United States. *Diabetes Care, 27*(12), 2806-2812.

Gruenberg, E.M. (1977). The failures of success. *Milbank Memorial Fund Quarterly/Health and Society, 55,* 3-24.

Hakama, M., Coleman, M.P., Alexe, D.M., and Auvinen, A. (2008). Cancer screening: Evidence and practice in Europe 2008. *European Journal of Cancer, 44*(10), 1404-1413.

Health and Retirement Study. (2006). *2004 HRS Core.* Final, v.1.0 (data file). Available http://hrsonline.isr.umich.edu/ [accessed January 2009].

Human Mortality Database. (2009). *Life Tables* (data file). University of California Berkeley, and Max Planck Institute for Demographic Research (Germany). Available http://www.mortality.org [accessed March 2009].

Iburg, K., Salomon, J.A., Tandon, A., and Murray, C.J.L. (2001). *Cross-Population Comparability of Physician-Assessed and Self-Reported Measures of Health: Evidence from the Third National Health and Nutrition Examination Survey.* Discussion Paper No.14. Available http://www.who.int/healthinfo/paper14.pdf [accessed November 2009].

Jemal, A., Ward, E., Hao, Y., and Thun, M. (2005). Trends in the leading causes of death in the United States, 1970-2002. *Journal of the American Medical Association, 294*(10), 1255-1259.

Kapteyn, A., Smith, J.P., and van Soest, A. (2007). Vignettes and self-reports of work disability in the United States and the Netherlands. *American Economic Review, 97*(1), 461-473.

Lafortune, G., Balestat, G., and the Disability Study Expert Group Members. (2007). *Trends in Severe Disability Among Elderly People: Assessing the Evidence in 12 OECD Countries and the Future Implications.* Working Paper No. 26. Available http://www.oecd.org/dataoecd/13/8/38343783.pdf [accessed March 2009].

Mantel-Teeuwisse, A.K., Klungel, O.H., Verschuren, W.M., Porsius, A.J., and de Boer, A. (2002). Time trends in lipid lowering drug use in the Netherlands. Has the backlog of candidates for treatment been eliminated? *British Journal of Clinical Pharmacology, 53,* 379-385.

Manton, K.G. (1982). Changing concepts of morbidity and mortality in the elderly population. *Milbank Memorial Fund Quarterly/Health and Society, 60,* 183-244.

Marmot, M., Banks, J., Blundell, R., Lessof, C., and Nazroo, J. (Eds.). (2007). *Health, Wealth, and Lifestyles of the Older Population in England: The 2002 English Longitudinal Study of Aging.* Report No. P2058. London, England: Institute for Fiscal Studies, National Center for Social Research.

Melzer, D., Lan, T.Y., Tom, B.D.M., Deeg, D.J.H., and Guralnik, J. (2004). Variation in thresholds for reporting mobility disability between national population subgroups and studies. *Journal of Gerontology: Medical Sciences, 59A*(12), 1295-1303.

Michaud, P., van Soest, A., and Andreyeva, T. (2007). Cross-country variation in obesity patterns among older Americans and Europeans. *Forum for Health Economics and Policy, 10*(2), Article 8.

Ministry of Health, Labour and Welfare of Japan. (2006). *National Health and Nutrition Survey Report, 2004.* (In Japanese). Tokyo, Japan: Daiichi Shuppan.

Nihon University Japanese Longitudinal Study of Aging. (2009). *Nihon University Japanese Longitudinal Study of Aging.* Available http://www.usc.edu/dept/gero/CBPH/nujlsoa/ [accessed February 19, 2009].

Okura, Y., Urban, L., Mahoney, D., Jacobsen, S., and Rodeheffer, R. (2004). Agreement between self-report questionnaires and medical record data was substantial for diabetes, hypertension, myocardial infarction and stroke but not for heart failure. *Journal of Clinical Epidemiology, 57,* 1096-1103.

Organisation for Economic Co-operation and Development. (2008). *OECD Health Data 2008* (Version 06/28/2008) [Statistics]. Available http://new.sourceoecd.org [accessed October 8, 2008].

Parikh, N.I., Gona, P., Larson, M.G., Fox, C.S., Benjamin, E.J., Murabito, J.M., O'Donnell, C.J., Vasan, R.S., Levy, D. (2009). Long-term trends in myocardial infarction incidence and case fatality in the National Heart, Lung, and Blood Institute's Framingham Heart Study. *Circulation, 10,* 1203-1210.

Primatesta, P., Brookes, M., and Poulter, N.R. (2001). Improved hypertension management and control: Results from the health survey for England 1998. *Hypertension, 38,* 827-832.

Quinn, M.J. (2003). Cancer trends in the United States: A view from Europe. *Journal of the National Cancer Institute, 95*(17), 1258-1261.

Rabin, B.A., Boehmer, T.K., and Brownson, R.C. (2007). Cross-national comparison of environmental and policy correlates of obesity in Europe. *European Journal of Public Health, 17*(1), 53-61.

Reed, D.M. (1990). The paradox of high risk of stroke in population with low risk of coronary heart disease. *American Journal of Epidemiology, 131*(4), 579-588.

Reynolds, S.L., Hagedorn, A., Yeom, J., Saito, Y., Yokoyama, E., and Crimmins, E.M. (2008). A tale of two countries—the United States and Japan: Are differences in health due to differences in overweight? *Journal of Epidemiology, 18,* 280-290.

Schoeni, R.F., Liang, J., Bennett, J., Sugisawa, H., Fukaya, T., and Kobayashi, E. (2006). Trends in old-age functioning and disability in Japan, 1993-2002. *Population Studies, 60*(1), 39-53.

Seeman, T., Merkin, S.S., Crimmins, E.M., and Karlamangla, A. (2010). Disability trends among older Americans: National Health and Nutrition Examination Surveys, 1988-1994 and 1999-2004. *American Journal of Public Health, 100*(1), 100-107.

Statistics Canada. (2010). *CANSIM,* Table 105-0501. No. 82-221-X. [Statistics]. Available http://www.statcan.gc.ca [accessed July 7, 2009].

Walley, T., Folino-Gallo, P., Stephens, P., and Van Ganse, E. (2005). Trends in prescribing and utilization of statins and other lipid lowering drugs across Europe 1997-2003. *British Journal of Clinical Pharmacology, 60*(5), 543-551.

Wang, Y.R., Alexander, G.C., and Stafford, R.S. (2007). Outpatient hypertension treatment, treatment intensification, and control in Western Europe and the United States. *Archives of Internal Medicine, 167,* 141-147.

Wareham, N.J., and O'Rahilly, S. (1998). The changing classification and diagnosis of diabetes: New classification is based on pathogenesis, not insulin dependence. *British Medical Journal, 317*(7155), 359-360.

Wolf-Maier, K., Cooper, R.S., Banega, J.R., Giampaoli, S., Hense, H.W., Joffres, M., Kastarinen, M., Poulter, N., Primatesta, P., Rodríguez-Artalejo, F., Stegmayr, B., Thamm, M., Tuomilehto, J., Vanuzzo, D., and Vescio, F. (2003). Hypertension prevalence and blood pressure levels in 6 European countries, Canada, and the United States. *Journal of the American Medical Association, 289*(18), 2363-2369.

World Health Organization. (2009). *WHO Global InfoBase Online* [Statistics]. Available https://apps.who.int/infobase/report.aspx [accessed January 2009].

Part II

Identifying Causal Explanations

4

Contribution of Smoking to International Differences in Life Expectancy

Samuel H. Preston, Dana A. Glei, and John R. Wilmoth

INTRODUCTION[1]

Cigarette smoking increases the risk of dying from many different causes of death. According to the criteria used by the U.S. surgeon general for establishing a causal relationship, these causes include lung cancer, many other forms of cancer, cerebrovascular disease, chronic obstructive pulmonary disease, and coronary heart disease (U.S. Surgeon General, 2004).

The most persuasive data identifying the mortality risks associated with smoking have been drawn from prospective cohort studies that compare the death rates of current smokers and former smokers with the death rates of those who never smoked regularly. The largest such study, the Cancer Prevention Study II (CPS-II), has tracked mortality among a cohort numbering 1.2 million individuals when the study began in 1982. Participants are volunteers recruited by the American Cancer Society and are more likely to be white, middle class, and college-educated than the U.S. population as a whole (Thun et al., 1997).

Although highly informative, the cohort studies are subject to several biases. Perhaps most important, imprecise classification of smoking status among participants reduces the measured impact of smoking on mortality. Smoking behavior often varies over time, whereas in cohort studies smoking status is typically identified at baseline and assumed constant thereafter. Movement of current smokers or nonsmokers out of their baseline category during the course of the study will downwardly bias the estimated hazard from smoking. Correction for this bias among a subsample of CPS-II par-

---

[1] Introductory sections of this paper draw on Preston, Glei, and Wilmoth (2010).

ticipants whose smoking behavior was followed up in 1994 substantially raised the estimated risk of smoking (Taylor et al., 2002). Furthermore, the smoking categories themselves impose a rigid frame on what can be blurry patterns of behavior. For example, CPS-II includes among "lifetime nonsmokers" persons who had smoked but who had not reported themselves as smoking daily for at least a year (Leistikow et al., 2008).

Cohort studies have also been used to estimate the number of deaths in a *population* that are attributable to smoking. This calculation is conventionally made by comparing the actual number of deaths in a particular age-sex group in the population with the number that would have occurred if everyone had had the death rates of lifetime nonsmokers in that category. Based on CPS-II results, Mokdad et al. (2004) used this method to estimate that 435,000 deaths were attributable to smoking in the United States in 2000. There was no control for potentially confounding variables in smoker's estimated risk. Using a nationally representative sample drawn from the National Health Interview Survey and controlling for many confounding factors, Rogers et al. (2005) estimated that 338,000 U.S. deaths were attributable to smoking in 2001. The wide range of existing estimates illustrates the inherent difficulty of this type of analysis and gives some indication of the uncertainty associated with all such estimates (including those presented here).

While the number of deaths attributable to smoking can be estimated directly from cohort studies, such studies are not available in many populations for which attributable risk estimates are sought. In 1992, Peto, Lopez, and colleagues developed an ingenious method for filling this gap (Peto et al., 1992). The method "borrows" the relative risks of cause-specific mortality for current smokers versus nonsmokers from CPS-II and applies them to the population of interest. Rather than applying them to the distribution of the population by smoking status, they instead used observed death rates from lung cancer as an indicator of the population's cumulative smoking exposure, which may be a more reliable index of the cumulative damage from smoking than directly measured smoking behavior based on self-report.

Having selected lung cancer death rates as the indicator of the cumulative damage from smoking, Peto et al. then translated observed lung cancer death rates for a given population into an estimate of the smoking impact ratio by referring to the difference between lung cancer death rates for smokers and nonsmokers in CPS-II. This scalar is then used to adjust the cause-specific relative risks for smokers versus nonsmokers from CPS-II in order to derive a population-specific estimate of the risk attributable to smoking for other smoking-related causes of death. Clearly, their approach is heavily dependent on the assumption that CPS-II estimates of lung cancer death rates for smokers and nonsmokers and relative risks for other causes of death can be applied (with some adjustment) to other countries and across time (Sterling, Rosenbaum, and Weinkam, 1993). Furthermore, because smokers are self-selected, some of the mortality differential between smokers and nonsmokers may be attributable to confounding with other risk factors. Thus, to avoid overstating the impact of smoking, Peto et al. rather arbitrarily halved the CPS-II relative excess risks for causes other than lung cancer. More recent applications of the method have lowered the reduction to 30 percent (Ezzati and Lopez, 2003). More recently still, researchers have adjusted directly for confounding factors (Ezzati et al., 2005; Danaei et al., 2009). Rostron and Wilmoth (forthcoming) modified the Peto-Lopez approach by using more refined age intervals and adjusting the baseline level of lung cancer mortality.

Staetsky (2009) has applied the Peto-Lopez method to trends in women's mortality above age 65 between 1973-1975 and 1995-1997. She found that a substantial fraction of the slowdown in women's mortality improvements in the United States, Denmark, and the Netherlands relative to France and Japan is attributable to smoking.

We have developed an alternative to the Peto-Lopez method for calculating deaths attributable to smoking in high-income countries (Preston, Glei, and Wilmoth, 2010). As they do, we use lung cancer mortality as the basic indicator of the damage caused by smoking in a particular population. However, we do not rely on the relative risks from CPS-II or any other study. Instead, we investigate the macro-level statistical association between lung cancer mortality and mortality from all other causes of death in a data set of 21 countries covering the period 1950 to 2007. This approach is motivated by the expectation that lung cancer mortality is a reliable indicator of the damage from smoking and that such damage has left a sufficiently vivid imprint on other causes of death that it is identifiable in country-level data. A related approach has been applied to subnational time-series data for various cancers (Leistikow and Tsodikov, 2005; Leistikow et al., 2008).

We apply this method to data from 21 high-income countries and estimate the proportion of deaths at ages 50+ that are attributable to smoking. We then estimate the impact of removing these deaths from a population's mortality profile on life expectancy at age 50 and on international variation therein.

METHODS

Modeling Strategy[2]

The model that we use for estimating the impact of smoking on mortality is based on the assumption that lung cancer mortality is a good proxy

---

[2]The model was introduced by Preston, Glei, and Wilmoth (2010); we repeat the description here for completeness.

for the impact of smoking on mortality from other causes. Specifically, we assume that, after adjusting for sex and age, smoking is the only source of variation in lung cancer death rates in the populations under consideration. This assumption is also used in the Peto-Lopez model and is justified by evidence suggesting that changes in lung cancer rates result primarily from the history of smoking behavior (Brennan and Bray, 2002; Haldorsen and Grimsrud, 1999; Lopez, 1995; Preston and Wang, 2006). The assumption that smoking is the overwhelming factor accounting for variation in lung cancer mortality is further justified by estimates that, among men ages 30 and older in industrialized countries in 2000, 91-92 percent of lung cancer deaths are attributable to smoking; for women, the corresponding percentages are 70-72 percent (Ezzati and Lopez, 2003).

We use negative binomial regression to model mortality at ages 50-54, 55-59, ..., 80-84 from causes other than lung cancer (M_O) as a function of lung cancer mortality (M_L) and other variables. Preliminary analyses indicated that variation in M_O was greater than would be present in a Poisson process, thus justifying the choice of a negative binomial model. A log-linear relationship is assumed between mortality and its predictors (thus, a unit increase in M_L is associated with a constant proportional increase in M_O). Additional justification of the functional form is presented in Annex 4A. The outcome variable is the number of deaths from causes other than lung cancer for a given country-year-age group divided by the number of person-years of exposure.

Data are available to apply the same model at ages 85+. When Preston, Glei, and Wilmoth (2009) included data for ages 85+, results showed a sharp rise in coefficients at older ages, particularly for women. This set of coefficients produced what was later determined to be an implausible increase with age in the proportion of deaths attributable to smoking among women in such high-smoking countries as the United States (Ho and Preston, 2009). Data at ages 85+ are more vulnerable to age misreporting, which has led the U.S. National Center for Health Statistics to make corrections of estimates at ages 85+ in U.S. life tables for 2000-2005 (E. Arias, personal communication, 2009, National Center for Health Statistics). Furthermore, the open-ended age interval is wider than others, creating the possibility that variation in age distributions may affect the 85+ death rate in a manner that is extraneous to actual mortality levels. And the increase with age in the number of conditions present at death may render cause-of-death assignments less precise. Accordingly, in this chapter, we fit the model using only data up to age 84.

Because the effects of smoking may differ between the sexes and because of sex differences in age patterns of mortality, we model mortality separately for men and women. The model includes country fixed effects as well as dummy variables representing age (50-54, ..., 80-84) and time (individual calendar years from 1950 to 2003). In addition to a set of dummies representing calendar year, we also include interactions between country and year (treated as linear) to allow for intercountry differences in the pace of mortality decline. We include an interaction between M_L and year of observation (treated as a linear variable), which may capture changes in the cause distribution of deaths, in the activity of confounding factors, or in the relative risks associated with smoking (e.g., Doll et al., 2004; Thun et al., 1997). Finally, we interact the smoking indicator with the set of age dummies to allow the association between M_L and M_O to vary across age. Previous studies have typically found that the relative risk of death for smokers versus nonsmokers declines with age (Thun et al., 1997).

Thus, we estimate the following model of ln M_O (technically, the log of its expected value) for each sex separately:

$$\ln M_O = \beta_a X_a + \beta_t X_t + \beta_c X_c + \beta_{ct}(t \times X_c) + \beta_L M_L + \beta_{Lt}(M_L \times t) + \beta_{La}(M_L \times X_a), \qquad (1)$$

where M_O is the death rate from causes other than lung cancer classified by age, sex, year of death, and country (or population); X_a is a set of dummy variables for each age group; X_t is a set of dummy variables for each calendar year; X_c is a set of dummy variables for each country; $(t \times X_c)$ denotes a set of interactions between calendar year (linear) and each country dummy; M_L is the death rate from lung cancer; $(M_L \times t)$ is an interaction between M_L and year; and finally, $(M_L \times X_a)$ represents M_L interacted with the age dummies.

Estimating the Attributable Fraction

To estimate the fraction of deaths attributable to smoking, we assume that in the absence of smoking, lung cancer rates (by sex and 5-year age group) would match those observed among individuals in the CPS-II study (1982-1988) who never smoked regularly (Thun et al., 1997). These rates are presented in Table 4-1. Lung cancer rates among other samples of nonsmokers in industrialized countries are generally similar (Doll et al., 1994; Enstrom, 1979). However, lung cancer mortality and incidence are substantially higher among nonsmokers in some parts of Asia, including China and Japan (Thun et al., 2008). No trend in lung cancer mortality among nonsmokers in the United States was observed over a 20-year period (Rosenbaum, Sterling, and Weinkam, 1998; U.S. Department of Health and Human Services, 1989). In some populations in which the prevalence of smoking is thought to have been very low, lung cancer rates were even lower than among nonsmokers in CPS-II. For example, rates of lung cancer among Spanish women ages 70 and older in 1951-1954 as estimated here

TABLE 4-1 Coefficients for Lung Cancer Death Rates in 2003 and Assumed Values of Lung Cancer Death Rates Among Nonsmokers

Age Group	Model Coefficients for Lung Cancer Death Rate (per 1,000) in 2003[a]		Assumed Lung Cancer Death Rates (per 1,000) Among Nonsmokers[b]	
	Men	Women	Men	Women
50-54	0.320	0.745	0.06	0.06
55-59	0.170	0.482	0.05	0.07
60-64	0.104	0.297	0.12	0.12
65-69	0.069	0.162	0.22	0.17
70-74	0.048	0.087	0.35	0.31
75-79	0.038	0.057	0.52	0.33
80-84	0.040	0.094	0.89	0.58
85+	0.042	0.080	0.87	0.61

[a]Based on a negative binomial regression model predicting mortality from causes other than lung cancer. For ages 50-54 through 80-84, the coefficients shown here correspond to values of β'_L as defined in the description of equation (3). Thus, a 0.001 change in the lung cancer death rate implies that the death rate for other causes combined is higher by a factor of $e^{\beta'_L}$ for the specified age-sex group in 2003, taking into account interactions with both age and calendar year. Each sex-specific model also includes dummy variables for country, calendar year, and age group as well as interactions between country and year (treated as linear). For ages 85+ (which were excluded when fitting the model), the coefficient is estimated as the mean of the coefficients for ages 70-74, 75-79, and 80-84.

[b]Based on observed lung cancer rates among persons in the 1982-1988 CPS-II who never smoked regularly (Thun et al., 1997).

SOURCES: The values are based on calculations by authors using data in the Human Mortality Database (accessed November 2009) and the World Health Organization Mortality Database (accessed December 2009).

(see below) are less than half the nonsmoker rates observed in the CPS-II. To the extent that we overestimate lung cancer death rates for nonsmokers, we will underestimate the fraction of deaths attributable to smoking and vice versa.

Our procedures lead to a particularly simple method of estimating the proportion of deaths attributable to smoking. For each country-year-sex-age group, we calculate the fraction of lung cancer deaths attributable to smoking as:

$$A_L = \frac{M_L - \lambda_L^N}{M_L}, \qquad (2)$$

where M_L is the observed lung cancer death rate and λ_L^N is the expected rate among nonsmokers. In cases in which $M_L - \lambda_L^N$ is negative, the value of A_L is set at 0. For mortality from other causes, we compare the number of deaths predicted by the negative binomial regression model under two assumptions about the lung cancer death rate: that it equals the observed level for the population or that it equals the level assumed for nonsmokers in the corresponding sex-age group. The difference between these two predicted numbers of deaths, divided by the prediction based on the observed level of lung cancer mortality, provides an estimate of the fraction attributable to smoking. This procedure is equivalent to implementing the following formula:

$$A_O = 1 - e^{-\beta'_L (M_L - \lambda_L^N)}, \qquad (3)$$

where $\beta'_L = \beta_L + (t - 1950)\beta_{Lt} + \beta_{La}$. Thus, the coefficient in this expression, β'_L, includes the main coefficient of M_L in equation (1) as well as any interactions between M_L and time (since 1950) or age. If $M_L - \lambda_L^N$ is positive (as it is in the large majority of cases), then A_O lies between 0 and 1.[3] If $M_L - \lambda_L^N$ is negative, we set the value to zero before computing A_O. Since ages 85+ were excluded when fitting the model, we estimate $\beta'_L(85+)$ as the average of $\beta'_L(70-74)$, $\beta'_L 75-79)$, and $\beta'_L(80-84)$.

Finally, the overall attributable fraction for deaths from all causes is a weighted average:

$$A = \frac{A_L D_L + A_O D_O}{D}, \qquad (4)$$

where D_L, D_O, and D represent the observed number of deaths from lung cancer, other causes, and all causes combined, respectively.

Validity and Robustness

In Preston, Glei, and Wilmoth (2010), we investigated the validity of this approach by applying it to specific causes of death in addition to the combination category, "all causes other than lung cancer." We observe the expected relationships for both men and women: lung cancer mortality is powerfully related to mortality from respiratory diseases across populations, strongly related to smoking-related cancers, positively but more weakly related to other cancers, and unrelated (or even slightly negatively related) to mortality from external causes. Previous approaches (e.g., Peto-Lopez) often estimate smoking-attributable mortality separately by groups of causes. Consequently, variation in coding practice across time and country may

---

[3] There are no cases in which β'_L is negative.

compromise the results.[4] By combining all causes other than lung cancer into one large group, our method is less sensitive to misclassification errors.

We also investigated the robustness of results to two alternative specifications of equation (1). The two alternatives are (1) the use of a second-degree polynomial rather than a set of dummy variables to represent the interaction between age and lung cancer mortality and (2) deletion of the variable representing trends in the relation between lung cancer mortality and mortality from other causes. In addition, we examined the sensitivity of the results to the exclusion of Hungary and Japan when fitting the model. Hungary is the only Eastern European country in our data set and exhibits excess mortality in middle adulthood similar to that observed in post-Soviet countries. Japan is the sole Asian country in our data set and has a very low level of mortality combined with a rapid increase in smoking prevalence, while nonsmokers' mortality from lung cancer in Japan may be higher than assumed in the present study. We determined that estimates of attributable risk produced by the method were robust to alternative specifications for men. They were less robust for women, the sex group on which smoking has left a lighter imprint (Preston, Glei, and Wilmoth, 2009). The sensitivity of results to alternative specifications among women was reduced by eliminating data for ages 85+.

Estimating the Effects of Smoking on e_{50}

To estimate the impact of removing smoking-attributable deaths on life expectancy at age 50 (e_{50}), we used period life table estimates from the Human Mortality Database (Human Mortality Database, 2009). These tables comprise national data on mortality rates by sex and age up to an open age interval of 110+. At very old ages (approximately 95+), the observed death rates have been smoothed, yielding more reliable estimates of underlying mortality conditions (Wilmoth et al., 2005, pp. 35-38). To estimate what e_{50} would be in the absence of smoking deaths, we multiplied each death rate (M_{sa}) for sex s at age a by the factor ($1 - A_{sa}$), where A_{sa} is the proportion of deaths attributable to smoking in the age interval that includes age a. We assumed that the same attributable fraction applies to all ages in each 5-year age group (50-54, . . . , 80-84) and in the open age interval (85+). Finally,

---

[4]For example, the proportion of deaths coded to ill-defined causes—which is often used as an indicator of coding reliability—ranged from 19 percent in France to 1.1 percent in the United States during 1955 (Glei, Meslé, and Vallin, Chapter 2, this volume). By 2004, this proportion had fallen to 6 percent in France compared with 1 percent in the United States. Given such variation in the level of ill-defined causes, the mixture of causes included in this category (and the extent to which smoking-related deaths are coded to this group) may have varied considerably across time and place.

we recalculated the sex-specific life table using these new age-specific death rates and following standard methods (Wilmoth et al., 2005).

Next, we decomposed gains in e_{50} between 1950 and 2003 into the contributions due to changes in smoking-attributable mortality versus other factors. First, we disaggregated the all-cause death rates (by sex and age) for each country in 1950 and 2003 into the part attributable to smoking ($M_{sa} \times A_{sa}$) and the part due to other factors ($M_{sa} \times (1 - A_{sa})$). Then, we decomposed the observed gains in e_{50} (1950-2003) into these two "causes" using the Pollard method (1988).

DATA

Death counts by cause of death are drawn from the World Health Organization Mortality Database (World Health Organization, 2009). All-cause death counts, exposure estimates, and death rates come from the HMD (2009). To estimate parameters of the statistical model, we used annual data by sex and 5-year age groups (50-54, . . . , 80-84) for 21 high-income countries since 1950. The data set used for this analysis contained 284.8 million deaths and 9.9 billion person-years of exposure. For each country-year-sex-age group, we apply the distribution of deaths by cause from the World Health Organization to the death counts and rates from the HMD to derive cause-specific death counts and rates.

RESULTS

Table 4-1 presents the estimated age- and sex-specific regression coefficients depicting the relationship between lung cancer death rates and mortality from other causes for 2003. As noted earlier, we estimate the coefficient for ages 85+ as the mean of coefficients for ages 70-74, 75-79, and 80-84. No clear age trend is evident for either sex in this set of three coefficients.

Each coefficient in the table indicates the proportionate effect of a 0.001 change in the lung cancer death rate on mortality from other causes of death. Since the model includes an interactive variable between lung cancer mortality and time and that variable has a significant (though small) positive coefficient, the relationship between lung cancer mortality and mortality from other causes of death has shifted from period to period. The coefficient for this interaction indicates a linear time trend (on a logarithmic scale) of 0.0003 for men and 0.0010 for women. Both coefficients, though very small, are statistically significant ($p < .001$). Thus, ceteris paribus, the predicted value of M_O corresponding to a particular value of M_L is estimated to increase by 1.5 percent for men and 5.1 percent for women over a 50-year period.

Attributable Risk Estimates

As described above, we estimate the number of lung cancer deaths that are attributable to smoking by comparing the actual number of deaths with the number that would have been observed if everyone had the lung cancer death rates of lifetime nonsmokers in CPS-II. To estimate the proportion of deaths from other causes attributable to smoking for a particular age-sex group, we use equation (3). Results of these calculations are shown in Table 4-2.

These estimates indicate that the attributable risk from smoking is much greater for men than for women. However, the risk for women, which was negligible in 1955, has been growing rapidly in most countries. France, Portugal, and Spain are exceptions where the imprint of smoking remains small for women; thus, more than a "Mediterranean diet" may be involved in the favorable mortality conditions among women in Spain and France

TABLE 4-2 Estimated Smoking-Attributable Fraction Among Deaths at Ages 50 and Older in 1955, 1980, 2003, by Sex and Country

Country	Men			Women		
	1955	1980	2003	1955	1980	2003
Australia	0.07	0.22	0.17	0.00	0.04	0.10
Austria	0.15	0.21	0.17	0.01	0.02	0.05
Belgium	0.09	0.30	0.27[a]	0.00	0.01	0.05[a]
Canada	0.07	0.22	0.24	0.01	0.06	0.19
Denmark	0.07	0.22	0.20	0.01	0.06	0.16
Finland	0.18	0.28	0.17	0.01	0.02	0.04
France	0.05	0.17	0.19	0.00	0.00	0.02
Hungary	0.07	0.22	0.30	0.01	0.05	0.13
Iceland	0.03	0.06	0.16	0.00	0.11	0.18
Ireland	0.04	0.17	0.19	0.02	0.07	0.14
Italy	0.04	0.20	0.23	0.00	0.01	0.04
Japan	0.01	0.11	0.20	0.00	0.03	0.09
Netherlands	0.10	0.32	0.26	0.00	0.01	0.09
New Zealand	0.08	0.21	0.17	0.00	0.06	0.12
Norway	0.02	0.09	0.16	0.00	0.01	0.07
Portugal	0.02	0.07	0.12	0.00	0.00	0.01
Spain	0.04	0.14	0.22	0.00	0.00	0.00
Sweden	0.03	0.10	0.09	0.00	0.02	0.06
Switzerland	0.09	0.19	0.16	0.00	0.01	0.04
United Kingdom	0.16	0.30	0.20	0.02	0.09	0.15
United States	0.08	0.23	0.22	0.01	0.08	0.20

[a]Estimates based on data from 2004 for Belgium.
SOURCES: Calculations by authors based on data in the Human Mortality Database (accessed November 2009) and the World Health Organization Mortality Database (accessed December 2009).

(Knoops et al., 2004). For men, trends in the attributable fraction are more mixed: the risk declined between 1980 and 2003 in 10 countries and rose in 11. In every country except Iceland, the attributable risk fraction for 2003 is greater for men than for women. In 2003, the largest estimated proportion of deaths above age 50 that is attributable to smoking occurred in Hungary among men (0.30) and in the United States among women (0.20). Annex 4B breaks down our estimates of deaths attributable to smoking into those attributable to lung cancer and those attributable to other causes of death.

It is possible that we have overestimated the impact of smoking on Japanese mortality because nonsmokers' death rates from lung cancer in Japan are higher than assumed here (Thun et al., 2008). In this regard, it is instructive to note that our results for Japanese men show lower attributable risk than that estimated from prospective studies. Katanoda et al. (2008) pool data from three Japanese prospective studies to estimate the smoking-attributable fraction. They estimate that 28 percent of deaths are attributable to smoking among men in a slightly younger age range, versus 20 percent for the present study. However, their estimate for women is 7 percent versus our estimate of 9 percent. Our high estimate for Japanese women is primarily attributable to very high lung cancer mortality above age 80, a phenomenon that seems likely to have an epidemiological source other than smoking (although passive smoke from coresidence with men and with a younger generation is a conceivable factor).[5]

Table 4-3 presents a comparison of the smoking-attributable fraction estimated by our model with the Peto-Lopez estimates for 2000, the latest year for which the Peto-Lopez method has been widely applied to data from developed countries (Peto et al., 2006). Peto-Lopez results pertain to ages 35+, whereas ours apply to ages 50+. Because deaths between ages 35 and 50 are few relative to deaths at ages 50+, the difference in age spans should have only a minor effect on the comparison (where such data exist, estimates of the attributable fraction for ages 35+ are typically no more than 1-2 percentage points higher than for ages 50+).

It is clear that the two methods produce very similar results for both men and women. This similarity pertains both to the level of attributable risk and to its international distribution. The correlation between the at-

---

[5]For example, among Japanese women in 2003, our estimates of the smoking-attributable fraction among the 5-year age groups from 50-54 to 75-79 ranges from 0.04 to 0.07 compared with 0.09 for ages 80-84 and 0.12 among ages 85+. Because ages 80+ account for a large proportion of all deaths (62 percent in this case), the overall attributable fraction is dominated by the higher values. In comparison, the estimated smoking-attributable fractions among their U.S. counterparts are 0.23-0.35 below age 80, 0.22 at ages 80-84, and 0.13 at ages 85+. Japanese women appear to have surprisingly high lung cancer rates at the oldest ages; for ages less than 80, the rates are much lower than for their U.S. counterparts (e.g., 0.6 versus 2.4 per 1,000 for ages 70-74, respectively), whereas the Japanese rates are nearly as high as the U.S. rates for ages 85+ (2.0 versus 2.2 per 1,000, respectively).

TABLE 4-3 Comparison of Smoking-Attributable Fraction in 2000, by Sex and Country

	Men		Women	
Country	Based on Model[a] (Ages 50+)	Peto-Lopez[b] (Ages 35+)	Based on Model[a] (Ages 50+)	Peto-Lopez[b] (Ages 35+)
Australia	0.18	0.20	0.10	0.11
Austria	0.17	0.19	0.06	0.06
Belgium	0.29[c]	0.31	0.04[c]	0.05
Canada	0.23	0.25	0.17	0.18
Denmark	0.21	0.25	0.17	0.20
Finland	0.18	0.18	0.04	0.04
France	0.19	0.21	0.01	0.02
Hungary	0.30	0.31	0.11	0.12
Iceland	0.13	N/A	0.18	N/A
Ireland	0.20	0.22	0.14	0.16
Italy	0.24	0.25	0.04	0.05
Japan	0.20	0.18	0.09	0.06
Netherlands	0.27	0.28	0.07	0.10
New Zealand	0.17	0.20	0.13	0.15
Norway	0.14	0.17	0.06	0.10
Portugal	0.11	0.15	0.01	0.01
Spain	0.21	0.25	0.00	0.00
Sweden	0.09	0.10	0.05	0.07
Switzerland	0.17	0.19	0.04	0.06
United Kingdom	0.22	0.23	0.14	0.16
United States	0.23	0.24	0.19	0.20

NOTE: N/A = data are not available.

[a]Estimates based on the model represent the fraction of all deaths at ages 50+.

[b]Estimates based on Peto et al. (2006; http://www.ctsu.ox.ac.uk/~tobacco/SMK_P5_6.pdf, accessed June 6, 2010) represent the fraction of all deaths at ages 35+.

[c]Estimates for Belgium are based on data for 1999.

SOURCES: Model estimates are based on calculations by authors using data in the Human Mortality Database (accessed November 6, 2009) and the World Health Organization Mortality Database (accessed December 24, 2009). Peto-Lopez estimates were derived from http://www.ctsu.ox.ac.uk/~tobacco/SMK_P5_6.pdf (accessed January 23, 2009). [Weighted estimates for ages 35+ were derived by the authors using data for ages 35-69 and 70+ from this source.]

tributable risk fractions for the two methods is 0.96 for men and 0.97 for women. Although both approaches use lung cancer mortality as an indirect measure of smoking histories, the procedures diverge sharply at that point. The Peto-Lopez approach exports the estimated relative risks among smokers by cause of death from the CPS-II study to other populations, whereas our approach is based entirely on macro-level statistical relationships. Because of the very different methodologies used, the highly consistent results help to support the validity of both approaches.

Effects of Smoking on Life Expectancy at Age 50

Table 4-4 shows the impact on life expectancy at age 50 (e_{50}) in 2003 of removing deaths attributed to smoking from age-specific death rates. In all cases e_{50} rises, by as little as 0.08 years among women in Spain and as much as 4.16 years among men in Hungary. Smoking has also substantially reduced e_{50} among men in Belgium (by 2.87 years), the Netherlands (2.58 years), the United States (2.52 years), and Canada (2.49 years). Among women, the greatest impact of smoking occurs in the United States (2.33 years), Denmark (2.12 years), and Canada (2.06 years). Relative to the average for women in other countries (shown at the foot of Table 4-4), the smoking histories of U.S. women have cost them an additional 1.31 years of life expectancy. U.S. women have a deficit of 1.08 years in observed life

TABLE 4-4 Life Expectancy at Age 50 (e_{50}) in 2003 Before and After Removal of Deaths Attributable to Smoking

	Men			Women		
Country	With Smoking	Without Smoking	Difference	With Smoking	Without Smoking	Difference
Australia	30.63	32.25	−1.63	34.59	35.61	−1.02
Austria	28.49	30.29	−1.80	33.13	33.77	−0.65
Belgium[a]	28.53	31.40	−2.87	33.40	34.08	−0.68
Canada	29.82	32.31	−2.49	33.85	35.91	−2.06
Denmark	27.77	29.89	−2.13	31.66	33.78	−2.12
Finland	27.98	29.68	−1.70	33.25	33.72	−0.47
France	28.83	31.01	−2.18	34.59	34.92	−0.33
Hungary	22.55	26.71	−4.16	29.15	30.79	−1.64
Iceland	30.95	32.42	−1.46	33.61	35.53	−1.92
Ireland	28.20	30.13	−1.92	32.04	33.51	−1.46
Italy	29.46	31.88	−2.41	34.19	34.64	−0.45
Japan	30.47	32.52	−2.05	36.66	37.41	−0.75
Netherlands	28.34	30.92	−2.58	32.55	33.69	−1.15
New Zealand	29.80	31.43	−1.63	33.26	34.65	−1.40
Norway	29.40	30.99	−1.59	33.39	34.41	−1.02
Portugal	27.69	29.04	−1.35	32.44	32.54	−0.09
Spain	29.00	31.39	−2.39	34.44	34.52	−0.08
Sweden	29.83	30.77	−0.95	33.66	34.51	−0.85
Switzerland	30.14	31.74	−1.60	34.48	35.04	−0.56
United Kingdom	28.62	30.67	−2.05	32.21	33.87	−1.66
United States	28.46	30.98	−2.52	32.25	34.58	−2.33
Non-U.S. average	28.83	30.87	−2.05	33.33	34.35	−1.02

[a]Estimates for Belgium based on 2004 data.
SOURCES: Calculations by authors based on data in the Human Mortality Database (accessed November 2009) and the World Health Organization Mortality Database (accessed December 2009).

expectancy compared with other countries. Thus, if we remove the effects of smoking, U.S. women hold a slight advantage (34.58 versus 34.35, a difference of 0.23 years). U.S. men's deficit in life expectancy of 0.37 years also reverses if smoking is removed, yielding an advantage of 0.11 years. So in both cases, U.S. life expectancy exceeds the mean for other countries when the effects of smoking are erased.

Additional light is shed on the relative position of U.S. life expectancy in Table 4-5. With smoking deaths included, women in the United States rank 17th out of 21 countries. When deaths attributable to smoking are excluded, the rank of U.S. women jumps to 9th. Correspondingly, the position for U.S. men improves from 15th to 12th. Their histories of heavy smoking are thus clearly implicated in the poor international rankings in e_{50} of U.S. men and women. In view of the disadvantaged position on many health indicators of the United States relative to England (Banks et al., 2006), it is noteworthy

TABLE 4-5 Effect of Removal of Smoking-Attributable Deaths on Ranking of e_{50} in 2003

Country	Men		Women	
	Rank Before Removal	Rank After Removal	Rank Before Removal	Rank After Removal
Australia	2	4	3	3
Austria	14	16	14	16
Belgium[a]	13	8	10	13
Canada	6	3	7	2
Denmark	19	18	20	15
Finland	18	19	13	17
France	11	10	2	6
Hungary	21	21	21	21
Iceland	1	2	9	4
Ireland	17	17	19	19
Italy	8	5	6	8
Japan	3	1	1	1
Netherlands	16	13	15	18
New Zealand	7	7	12	7
Norway	9	11	11	12
Portugal	20	20	16	20
Spain	10	9	5	10
Sweden	5	14	8	11
Switzerland	4	6	4	5
United Kingdom	12	15	18	14
United States	15	12	17	9

[a]Estimates for Belgium based on 2004 data.
SOURCES: Calculations by authors based on data in the Human Mortality Database (accessed November 2009) and the World Health Organization Mortality Database (accessed December 2009).

that men and women in the United States share similar rank with their counterparts in the United Kingdom before smoking deaths are removed but rank well above them after smoking deaths are accounted for.

Is it possible that lung cancer is overrecorded as a cause of death in the United States relative to coding tendencies typical of other countries, thus accounting for the unusually high estimates of attributable risk in the United States? Such a pattern does not appear likely in view of an international study that asked countries to record the underlying cause of death, using the International Statistical Classification of Diseases (ICD-9), for an identical set of 1,243 U.S. death certificates that mentioned cancer. Among the seven countries considered in this chapter and in the coding study, the United States and Canada were tied with the lowest proportion of these deaths that were attributed to lung cancer (Percy and Muir, 1989).

Canadians have also suffered from their histories of heavy smoking. Canadian men jump to third in international rankings while their female counterparts move to second when smoking deaths are removed. In contrast, Swedish men and Spanish women owe much of their favorable international ranking (in each case, fifth) to their histories of light smoking: when smoking deaths are excluded for all countries, they drop below the median in terms of e_{50}.

It is sometimes remarked that Japan is an anomaly because people in Japan smoke heavily yet the country enjoys an excellent ranking in life expectancy comparisons (Stellman et al., 2001). These results shed light on this issue. The removal of smoking deaths implies an increase in e_{50} among Japanese men (2.05 years) and women (0.75 years) that is similar to the average for all countries in Table 4-4. The increase for men actually improves Japan's ranking in Table 4-5 from third to first. So, according to our estimates, heavy smoking among Japanese men has in fact negatively affected their international ranking. Japanese women rank first both before and after the removal of deaths from smoking. These results are, of course, subject to the uncertainties noted above regarding lung cancer mortality among Japanese nonsmokers (Thun et al., 2008).

Changes in smoking patterns have also affected mortality *trends*. To demonstrate the impact on trends, we have decomposed mortality changes between 1950 and 2003 using a method developed by Pollard (1988). The two causes of death considered in the decomposition are smoking-attributable deaths and all other deaths. Table 4-6 presents the total gains in e_{50} between 1950 and 2003 and shows the estimated contribution of smoking changes to those gains.

Among women, increases in the damage from smoking reduced the gains in life expectancy in all countries. The biggest reductions occurred in the United States (1.58 years), Denmark (1.48), Iceland (1.47), and Canada (1.39). The gain in U.S. women's life expectancy trailed the mean gain of

TABLE 4-6 Gains in e_{50} During 1950-2003 and Amount of Gain Attributable to Changes in Smoking and Other Factors

	Men			Women		
		Contribution due to:			Contribution due to:	
Country	Total Gain in e_{50}	Smoking	Other Factors	Total Gain in e_{50}	Smoking	Other Factors
Australia	7.88	−0.37	8.25	7.95	−0.67	8.61
Austria	5.85	0.86	4.98	6.73	−0.34	7.07
Belgium	5.42	−0.63	6.05	6.80	−0.47	7.27
Canada	5.89	−0.99	6.88	7.06	−1.39	8.44
Denmark	2.58	−0.93	3.51	4.97	−1.48	6.45
Finland	6.97	1.08	5.89	8.16	−0.13	8.29
France	6.34	−1.06	7.40	8.13	−0.22	8.35
Hungary	−1.09	−2.83	1.74	3.40	−1.15	4.55
Iceland	4.71	−0.81	5.52	5.03	−1.47	6.50
Ireland	5.14	−0.94	6.08	7.15	−0.91	8.06
Italy	5.85	−1.18	7.03	8.29	−0.29	8.57
Japan	9.48	−0.92	10.40	12.74	−0.31	13.05
Netherlands	2.54	−1.07	3.61	5.63	−0.89	6.51
New Zealand	6.11	−0.34	6.45	6.47	−1.01	7.48
Norway	2.52	−1.12	3.64	4.76	−0.82	5.57
Portugal	4.93	−0.77	5.70	5.95	−0.08	6.03
Spain	7.22	−1.28	8.51	9.40	−0.06	9.45
Sweden	4.58	−0.44	5.02	6.96	−0.56	7.51
Switzerland	7.03	0.07	6.96	8.47	−0.39	8.86
United Kingdom	6.22	0.51	5.71	6.03	−0.90	6.93
United States	5.82	−0.82	6.64	5.70	−1.58	7.28
Non-U.S. average	5.31	−0.66	5.97	7.00	−0.68	7.68

NOTES: 1951-2003 for Iceland, Italy, Norway, Spain, Sweden, and Switzerland; 1952-2003 for Denmark and Finland; 1954-2004 for Belgium; 1955-2003 for Austria, Hungary, and Portugal.
SOURCES: Calculations by authors based on data in the Human Mortality Database (accessed November 2009) and the World Health Organization Mortality Database (accessed December 2009).

other countries by 1.30 years. Our results suggest that most of this shortfall (0.90 of 1.30 years, or 69 percent) is attributable to the greater impact of smoking among U.S. women. Thus, these results reinforce those of Tables 4-4 and 4-5 in showing that smoking has had a major, adverse impact on the relative position of U.S. women's mortality. In contrast, changes in smoking among women in Spain and Portugal have had very little effect on life expectancy to date—less than 0.10 years. Our results for women are thus broadly consistent with those of Staetsky (2009), who applied the Peto-Lopez method to a smaller set of countries over a shorter time period and age range.

The picture for men is less systematic. In four early-smoking countries including the United Kingdom, reductions in smoking-attributable mortality during the period actually served to increase male life expectancy. In the remainder, gains in life expectancy were reduced by changes in smoking, by as much as 2.83 years in Hungary.

It may appear odd that smoking reduced gains in life expectancy by slightly less for men than for women in Table 4-6. One reason is related to differences in the timing of the smoking epidemic. Among men, smoking already had made a substantial impact by 1955, whereas it had virtually no effect for women (Table 4-2). Since then, the effects of smoking grew among both sexes, but recently have begun to decline among men in many countries. In contrast, the impact of smoking grew rapidly throughout the period among women in every country. Thus, over this period, the trends for men capture the latter part of the smoking epidemic (including the waning), whereas the trends for women capture the escalating portion. Another part of the explanation is that male mortality from nonsmoking causes is much higher than female mortality. As a result, a death attributable to smoking at age 70, for example, has a much bigger impact on women's life expectancy than on men's. Thus, the rise in smoking among women is in a sense being weighted more heavily in its impact on life expectancy in Table 4-6 than if the same increase had occurred among men.

According to Table 4-6, gains in life expectancy among U.S. men outpaced those of other countries by an average of 0.51 years (5.82 minus 5.31) between 1950 and 2003. Without the changes in mortality induced by smoking, which include both increases and decreases, the U.S. gain would have been greater by 0.67 years (6.64 minus 5.97). Thus, consistent with Tables 4-4 and 4-5, Table 4-6 shows that smoking has produced a modest deterioration in the position of U.S. men in international comparisons of life expectancy.

A more detailed assessment of the impact of smoking on trends in U.S. life expectancy is possible by computing the effects of smoking annually. Figure 4-1 demonstrates the actual evolution of e_{50} in the United States since 1950 and presents our estimates of what the trend would have looked like without smoking-attributable deaths. The discrepancy between the two series for men widened steadily from 0.7 years in 1950 to 3.1 years in 1990 but has since begun a slow contraction (to 2.5 years in 2005). In contrast, the discrepancy between the two series for women began to widen rapidly after 1975 and has continued to grow, reaching 2.3 years by 2005.

The earlier impact of smoking on male mortality and the catch-up phase for women has produced a striking pattern of sex mortality differentials. Figure 4-2 shows the observed trend in the difference between female and male life expectancy at age 50. The hill-shaped pattern begins at a difference just under 4 years, rises to a peak of nearly 6 years, and then declines

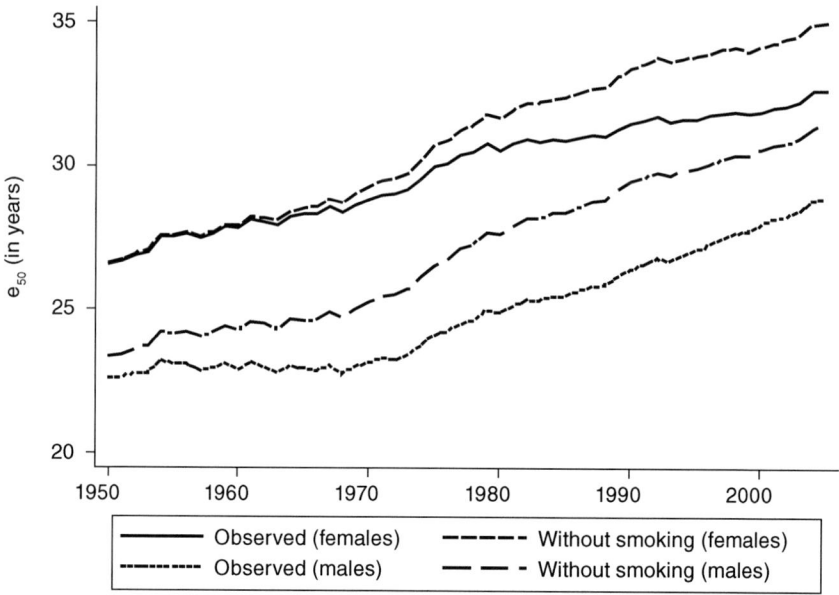

FIGURE 4-1 U.S. trends in observed e_{50} and estimated e_{50} without smoking by sex.
SOURCE: Calculations by authors based on data in the Human Mortality Database (accessed November 2009) and the World Health Organization Mortality Database (accessed December 2009).

to just below its starting value by 2005. This hill appears to be primarily attributable to smoking; we estimate that, without smoking deaths, the sex difference in e_{50} would have remained within the narrower range of 3.3-4.2 years.

The Future

If we are correct that smoking has played an important role in international levels and trends in mortality at ages 50+, then elements of the future come into clearer focus. The smoking epidemic among men has receded in nearly all industrialized countries (Forey et al., 2006; Glei, Meslé, and Vallin, Chapter 2, in this volume). According to Table 4-2, smoking-attributable mortality is already declining sharply among men in several countries (Australia, Finland, the Netherlands, United Kingdom), and it has stabilized in the United States. In view of the lag between smoking behavior and smoking-attributable mortality, it is reasonable to expect that men in nearly all the study countries will benefit from reductions in the smoking-attributable fraction of deaths, thereby boosting life expectancy. Among

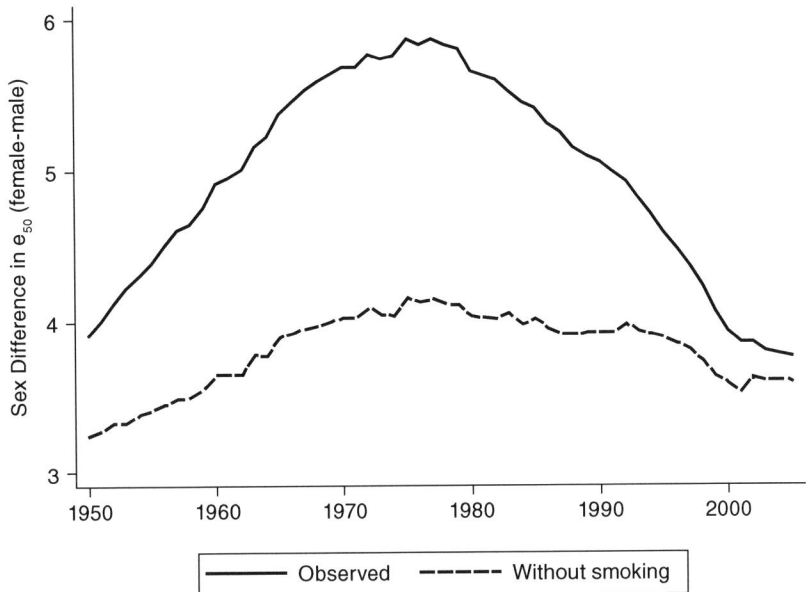

FIGURE 4-2 U.S. trends in the observed sex difference in e_{50} and the estimated sex difference without smoking.
SOURCE: Calculations by authors based on data in the Human Mortality Database (accessed November 2009) and the World Health Organization Mortality Database (accessed December 2009).

women, however, a later uptake of smoking has produced an upsurge in smoking-attributable deaths that is readily apparent in Table 4-2. In most countries in this study, the prevalence of smoking among women has begun to decline, albeit much later than for men. But the effects of earlier increases have been playing a more powerful role in women's mortality profiles and are likely to continue doing so for some time to come. One set of mortality projections that takes explicit account of smoking patterns projects a very rapid reduction in men's mortality at ages 50+ in the United States between now and 2034, while projected improvements among women remain much slower (Wang and Preston, 2009). The narrowing of sex differentials would continue a pattern that has been observed since 1980 and that is also heavily dependent on smoking differences between the sexes, as suggested in Figure 4-2.

For the past half-century, smoking has played a major role in mortality trends and differentials, both among nations and between the sexes. Welcome declines in smoking in most industrialized countries suggest that the imprint of smoking will recede over the next half-century, but the recession is likely to be slower for women than for men.

ACKNOWLEDGMENTS

We are grateful to the National Institute on Aging grants 1-R03-AG031310 and R01-AG11552 and to the Social Security Administration for support of this project.

REFERENCES

Banks, J., Marmot, M., Oldfield, Z., and Smith, J.P. (2006). Disease and disadvantage in the United States and in England. *Journal of the American Medical Association, 295*(17), 2037-2045.

Brennan, P., and Bray, I. (2002). Recent trends and future directions for lung cancer mortality in Europe. *British Journal of Cancer, 87*(1), 43-48.

Danaei, G., Ding, E.L., Mozaffarian, D., Taylor, B., Rehm, J., Murray, C.J., et al. (2009). The preventable causes of death in the United States: Comparative risk assessment of dietary, lifestyle, and metabolic risk factors. *PLoS Medicine, 6*(4), e1000058. [doi:10.1371/journal.pmed.1000058.]

Doll, R., Peto, R., Boreham, J., and Sutherland, I. (2004). Mortality in relation to smoking: 50 years' observations on male British doctors. *British Medical Journal (Clinical Research Ed.), 328*(7455), 1519. [doi:10.1136/bmj.38142.554479.AE].

Doll, R., Peto, R., Wheatley, K., Gray, R., and Sutherland, I. (1994). Mortality in relation to smoking: 40 years' observations on male British doctors. *British Medical Journal (Clinical Research Ed.), 309*(6959), 901-911.

Enstrom, J.E. (1979). Rising lung cancer mortality among nonsmokers. *Journal of the National Cancer Institute, 62*(4), 755-760.

Ezzati, M. (2004). How can cross-country research on health risks strengthen interventions? Lessons from INTERHEART. *Lancet, 364*(9438), 912-914.

Ezzati, M., and Lopez, A.D. (2003). Estimates of global mortality attributable to smoking in 2000. *Lancet, 362*(9387), 847-852.

Ezzati, M., Henley, S.J., Thun, M.J., and Lopez, A.D. (2005). Role of smoking in global and regional cardiovascular mortality. *Circulation, 112*(4), 489-497.

Forey, B., Hamling, J., Lee, P., and Wald, N. (Eds.). (2002). *International Smoking Statistics: A Collection of Historical Data from 30 Economically Developed Countries*. Oxford, England: Oxford University Press.

Haldorsen, T., and Grimsrud, T.K. (1999). Cohort analysis of cigarette smoking and lung cancer incidence among Norwegian women. *International Journal of Epidemiology, 28*(6), 1032-1036.

Ho, J., and Preston, S. (2009). *U.S. Mortality in an International Context: Age Variations*. Population Studies Center Working Paper 09-04. Philadelphia: University of Pennsylvania.

Human Mortality Database. (2009). *HMD Main Menu*. Available: http://www.mortality.org [accessed November 2009].

Jee, S.H., Suh, I., Kim, I.S., and Appel, L.J. (1999). Smoking and atherosclerotic cardiovascular disease in men with low levels of serum cholesterol: The Korea medical insurance corporation study. *Journal of the American Medical Association, 282*(22), 2149-2155.

Katanoda, K., Marugame, T., Saika, K., Satoh, H., Tajima, K., Suzuki, T., et al. (2008). Population attributable fraction of mortality associated with tobacco smoking in Japan: A pooled analysis of three large-scale cohort studies. *Journal of Epidemiology/Japan Epidemiological Association, 18*(6), 251-264.

Knoops, K.T., de Groot, L.C., Kromhout, D., Perrin, A.E., Moreiras-Varela, O., Menotti, A., et al. (2004). Mediterranean diet, lifestyle factors, and 10-year mortality in elderly European men and women: The HALE project. *Journal of the American Medical Association, 292*(12), 1433-1439.

Leistikow, B.N., and Tsodikov, A. (2005). Cancer death epidemics in U.S. black males: Evaluating courses, causation, and cures. *Preventive Medicine, 41*(2), 380-385.

Leistikow, B.N., Kabir, Z., Connolly, G.N., Clancy, L., and Alpert, H.R. (2008). Male tobacco smoke load and non-lung cancer mortality associations in Massachusetts. *BMC Cancer, 8,* 341.

Liu, B.Q., Peto, R., Chen, Z.M., Boreham, J., Wu, Y.P., Li, J.Y., et al. (1998). Emerging tobacco hazards in China: 1. Retrospective proportional mortality study of one million deaths. *British Medical Journal (Clinical Research Ed.), 317*(7170), 1411-1422.

Lopez, A.D. (1995). The lung cancer epidemic in developed countries. In A.D. Lopez, G. Caselli, and T. Valkonen (Eds.), *Adult Mortality in Developed Countries: From Description to Explanation* (pp. 111-134). Oxford, England: Clarendon Press.

McCullagh, P., and Nelder, J.A. (1989). *Generalized Linear Models* (2nd ed.). Boca Raton, FL: CRC Press.

Mokdad, A.H., Marks, J.S., Stroup, D.F., and Gerberding, J.L. (2004). Actual causes of death in the United States, 2000. *Journal of the American Medical Association, 291*(10), 1238-1245.

Percy, C., and Muir, C. (1989). The international comparability of cancer mortality data. Results of an international death certificate study. *American Journal of Epidemiology, 129*(5), 934-946.

Peto, R., Lopez, A.D., Boreham, J. and Thun, M. (2006). *Mortality from Smoking in Developed Countries 1950-2000 (2nd ed.).* Available http://www.ctsu.ox.ac.uk/~tobacco/ [accessed January 2009].

Peto, R., Lopez, A.D., Boreham, J., Thun, M., and Heath, C., Jr. (1992). Mortality from tobacco in developed countries: Indirect estimation from national vital statistics. *Lancet, 339*(8804), 1268-1278.

Pollard, J.H. (1988). On the decomposition of changes in expectation of life and differentials in life expectancy. *Demography, 25*(2), 265-276.

Preston, S.H., and Wang, H. (2006). Sex mortality differences in the United States: The role of cohort smoking patterns. *Demography, 43*(4), 631-646.

Preston, S.H., Glei, D.A., and Wilmoth, J.R. (2009). A new method for estimating smoking-attributable mortality in high-income countries. *International Journal of Epidemiology, 39*, 430-439.

Rogers, R.G., Hummer, R.A., Krueger, P.M., and Pampel, F.C. (2005). Mortality attributable to cigarette smoking in the United States. *Population and Development Review, 31*(2), 259-292.

Rosenbaum, W.L., Sterling, T.D., and Weinkam, J.J. (1998). Use of multiple surveys to estimate mortality among never, current, and former smokers: Changes over a 20-year interval. *American Journal of Public Health, 88*(11), 1664-1668.

Rostron, B., and Wilmoth, J.R. (forthcoming). Estimating the effect of smoking on slowdowns in mortality declines in developed countries. Submitted to *Demography*.

Staetsky, L. (2009). Diverging trends in female old-age mortality: A reappraisal. *Demographic Research, 21*(30), 885-914. [doi:10.4054/DemRes.2009.21.30].

Stellman, S.D., Takezaki, T., Wang, L., Chen, Y., Citron, M.L., Djordjevic, M.V., et al. (2001). Smoking and lung cancer risk in American and Japanese men: An international case-control study. *Cancer Epidemiology, Biomarkers and Prevention: A Publication of the American Association for Cancer Research, cosponsored by the American Society of Preventive Oncology, 10*(11), 1193-1199.

Sterling, T.D., Rosenbaum, W.L., and Weinkam, J.J. (1993). Risk attribution and tobacco-related deaths. *American Journal of Epidemiology, 138*(2), 128-139.

Taylor, D.H., Jr., Hasselblad, V., Henley, S.J., Thun, M.J., and Sloan, F.A. (2002). Benefits of smoking cessation for longevity. *American Journal of Public Health, 92*(6), 990-996.

Thun, M.J., Day-Lally, C., Myers, D.G., Calle, E.E., Flanders, W.D., Zhu, B., et al. (1997). Trends in tobacco smoking and mortality from cigarette use in cancer prevention studies I (1959 through 1965) and II (1982 through 1988). In D.M. Burns, L. Garfinkel, and J.M. Samet (Eds.), *Changes in Cigarette-Related Disease Risks and Their Implications for Prevention and Control, Smoking and Tobacco Control* (pp. 305-382). NIH publication 97-4213. Bethesda, MD: Cancer Control and Population Sciences, National Cancer Institute, U.S. National Institutes of Health.

Thun, M.J., Hannan, L.M., Adams-Campbell, L.L., Boffetta, P., Buring, J.E., Feskanich, D., et al. (2008). Lung cancer occurrence in never-smokers: An analysis of 13 cohorts and 22 cancer registry studies. *PLoS Medicine, 5*(9), e185. [doi:10.1371/journal.pmed.0050185.]

U.S. Department of Health and Human Services. (1989). *Reducing the Health Consequences of Smoking: 25 Years of Progress. A Report of the Surgeon General.* (DHHS Publication (CDC) 89-8411). Public Health Service, Centers for Disease Control, Center for Chronic Disease Prevention and Health Promotion, Office on Smoking and Health. Rockville, MD: Author.

U.S. Surgeon General. (2004). *The Health Consequences of Smoking: A Report of the Surgeon General.* Washington, DC: U.S. Department of Health and Human Services, Centers for Disease Control and Prevention, National Center for Chronic Disease Prevention and Health Promotion, Office on Smoking and Health.

Wang, H., and Preston, S.H. (2009). Forecasting United States mortality using cohort smoking histories. *Proceedings of the National Academy of Sciences of the United States of America, 106*(2), 393-398. [doi:10.1073/pnas.0811809106.]

Wilmoth, J.R., et al. (2005). *Methods Protocol for the Human Mortality Database.* Available: http://www.mortality.org/Public/Docs/MethodsProtocol.pdf [accessed December 2005].

World Health Organization. (2009). *Detailed Data Files of the WHO Mortality Database.* Available: http://www.who.int/whosis/mort/download/en/index.htm [accessed December 2009].

Yusuf, S., Hawken, S., Ounpuu, S., Dans, T., Avezum, A., Lanas, F., et al. (2004). Effect of potentially modifiable risk factors associated with myocardial infarction in 52 countries (the INTERHEART study): Case-control study. *Lancet, 364*(9438), 937-952.

ANNEX 4A

DEVELOPMENT OF THE STATISTICAL MODEL

Our approach begins with an assumption about how smoking affects mortality from lung cancer for persons in a particular age-sex group in a certain population:

$$M_L = \lambda_L^N (1 + \theta), \tag{A1}$$

where M_L is the observed death rate from lung cancer, λ_L^N is the nonsmokers' death rate from lung cancer, and $1 + \theta$ is the proportionate factor by which mortality is raised in the group relative to what it would be if everyone were a lifetime nonsmoker. Thus, any departure of lung cancer mortality in the population from that of nonsmokers is assumed to be attributable to smoking. θ is used as a measure of the mortality damage caused by the prevalence, duration, and intensity of smoking. θ and λ_L^N are assumed to vary by age and sex in any population. λ_L^N is assumed to be fixed across populations for a particular age-sex group, whereas θ is assumed to vary with the smoking behavior of the population.

In the case of mortality from causes other than lung cancer (M_O), we assume that θ, the measure of damage from smoking in equation (A1), also captures the effect of smoking on other causes of death. However, that damage is only one of many factors that affect mortality, which we express as a standard hazards model. That is, the log of M_O is assumed to be a linear function of the predictors, including the damage from smoking:

$$\ln(M_O) = \sum \beta_i X_i + \beta_\theta \theta \text{ or } M_O = \exp\left(\sum_i \beta_i X_i + \beta_\theta \theta\right), \tag{A2}$$

where X_i represents the set of other predictors (which may be observed quantities or transformations thereof), β_i denotes the set of corresponding coefficients, and β_θ is the coefficient associated with θ. Evidence in support of the proportionality assumption embedded in the hazards model for smoking has been presented for cardiovascular diseases. In particular, Ezzati et al. (2005) cite several studies in support of the constancy across populations of smokers' relative risk of cardiovascular death (Ezzati, 2004; Jee et al., 1999; Liu et al., 1998; Yusuf et al., 2004).

From (A1), we can solve for θ as follows:

$$\theta = \frac{M_L - \lambda_L^N}{\lambda_L^N} = \frac{1}{\lambda_L^N} M_L - 1 \tag{A3}$$

Substituting (A3) into (A2), we obtain:

$$M_O = \exp\left(\sum_i \beta_i X_i + \frac{\beta_\theta}{\lambda_L^N} M_L - \beta_\theta\right), \text{ or} \tag{A4}$$

$$\ln M_O = \sum_i \beta_i X_i + \frac{\beta_\theta}{\lambda_L^N} M_L - \beta_\theta \tag{A5}$$

With these assumptions, the log of M_O will be a linear function of M_L. The implied coefficient for M_L,

$$\frac{\beta_\theta}{\lambda_L^N},$$

goes up with β_θ (the effect of θ on M_O) and down with λ_L^N (because a larger value of λ_L^N implies that less mortality damage is being done by smoking for a given value of M_L). This analysis motivates our choice to use M_L itself as the measure of the damage caused by smoking in a model of mortality due to causes other than lung cancer. Since θ is a linear function of M_L (and vice versa), either quantity could be used for estimating the final model, with no difference for any of the results that interest us here.

Thus, within the framework of generalized linear models (McCullagh and Nelder, 1989), we assume a negative binomial probability distribution of observed death counts in order to estimate the following model of $\ln M_O$ (or, technically, the log of its expected value) for each sex separately:

$$\ln M_O = \beta_a X_a + \beta_t X_t + \beta_c X_c + \beta_{ct}(t \times X_c) + \beta_L M_L + \beta_{Lt}(M_L \times t) + \beta_{La}(M_L \times X_a), \tag{A6}$$

where M_O is the death rate from causes other than lung cancer classified by age, sex, year of death, and country (or population); X_a is a set of dummy variables for each age group; X_t is a set of dummy variables for each calendar year; X_c is a set of dummy variables for each country; $(t \times X_c)$ denotes a set of interactions between calendar year (linear) and each country dummy; M_L is the death rate from lung cancer; $(M_L \times t)$ is an interaction between M_L and year (linear); and finally, $(M_L \times X_a)$ represents M_L interacted with the age dummies.

To estimate the fraction of deaths attributable to smoking, one may exponentiate both sides of equation (A6) to obtain a predicted value of M_O given M_L, the observed lung cancer death rate. We estimate what M_O would have been in the absence of smoking by substituting λ_L^N, the assumed lung cancer death rate among nonsmokers, in place of M_L. We then divide the difference between these two expressions by the model's prediction of M_O. This last expression can be simplified to yield equation (3) of the main text.

ANNEX 4B

Smoking-Attributable Deaths Due to Lung Cancer and Other Causes (in absolute numbers and as a percentage of deaths from all causes), by Sex and Country, Ages 50+, 2003

Smoking-Attributable Deaths due to:	Men					
	Lung Cancer		Other Causes		All Causes	
Country	N	% of All Deaths	N	% of All Deaths	N	% of All Deaths
Australia	3,751	6.2	6,473	10.7	10,224	16.9
Austria	1,963	6.1	3,540	11.0	5,503	17.1
Canada	8,849	8.6	15,485	15.1	24,334	23.8
Denmark	1,636	6.5	3,441	13.6	5,077	20.1
Finland	1,194	5.6	2,465	11.5	3,659	17.1
France	17,290	6.9	29,459	11.8	46,749	18.7
Hungary	5,020	8.2	13,539	22.2	18,558	30.4
Iceland	46	5.6	87	10.4	133	15.9
Ireland	847	6.4	1,735	13.1	2,582	19.5
Italy	22,635	8.4	40,032	14.9	62,667	23.3
Japan	35,475	6.9	67,658	13.2	103,133	20.0
Netherlands	5,451	8.6	11,027	17.4	16,478	25.9
New Zealand	704	5.7	1,363	11.1	2,067	16.8
Norway	1,012	5.4	1,945	10.3	2,958	15.6
Portugal	2,013	4.0	3,934	7.9	5,947	12.0
Spain	13,968	7.7	25,108	13.9	39,076	21.6
Sweden	1,382	3.2	2,514	5.9	3,896	9.1
Switzerland	1,641	5.9	2,701	9.7	4,343	15.6
United Kingdom	17,162	6.4	37,421	14.1	54,583	20.5
United States	77,286	7.6	148,216	14.5	225,502	22.1

SOURCES: Calculations by authors based on data in the Human Mortality Database (accessed November 2009) and the World Health Organization Mortality Database (accessed December 2009).

CONTRIBUTION OF SMOKING TO INTERNATIONAL DIFFERENCES 131

Women					
Lung Cancer		Other Causes		All Causes	
N	% of All Deaths	N	% of All Deaths	N	% of All Deaths
1,742	2.9	4,524	7.6	6,266	10.5
590	1.5	1,549	3.9	2,138	5.3
5,702	5.5	13,974	13.4	19,676	18.9
1,186	4.4	3,155	11.6	4,341	16.0
291	1.2	791	3.3	1,082	4.5
2,047	0.8	3,305	1.3	5,352	2.1
1,671	2.7	6,383	10.3	8,054	13.0
49	5.5	106	12.1	155	17.6
459	3.4	1,477	11.1	1,936	14.5
3,314	1.2	9,580	3.3	12,894	4.5
8,705	2.0	31,475	7.1	40,180	9.0
1,856	2.7	4,318	6.2	6,173	8.9
456	3.5	1,118	8.6	1,574	12.2
499	2.4	1,015	4.8	1,514	7.2
108	0.2	200	0.4	308	0.6
298	0.2	415	0.2	713	0.4
888	1.9	2,075	4.5	2,963	6.4
459	1.5	886	2.8	1,345	4.3
10,817	3.5	37,062	12.0	47,879	15.5
55,331	4.8	169,840	14.8	225,171	19.7

5

Divergent Patterns of Smoking Across High-Income Nations

Fred Pampel

Tobacco use in high-income nations is notable in two ways. First, despite intense and in many ways successful public health campaigns, average cigarette use remains stubbornly high. Second, there is considerable diversity in the prevalence and intensity of tobacco use across nations. Given the clear connection between tobacco use and premature death, both characteristics have the potential to affect current and future mortality trajectories.

First, smoking remains high enough to affect mortality for some time to come. In brief review, after rising during the decades before 1970 in most high-income nations, per capita cigarette consumption fell by 9 percent from 1970 to 1990 (World Health Organization, 1997, pp. 15, 23). Since then, public health efforts have moved beyond initial antitobacco policies that relied on public service ads, bans on certain types of advertising, and warning labels on tobacco product packaging. Policies now focus on more stringent restrictions, such as bans on indoor smoking in bars, restaurants, and workplaces; steep increases in tobacco taxes and cigarette prices; and strict enforcement of limits on sales to minors and tobacco company promotions (Davis et al., 2007; Eriksen and Cerak, 2008).

Smoking prevalence in the new policy environment has continued to decline in the United States (Rock et al., 2007), and the drop from 44.1 for men and 31.5 for women in 1970 (U.S. Department of Health and Human Services, 2001, p. 36) to 23.1 for men and 18.3 for women in 2008 (Dube et al., 2009) represents a major public health accomplishment (Warner, 2005). At the same time, however, the rate of decline has slowed over the past decade in the United States (Mendez and Warner, 2004); the most recent figures even show a small increase in prevalence (19.8 to 20.6 percent) from

2007 to 2008 (Dube et al., 2009). More generally, cigarette use persists at frustratingly high levels in all high-income nations. Using figures circa 2000, the *Tobacco Atlas* (Mackay, Eriksen, and Shafey, 2006) reports that about 35 percent of men and 22 percent of women in developed nations smoke; Cutler and Glaeser (2006) report that in 17 European nations an average of 30 percent smoke.

The persistence of smoking relates closely to socioeconomic status (SES) differences in health behaviors. The decline in smoking has proceeded fastest among high-SES groups, leaving disadvantaged groups as the primary users of cigarettes (Pampel, 2005). Of the components of SES, education proves a stronger predictor of smoking than occupation or income, although higher levels of all three are associated with lower smoking (Barbeau, Krieger, and Soobader, 2004; Huisman, Kunst, and Mackenbach, 2005a). For example, analysis of the 2006 U.S. National Health Interview Survey shows that odds ratios of smoking equal 3.7 for high school dropouts relative to college graduates, 2.2 for laborers and farmers relative to professionals and managers, and 2.6 for the lowest income quartile relative to the highest income quartile. Rock et al. (2007) report that 43.5 percent of those with 9 to 11 years of education smoke, compared with 10.0 percent of those with an undergraduate degree and 7.3 percent of those with a graduate degree. Even among the most educated, the low rates still translate into millions of smokers. Among the less educated, the problem is considerably worse and has led to government efforts in the United States to focus on eliminating SES disparities in smoking (Fagan et al., 2004).[1]

Second, high-income nations show considerable diversity around the average. Despite similarly high levels of economic development compared with the rest of the world and educated populations largely familiar with the harm of tobacco, the high-income nations of Western Europe plus Australia, Canada, Japan, New Zealand, and the United States differ in the prevalence and intensity of use. For example, according to figures from Cutler and Glaeser (2006) for the European Union, smoking rates range from 19 and 21 percent in Sweden and Portugal, respectively, to 34 percent in Spain, 35 percent in Germany, and 38 percent in Greece. The *Tobacco Atlas* (Mackay et al., 2006) reports smoking percentages of 17 percent in Sweden, 20 percent in Portugal, 32 percent in Germany, 32 percent in Spain, and 38 percent in Greece. That is, smoking is at least twice as common in some

---

[1]The stronger influence of education stems in part from its stability over the life course; it changes less than occupation and income from adolescence and young adulthood, when most people start to smoke. Even at that, the effects of education are complex. Youth often make decisions to smoke or not smoke before they complete their education, suggesting that the SES background of parents affects the smoking behavior of their children or that latent traits of youth affect both healthy behavior and educational attainment. In addition, learning that occurs during higher levels of education can prevent later starting and foster quitting.

ations as in others. And the levels do not vary simply by region. Sweden and Portugal are similarly low, whereas Germany and Spain are similarly high. English-speaking nations outside Europe have relatively low smoking rates (22 and 20 percent in the United States and Canada, respectively).

Gender complicates the picture. According to the *Tobacco Atlas*, the gap in male prevalence between Sweden (17 percent) and Greece (47 percent) reaches 30 percent; that between Sweden and Germany (37 percent) reaches 20 percent. For women, the gaps are smaller but still substantial. Lower levels of 10 percent in Portugal and 18 percent in Sweden contrast with higher levels of 28 percent in Germany, 28 percent in the Netherlands, and 29 percent in Greece. The United States shows similar prevalence among men (24 percent) and women (19 percent), whereas Japan has a huge gap between men (47 percent) and women (14 percent).

Differences in smoking between the United States and European nations generate particular interest. Throughout the 1950s, the United States had higher levels of cigarette consumption than other countries (Forey et al., 2002), perhaps because it was a major source of tobacco leaf, the location of many large tobacco companies, and the source of innovative and misleading advertising about the safety of smoking (Brandt, 2007). In more recent years, however, smoking among Americans has dropped faster than in Europe, particularly among men. Cutler and Glaeser (2006) highlight this change in their paper "Why Do Europeans Smoke More Than Americans?" As discussed below, their answer to the question—differences in beliefs about the harm of smoking—offers one of several explanations for country differences.

The addictive attractions of nicotine and widespread access to cigarettes certainly play a role in the persistence across countries. But for insight into the national differences, other factors relating to government policies, social patterns of smoking, beliefs, and the timing of adoption need to be considered. The next sections review explanations of the cross-national patterns of smoking and then examine variation in smoking prevalence among high-income nations.

AN EPIDEMIC OR DIFFUSION MODEL OF NATIONAL DIFFERENCES

Epidemiologists note that population changes in smoking take a form analogous to an epidemic that spreads from relatively small parts of a population to other parts and then eventually recedes (Lopez, 1995; Lopez, Collishaw, and Piha, 1994; Mackenbach, 2006). More than changes in level, the epidemic involves a diffusion process that changes the socioeconomic composition of the smoking population. In the early stages, smoking emerges first among high-SES groups, who are most open to innovations and have the resources to adopt them (Rogers, 2003). During the middle stages, smoking diffuses to the rest of the population but begins to decline among high-SES persons, who become concerned with health, fitness, and the harm of smoking and who separate themselves from other groups by rejecting smoking and other unhealthy lifestyles (Link, 2008). Like smoking decades earlier, the adoption of healthy lifestyles is itself an innovation that emerges after the spread of the epidemic and relates closely to SES (Pampel, 2005). In the later stages of the epidemic, smoking falls among all groups, but disparities widen as the decline occurs faster among high- than among low-SES groups.

Gender also plays a role: the diffusion process among women typically lags a few decades behind that among men (Lopez, 1995; U.S. Department of Health and Human Services, 2001, p. 135). Since men adopt cigarettes first, the earliest stage of the epidemic shows a rising gap between men and women. In the middle stage, smoking among men levels off while it rises more quickly among women (particularly young and high-status women), and the gap stops growing. In later stages, smoking declines faster among men than women, and the gap narrows. With women adopting smoking later, educational disparities in smoking tend to emerge less strongly than for men; among older women in particular, high-SES rather than low-SES groups tend to smoke (Pampel, 2001).

These status-based processes of change in cigarette smoking should produce diverse experiences and patterns across nations (Giskes et al., 2005; Huisman, Kunst, and Mackenbach, 2005b; Schaap et al., 2008). Nations that began the epidemic earlier and have had more time for smoking to diffuse through the population and recede should have lower smoking than nations that began the epidemic later. Furthermore, nations that began the epidemic earlier should show stronger SES disparities in smoking among men, as the diffusion process has had more time for low-SES groups to adopt smoking and high-SES groups to stop smoking. Because of the female lag in adoption, however, the patterns may be less clear among women.

Since smoking begins by adulthood for the vast majority of smokers, attitudes and behaviors at the time of a cohort's adolescence will shape later patterns of smoking (Preston and Wang, 2006; U.S. Department of Health and Human Services, 2001, p. 453). Older groups that entered adolescence during periods of growing cigarette use decades ago will reflect patterns at earlier stages of diffusion. High-SES groups should show relatively high rates of smoking, and SES disparities should be modest. Among younger age groups that entered adolescence during periods of declining cigarette use and later stages of diffusion, the predictions about levels and SES disparities should be stronger. Lower SES groups should show substantially higher rates of smoking, and SES disparities should be greater. Again, however, because the diffusion process began later and has proceeded less far for women, the size of SES disparities in smoking should prove smaller for women than for men.

Why did some nations start the epidemic earlier than others? Many culturally and historically specific circumstances affect the timing, but national income probably plays a role (Cutler and Glaeser, 2006; Pampel, 2007). Historically high levels of national income should foster early adoption and the spread of smoking because more people can afford tobacco. However, as national income further increases, another mechanism tends to lower smoking, particularly among high-SES groups. The growing longevity that accompanies economic growth makes the health costs of smoking greater and more obvious, and the costs come to outweigh any benefits. Thus, if historically high national income predicts the early start of the epidemic, it also predicts the early retreat of the epidemic in later decades. This prediction holds particularly for high-SES groups, who benefit most from health advances and greater longevity (Becker and Murphy, 1988; Cutler and Lleras-Muney, 2008; Murphy and Topel, 2006). For lower SES groups, the risks of premature mortality from causes other than smoking may limit the perceived harm of smoking (Lawlor et al., 2003). In short, historical economic conditions relate to the timing of adoption and current national differences in smoking.

Other explanations of differences across nations offer alternatives to the diffusion arguments:

- Prices: higher prices due largely to taxes may increase costs and reduce levels of smoking overall (Gallus et al., 2006), but particularly among economically disadvantaged groups (Farrelly and Bray, 1998; Levy, Mumford, and Compton, 2006; Townsend, 1987; Warner, 2000). Thomas et al. (2008, p. 234) conclude from a comprehensive review that "the balance of econometric evidence suggests that increasing the price of tobacco is more effective in reducing smoking in lower-income adults and those in manual occupations."
- Government regulations: by reducing opportunities to smoke and emphasizing the dangers of the habit, bans on smoking in public places may reduce prevalence, again particularly among low-SES service and factory workers most affected by the bans (Farrelly, Evans, and Sfekas, 1999; Moskowitz, Lin, and Hudes, 2000; Sorenson et al., 2004).
- Inequality: low inequality moderates relative deprivation and associated stress among low-SES groups and reduces the dependence on smoking as a way to cope with disadvantaged circumstances (Wilkinson, 1996).
- Beliefs: acceptance of evidence that smoking causes harm and beliefs about dangers of smoking reduce prevalence (Cutler and Glaeser, 2006).

Cross-national evidence for these arguments is thin, but micro-level or within-nation evidence suggests their potential influence at the macro level.

NATIONAL DIFFERENCES IN TOBACCO USE

The second edition and web update of *International Smoking Statistics* (ISS) (Forey et al., 2002, 2009) provide the most complete source of data on smoking across the high-income nations. The second edition compiles reported smoking prevalence from surveys done through 1995 in each of 21 nations. The web update includes figures through 2005, but for only half of the countries thus far. To maximize the number of countries with data, the analysis examines male and female smoking prevalence for the years from 1950 to 1995. Because the harm of smoking accumulates over several decades, data ending in 1995 can still help to explain current levels of mortality (and can be supplemented later with more recent figures available from other sources). Data before 1950 exist for too few nations to include in the analysis.

The ISS reports the percentage of current smokers among adult men and women but not the percentage of former or never smokers. Since quitting reduces mortality, the greater risks of death among current smokers make current prevalence a valuable measure. However, it is also true that grouping former and never smokers together misses information, as former smokers have higher mortality than never smokers. The ISS also reports the kind of question used in the survey. Questions varyingly refer to all tobacco products, manufactured cigarettes, total cigarettes, unspecified tobacco products, and unspecified cigarettes. Questions may also refer to all smoking, regular smoking, and unspecified smoking. Dummy variables created for each set of categories adjust for varying levels of smoking generated by different questions.

A pooled regression of nations and time points of the percentage male and percentage female smokers uses several determinants: 20 dummy variables for nation (United States omitted), 45 dummy variables for year (1995 omitted), 4 product dummy variables (the total cigarettes category omitted), and 2 frequency dummy variables (the all-smoking category omitted). The controls for year adjust for differences across nations in the number and timing of available surveys, and the controls for product and frequency adjust for the type of questions asked. The controls for year are needed in particular for the unbalanced structure of the pooled data. Although some nations have many more data points than others, the year dummy variables control for this imbalance by adjusting for the average trend (i.e., the level of smoking at each time point).

Table 5-1, which is based on this regression model, lists the adjusted smoking prevalence for each nation in two forms: first as a deviation from the omitted value for the United States and then as a percentage for all cigarettes and all smoking. For men, Australia, Finland, Sweden, and the United States have the lowest smoking rates, and Greece, Japan, and Spain have the highest ones. It is notable that, when percentages are averaged across all years, the United States has lower smoking than nearly all European nations. The patterns in the next columns, for female smoking, show quite different orderings. Women in Austria, Finland, Japan, and Portugal have the lowest smoking rates, and women in Denmark, Ireland, the Netherlands, and the United Kingdom have the highest ones. With a correlation across nations for men and women equaling −.23, the rankings by gender tend to be reversed. Those nations with low male smoking tend to have high female smoking (e.g., Sweden, United States), and those with high male smoking tend to have low female smoking (e.g., Japan, Portugal).

For purposes of calibrating the effect of smoking on mortality, however, prevalence measures alone may be misleading, as they do not reflect the intensity of smoking. Figures on cigarette consumption (number per year per adult) combine both the number of smokers and the number of cigarettes per smoker but do not separate smoking of men and women or count cigarettes smuggled or brought in from other countries. The columns listing mean cigarette consumption by nation again average figures for each nation from 1950 to 1995, both as deviations from the United States and as adjusted means. The low consumption in Finland, Portugal, and Sweden also shows in low prevalence, and the United Kingdom and the Netherlands are high on both consumption and prevalence measures. Yet several countries show large differences, and the correlation for all countries of cigarette consumption with the average of male and female prevalence equals only .39. Despite low to medium levels of prevalence, Australia, Canada, and the United States show high consumption. Conversely, Denmark, Norway, and Spain have medium to high prevalence but lower consumption.

One interpretation of the discrepancy is that some nations have relatively few smokers who consume many cigarettes per day, while others have more smokers who consume relatively few cigarettes per day. Alternatively, measurement error may greatly bias one of the measures. One way to check on their validity is to examine the relationships of the prevalence and consumption measures with lung cancer. The fact that about 87 percent of lung cancer deaths in the United States (Satcher, Thompson, and Kaplan, 2002) occur among smokers suggests that lung cancer rates can serve as a valid indicator of smoking. The more effective measure should better predict later mortality from a cause closely associated with smoking. The last columns of Table 5-1 present, for each nation, the age-standardized lung cancer rates for men and women in 2000, calculated from the World Health Organiza-

TABLE 5-1 Average Smoking Measures for Males and Females Among 21 High-Income Nations, 1950-1995

Nation	N Data Points	Male Prevalence[a] Difference vs. U.S.	Male Prevalence[a] Adjusted Mean	Female Prevalence[a] Difference vs. U.S.	Female Prevalence[a] Adjusted Mean	Cigarettes Sold per Adult Difference vs. U.S.	Cigarettes Sold per Adult Adjusted Mean	Lung Cancer Mortality (Age Standardized) Male	Lung Cancer Mortality (Age Standardized) Female
Australia	41	0.2	36.8	-0.3	26.7	-10.0**	78.3	103.4	51.8
Austria	20	2.7	39.3	-9.5***	17.5	-35.0***	53.3	114.2	39.9
Belgium	42	8.2***	44.8	-4.8***	22.2	-21.7***	66.6	213.2	35.6
Canada	74	4.2**	40.8	2.7**	29.7	-4.2	84.1	137.7	86.6
Denmark	119	7.3***	43.9	12.3***	39.3	-36.7***	51.6	140.4	93.6
Finland	86	-2.8*	33.8	-10.6***	16.5	-44.5***	43.8	110.4	29.1
France	88	10.5***	47.1	-2.0*	25.0	-36.3***	52.0	134.6	24.2
Germany	93	6.4***	43.0	-4.8***	22.3	-31.8***	56.5	129.9	36.7
Greece	22	21.1***	57.7	-4.8***	22.2	-22.5***	65.8	150.3	27.8
Ireland	39	6.2***	42.8	6.0***	33.1	-13.1***	75.2	125.5	72.7
Italy	36	8.4***	45.0	-5.6***	21.4	-41.8***	46.5	149.4	31.7
Japan	47	28.2***	64.8	-14.8***	12.2	-17.0***	71.4	104.6	36.2
Netherlands	75	10.6***	47.2	7.4***	34.4	-14.0***	74.3	166.3	52.9
New Zealand	19	4.0*	40.6	5.6***	32.7	-18.8***	69.6	102.7	63.0
Norway	85	3.0*	39.6	5.0***	32.0	-45.0***	43.3	95.1	52.6
Portugal	26	5.1**	41.7	-18.2***	8.8	-44.2***	44.1	85.1	17.4
Spain	30	16.3***	52.9	-6.0***	21.1	-30.6***	57.7	140.2	15.8
Sweden	80	-5.1***	31.5	0.7	27.8	-49.3***	39.0	65.7	43.9
Switzerland	27	2.6	39.2	-1.2	25.8	-17.6***	70.7	107.6	36.6
United Kingdom	99	8.7***	45.3	9.4***	36.4	-16.1***	72.2	128.6	74.7
United States	35	0.0	36.6	0.0	27.0	0.0	88.3	147.7	95.1

[a]Controlling for year, product type, and frequency.
*p < .05, **p < .01, ***p < .001 (compared to value for United States).
SOURCE: Author's calculations from *International Smoking Statistics* and World Health Organization mortality database.

tion database (2009).² Sweden has the lowest lung cancer rate among men, and Belgium the highest. Spain and Portugal have the lowest rate among women, and the United States and Denmark have the highest.

To summarize the relationships, the top rows of Table 5-2 list the correlations between the measures of smoking and the age-standardized lung cancer rates. The correlations of the male lung cancer rate with male prevalence and cigarette consumption equal only .275 and .365. However, one outlying case greatly affects the male correlations. Japan has average male smoking of 65 percent, by far the highest, but is sixth lowest on lung cancer. This oddity attenuates the relationship. The same correlations with Japan omitted equal .506 and .398. For women, who are not affected strongly by outliers, the correlations of the female lung cancer rate with female prevalence and cigarette consumption equal .719 and .541. The correlations are higher for women than men, but both genders show the usefulness of prevalence.³ Still, the correlations are small given the strong relationship between smoking and lung cancer at the individual level. The crude measures of prevalence miss much about former smoking, years smoked, intensity of inhalation, and exposure to fumes that weakens the observed aggregate relationships between smoking and lung cancer.

NATIONAL DIFFERENCES IN TRENDS

Along with average levels across nations, differences in the rate of decline in smoking may influence current levels of smoking-related mortality. In describing the trends, it helps to focus on the last 25 years, from 1970 to 1995, when all the nations have complete data. With sparser data before 1970, nations have different starting points for the trends and comparisons become biased. For the shorter time period, regressions of male and female prevalence on a year quadratic with controls for nation, product type, and frequency measures show a nearly linear downward trend in prevalence for both men and women (see Figure 5-1).⁴ Prevalence decreases on average by 9.0 percentage points per decade among men and 2.3 percentage points per decade among women. Male smoking still exceeds female smoking prevalence, but the greater rate of decline among men leads to converging levels. Adjusted for controls, levels in 1970 of 57.8 and 31.9 for men and women fall to 34.9 and 26.1 in 1995. The decline in cigarette consumption differs

---

²The age-standardized lung cancer rate closely matches the percentage of smoking-attributed deaths in 2000 obtained from the methods of Peto et al. (1994) and available from Shafey, Dolwick, and Guindon (2003). The correlation for men across the 21 nations equals .968.

³Correlations do not change appreciably when figures are used for specific years (e.g., 1970 to 1974) rather than the average from 1950 to 1995.

⁴Use of the longer period and fewer nations likewise shows a linear downward trend for men but reveals a rise in female smoking during the 1950s and 1960s rather than a steady drop.

TABLE 5-2 Relationships of 2000 Age Standardized Lung Cancer Mortality Rates with Measures of Smoking Prevalence, Cigarette Consumption, and Change

	Male Lung Cancer Rate				Female Lung Cancer Rate
Level Measures Bivariate Correlations	All Nations	No Japan	All Nations	No Japan	All Nations
Male Prevalence	0.275	0.506*			
Female Prevalence					0.719*
Cigarette Consumption			0.365	0.398	0.541*

	Male Lung Cancer Rate				Female Lung Cancer Rate
Level and Change Multivariate Standardized	All Nations	No Japan	All Nations	No Japan	All Nations
Male Prevalence	0.269	0.495*			
Male Change	−0.184	−0.156			
Female Prevalence					0.513*
Female Change					−0.330
Cigarette Consumption			0.499	0.667*	0.214
Cig. Consumption Change			0.224	0.405	−0.547*
N	21	20	21	20	21	21

*p < .05.
SOURCE: Author's calculations from *International Smoking Statistics* and World Health Organization mortality database.

only slightly from the decline in prevalence. As also graphed in Figure 5-1, it shows some increase in the early 1970s before a nearly linear decline to a 1995 level of 44.2 cigarettes per adult per year.

Nations vary significantly in the extent of the downward trend, but the rate of change has limited influence on the age-standardized lung cancer rates in 2000. Table 5-2 examines simple regressions of the lung cancer rates on both the average prevalence and the average rate of change to compare the effects of level and trend in smoking. For men, prevalence has a larger net effect on lung cancer than does the trend (particularly with Japan omitted). The effect of trend is small and *negative*. For women, the same pattern emerges: prevalence has a positive effect, but trend has a negative effect. Obviously, there is spuriousness here. That those countries with the greatest drop have the highest lung cancer suggests that the drop occurs at later stages of the epidemic, after mortality has peaked. This pattern shows in cigarette consumption as well. The level of consumption has stronger

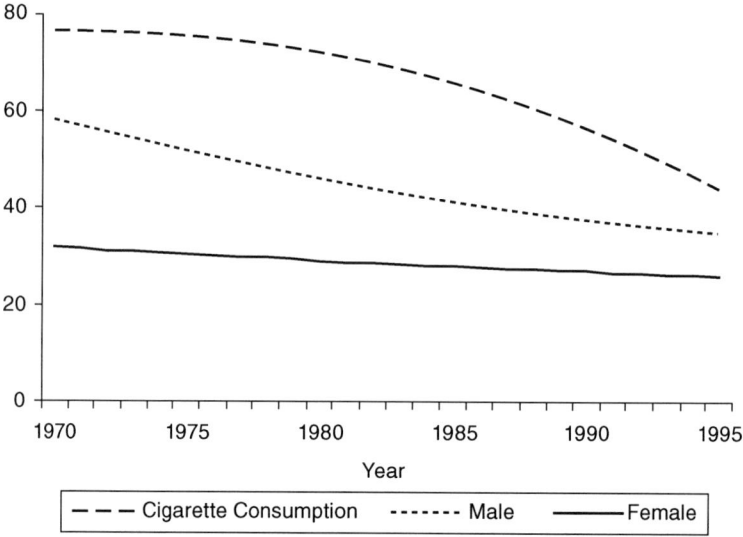

FIGURE 5-1 Adjusted trends in male prevalence (%), female prevalence (%), and cigarette consumption (number per adult).
SOURCE: Author's calculations from *International Smoking Statistics* (Forey et al., 2002).

effects, while the trend has mixed effects, positive for men and negative for women. Although none of the measures of smoking prove ideal in predicting subsequent mortality, the prevalence measures work well and distinguish between male and female smoking. The next step is to explain national patterns in these measures.

SOURCES OF NATIONAL DIFFERENCES: AGGREGATE CORRELATIONS

According to the epidemic or diffusion model, greater national income and a later stage of diffusion should lead to lower prevalence and greater decline of smoking. A simple test of these claims is to correlate past characteristics with subsequent patterns of smoking. I use two measures to predict smoking prevalence during the 1970 to 1995 period. First, gross domestic product (GDP) per capita in 1950 (20 years before the first year of the smoking data and 45 years before the last year) measures the resources available for an early start to the epidemic. An early start to the epidemic should lead in subsequent decades to a decline in smoking among men and an increase among women, while a later start should lead to high levels among men and low levels among women. Thus, nations with high income earlier in the 20th century will have lower smoking and greater decline among men but higher smoking and a smaller decline among women. Second, a measure of cigarette consumption per capita in 1950 also reflects the stage of diffusion. Nations with high consumption earlier in the century will have advanced farther in the rising part of the epidemic and therefore will have lower prevalence and a greater drop in more recent years for men but not for women. These diffusion-based predictions run counter to a null hypothesis of persistence in relative position—that nations with the highest past smoking will have the highest levels today.

The correlations of the 1950 variables with the average prevalence for 1970 to 1995 fit the diffusion predictions (see Table 5-3). Measures of the stage of the epidemic are correlated negatively with male prevalence and positively with female prevalence. For men, nations with high GDP and cigarette consumption early on have low smoking later on; for women, whose smoking follows that of men after a lag, high GDP and cigarette consumption in the past lead later to high smoking among women and gender convergence in smoking. Conversely, low GDP and cigarette consumption in the past and a late start to the epidemic lead to high male smoking and low female smoking.

For changes over time, the results are less clear but still revealing (bottom panel of Table 5-3). For men, the stage of diffusion appears to have little influence, perhaps because all nations have advanced far enough for male smoking to fall from previous levels. For women, however, the correlations

TABLE 5-3 Correlations of Smoking Level and Trend Measures with Gross Domestic Product (GDP) and Cigarette Consumption in 1950

	Prevalence		Cig. Cons.	GDP 1950	ln GDP 1950	Cig. Cons. 1950
	Male	Female				
Male Prevalence	1.00					
Female Prevalence	−0.17	1.00				
Cig. Cons.	0.04	0.31	1.00			
GDP 1950	−0.57**	0.62**	0.42*	1.00		
ln GDP 1950	−0.58**	0.68***	0.35	0.98***	1.00	
Cig. Cons. 1950	−0.35	0.41	0.79***	0.56**	0.53*	1.00
	Trend		Cig. Cons. Trend	GDP 1950	ln GDP 1950	Cig. Cons. 1950
	Male	Female				
Male Trend	1.00					
Female Trend	0.57**	1.00				
Cig. Cons. Trend	0.23	0.75***	1.00			
GDP 1950	−0.09	−0.68***	−0.69***	1.00		
ln GDP 1950	−0.13	−0.70***	−0.72***	0.98***	1.00	
Cig. Cons. 1950	−0.03	−0.51*	−0.76***	0.56**	0.53*	1.00

*p < .05, **p < .01, ***p < .001.
SOURCE: Author's calculations from *International Smoking Statistics*.

between stage of diffusion and trend are negative. This means that nations farther along in the epidemic earlier in the century show greater drops in female smoking. That these nations on average have both higher prevalence and a greater drop again fits the predictions. Late-stage nations have given women more time to reach higher levels of smoking and begin to decline. For early-stage nations, smoking among women has neither reached the higher levels of late-stage nations nor declined much.

What else might explain the historical differences? It's not apparent that historical differences across nations in government regulation of business or welfare support of the population can explain the differences. Both free-market nations like the United States and social democratic nations like Sweden have low male smoking, while egalitarian nations like the Netherlands and inegalitarian nations like Greece have high smoking. The economic and political environments of individual nations certainly affect smoking, but not in ways that easily account for the patterns. Thus far, the results seem to support the diffusion hypothesis.

SOURCES OF NATIONAL DIFFERENCES: INDIVIDUAL DATA

Eurobarometer 2006

Even were updated figures on men and women for more recent years available from *International Smoking Statistics*, other sources of data that distinguish smoking by SES are needed to fully test the arguments. The various theories of national differences make competing predictions about SES disparities in smoking as well as levels of smoking. To move beyond aggregate data and test the SES predictions, I examine a recent data source with individual-level data on smoking. The Eurobarometer (EB) 66.2 survey, done in October-November 2006, asks about sociodemographic characteristics and smoking of nationally representative samples in 31 nations (or national regions, such as Northern Ireland and East Germany) that belong to or are being considered for membership in the European Union (International Data Resource Center, 2006). Along with the high-income Western European nations, the survey includes many former Communist nations, Malta, the Republic of Cyprus, and the Turkish Cypriot Community. The surveys use multistage probability samples of typically 1,000 respondents (but fewer for small nations like Luxembourg and national regions like Northern Ireland). I focus on adults ages 26 to 64. Younger persons have not had time to complete school and establish a position in the socioeconomic hierarchy, and older persons may be sufficiently affected by smoking-related mortality as to attenuate the disparities. Annex A provides additional details about the Eurobarometer measures.

With questions on whether each individual currently smokes or formerly smoked, the survey allows for comparisons across countries of the level of smoking not only among men and women but also among low- and high-SES groups. The diffusion theory predicts that nations at later stages should have lower levels of male smoking and higher levels of female smoking, but it also makes predictions about the distribution of smoking. Nations at later stages should show larger SES disparities in smoking, particularly among men and less so for women. Other arguments predict that taxes and regulations will lower smoking. Although specifying different causes of low rates of smoking, the two groups of arguments predict similarly low rates of smoking among the same set of mostly northern nations with a long history of smoking and strong antitobacco policies. However, the tax and regulation arguments differ from the diffusion arguments in regard to SES disparities in smoking. Advocates say that higher taxes and greater restrictions affect low-SES groups most attuned to prices, least influenced by scientific information, and more focused on current health than future health. Nations with these policies should show smaller rather than larger SES disparities in smoking.

National Differences

Table 5-4 first presents the percentage of male and female smokers ages 25-64 for each nation from the Eurobarometer. The addition of the many Eastern and Southern European nations to the 21 studied previously affirms points about levels and variation in smoking. First, smoking prevalence in 2006—after decades of knowledge about the harm of smoking and more recent changes in policies to restrict smoking and make it more expensive—remains high. The mean levels equal 40.6 percent for men and 28.5 percent for women. Cyprus, Hungary, Latvia, Lithuania, and Romania contribute to the high mean for men. But figures show that 40.1 percent of men smoke in West Germany, 40.9 percent in Italy, 45.5 percent in Spain, and 59.1 percent in Greece. Only in Sweden does the level fall below 20 percent. Female smoking is lower than for men, but in many countries more than one-third of women smoke (Bulgaria, Great Britain, Greece, Hungary, Northern Ireland, Poland, and Spain). Nations with the lowest female smoking rates, such as Latvia, Malta, and Portugal, are probably on the upswing in adoption rather than the downswing of rejection.

The range in smoking rates is large as well. For men, it goes from 14.0 percent in Sweden to 59.1 percent in Greece. For women, it goes from 17.2 percent in Portugal to 40.7 percent in Greece. On average, men are 47 percent more likely to smoke than women, but again there is much variation. Men are 41 percent less likely to smoke than women in Sweden but 180 percent more likely in Latvia.[5]

---

[5]These figures represent high-end estimates of prevalence. They include smokers of both manufactured and hand-rolled cigarettes. If manufactured cigarettes only are included, the mean for men falls from 40.6 to 37.3. If only regular smokers are included, the mean for men

TABLE 5-4 Percentage Current Smokers and Ratios for Men to Women and for Low- to High-Education Groups by Country: Eurobarometer 2006 (ages 25-64)

Country	Gender			Male Education			Female Education		
	Male	Female	Ratio	Low[a]	High[b]	Ratio	Low[a]	High[b]	Ratio
Sweden	14.0	23.6	0.59	12.6	14.1	0.90	44.2	20.0	2.21
Netherlands	26.6	28.1	0.95	32.1	24.8	1.30	33.2	23.3	1.42
Slovenia	27.2	25.3	1.07	22.9	27.5	0.83	23.6	22.1	1.07
Luxembourg	29.0	25.8	1.12	33.4	16.9	1.98	21.6	18.0	1.20
Belgium	29.7	24.8	1.20	29.0	29.1	0.99	18.6	18.3	1.02
Ireland	31.6	31.3	1.01	50.0	16.7	3.00	54.5	19.4	2.81
Finland	31.7	23.9	1.33	55.0	28.0	1.97	40.0	19.4	2.06
Malta	31.8	21.6	1.47	38.0	21.0	1.81	15.8	16.3	0.97
Denmark	36.0	31.0	1.16	47.1	34.5	1.37	51.7	28.9	1.79
Slovakia	36.6	23.2	1.58	49.3	27.4	1.79	26.3	18.5	1.42
Northern Ireland	37.3	37.9	0.98	42.1	13.3	3.16	51.7	13.0	3.98
Germany East	37.8	31.0	1.22	27.9	22.2	1.26	54.6	15.8	3.46
Great Britain	37.8	35.5	1.07	52.6	25.5	2.06	46.9	18.8	2.49
France	38.8	29.2	1.33	49.2	35.2	1.40	21.0	24.0	0.87
Portugal	38.8	17.2	2.25	42.1	30.0	1.40	11.5	13.6	0.85
Germany West	40.1	30.5	1.32	56.4	29.2	1.93	27.8	21.9	1.27
Czech Republic	40.5	25.9	1.56	100.0	35.6	2.81	41.6	23.5	1.77
Italy	40.9	24.1	1.69	35.9	42.7	0.84	24.9	25.8	0.97
Austria	41.5	28.4	1.46	46.6	32.7	1.42	31.4	20.4	1.54
Croatia	44.0	29.8	1.48	58.0	36.3	1.60	20.5	28.2	0.73
Spain	45.5	34.7	1.31	44.0	40.0	1.10	32.8	31.2	1.05
Estonia	46.0	31.9	1.44	68.5	38.5	1.78	38.5	27.3	1.41
Bulgaria	46.4	35.0	1.33	50.0	40.8	1.22	35.0	32.9	1.06
Poland	47.0	36.2	1.30	66.9	38.8	1.72	37.2	33.2	1.12
Romania	48.7	23.8	2.04	39.8	52.5	0.76	4.7	33.2	0.14
Cyprus (TCC)	51.8	27.6	1.88	51.6	48.1	1.07	21.8	26.1	0.84
Hungary	52.5	38.2	1.37	75.2	31.9	2.36	47.4	29.0	1.63
Cyprus (Republic)	55.9	21.8	2.56	58.4	61.8	0.94	18.7	31.3	0.60
Lithuania	57.2	24.0	2.38	49.5	44.4	1.12	15.4	17.7	0.87
Latvia	57.3	20.4	2.80	63.3	47.3	1.34	32.2	14.9	2.16
Greece	59.1	40.7	1.45	52.5	58.9	0.89	27.3	40.3	0.68
Mean	40.6	28.5	1.47	48.4	33.7	1.55	31.4	23.4	1.47
SD	10.4	5.8	0.49	16.7	12.2	0.63	13.3	6.8	0.80

[a]Finished school before age 15.
[b]Finished school after age 19.
SOURCE: Data from Eurobarometer 2006.

falls from 40.6 to 36.2. The drops of 3 to 4 percent lower the estimates but may understate the risks. Hand-rolled cigarettes, even if smoked less often than readily available manufactured cigarettes, lack filters that reduce the harm of tobacco smoke. Occasional smokers have lower health risks than regular smokers, but experts say that any level of smoking is dangerous. For that reason, it makes sense to include all types of cigarette smoking in the measure of prevalence.

The results by SES reveal additional variation across countries. Table 5-4 lists smoking among those with low education (finished school before age 15) and high education (finished school after age 19) and then lists the ratio. The mean ratio of 1.55 for men indicates higher smoking among low-education groups. The male ratios reach 2.06, 3.00, and 3.16 in Great Britain, Ireland, and Northern Ireland, respectively, but fall below 1.00 in Belgium, Greece, Italy, Cyprus (Republic), Slovenia, Romania, and Sweden. The mean ratio for women is only slightly lower than for men but has a larger standard deviation. Northern Ireland again shows much greater smoking among less educated persons, but several other nations show greater smoking among more educated persons. The ratio equals only 0.14 in Romania, 0.60 in Cyprus (Republic), and 0.68 in Greece. However, these ratios are not age-adjusted and may confound low education with old age; multivariate, multilevel analysis to follow examines education effects with controls for age and other variables.

Individual-Level Models

To start, consider the individual-level relationships with smoking when averaged across all nations. Using available measures from the Eurobarometer and multilevel estimation from HLM 6.08 (Raudenbush et al., 2004), Table 5-5 presents the logistic regression coefficients relating current smoking to individual measures. Of special interest, education and occupational ranking lower smoking for both men and women, and goods owned lower smoking for men. However, as the variance components show, the effects of these three variables differ significantly across nations, and the negative coefficients may hide substantial diversity in SES effects.

As suggested by diffusion arguments, the negative effects of the SES measures emerge stronger among younger persons than older persons. Without presenting more tables, results from adding interaction terms of age by education, occupation, and goods owned offer some insights. The positive effects of the interaction terms show that as age increases, the negative effects of the SES variables moderate. Thus, younger age groups entering adulthood at later stages of diffusion show stronger SES disparities, whereas older age groups entering adulthood many decades ago during earlier stages of diffusion show weaker SES disparities.

Aggregate Influences

Table 5-6 examines a different set of determinants. It lists effects of several aggregate variables on the nation-specific intercept (or level of smoking at the means for all the individual-level variables) and the nation-specific slopes for education, occupation, and goods owned. The table contains eight

TABLE 5-5 Unstandardized Coefficients and t Statistics from Multilevel Logistic Regression of Current Smoking on Individual Predictors

Predictors	Males b t	Variance Components	Females b t	Variance Components
Age	0.107*** 6.442		0.098*** 3.916	
Age^2	−0.001*** −7.615		−0.001*** −4.729	
Urban	0.101* 2.429		0.193*** 5.568	
Married	−0.410*** −8.555		−0.652*** −10.824	
Out of School	0.569 1.891		1.178*** 4.118	
Education[a]	−0.060*** −4.069	0.003**	−0.085*** −5.381	0.010***
Reports Job	0.132 0.509		0.289* 2.511	
Occupation[b]	−0.053*** −5.790	0.001*	−0.031** −2.653	0.006***
Goods Owned[c]	−1.115*** −6.889	0.439**	−0.032 −0.253	1.127***
Intercept	−0.442*** −7.415	0.104***	−0.988*** −19.187	0.070***
N persons	7643		10175	
N nations	31		31	

[a]For those out of school.
[b]For those reporting a job.
[c]Proportion of nine household items owned.
*p < .05, **p < .01, ***p <.001.
SOURCE: Data from Eurobarometer 2006.

Descriptive Statistics			
Males Mean	Females Mean	All Min	All Max
45.39	45.09	26	64
2181.20	2152.31	6776	4096
1.89	1.89	1	3
0.65	0.65	0	1
0.99	0.99	0	1
6.21	5.93	0	10
0.99	0.93	0	1
5.93	5.53	0	12
0.69	0.67	0	1

TABLE 5-6 Unstandardized Coefficients and t Statistics from Multilevel Logistic Regression of Current Smoking Intercepts and Slopes on Level-2 Predictors

Level-2 Predictors	Level-1 Male Intercept and Slopes as Outcomes			
	Intercept	Education	Occupation	Goods Owned
Logged GDP per Capita				
b	−0.115**	−0.013	−0.004	−0.020
t	−2.555	−0.712	−0.430	−0.112
Gini Coefficient of Income Inequality				
b	0.114*	0.014	0.000	0.039
t	1.980	0.954	0.039	0.260
Ex-Communist Nations (=1)				
b	0.041	−0.012	−0.008	−0.153
t	0.700	−0.703	−0.933	−0.974
Tobacco Control Scale[a]				
b	−0.115**	−0.019	−0.002	−0.386***
t	−2.309	−1.242	−0.165	−3.082
Smoking Ban Scale[a]				
b	−0.114**	−0.004	0.009	−0.138
t	−2.291	−0.287	1.006	−0.689
Cigarette Price Scale[a]				
b	−0.045	−0.006	−0.002	−0.215
t	−0.879	−0.428	−0.131	−1.792
Current M/F Ratio[b]				
b	0.177***	0.023**	0.011	0.204*
t	2.909	2.767	0.964	1.950
Ever M/F Ratio[b]				
b	0.210***	0.025**	0.011	0.247**
t	4.057	2.473	1.171	2.146

[a]Scales from Joosens and Raw (2006) with values ranging from 26 to 74 for tobacco control, 1 to 21 for smoking ban, and 7 to 30 for cigarette price

[b]Percentage male current or ever smokers as a ratio to percentage female current or ever smokers, with high score indicating early stage of diffusion.

*p < .10, **p < .05, ***p < .01.
SOURCE: Data from Eurobarometer 2006.

Level-1 Female Intercept and Slopes as Outcomes			
Intercept	Education	Occupation	Goods Owned
−0.001	−0.044***	−0.040***	−0.566***
−0.016	−2.966	−3.003	−3.703
−0.026	0.024	0.021	0.288
−0.393	1.415	1.488	1.669
0.023	0.005	0.015	0.206
0.437	0.294	1.038	1.103
0.051	−0.043**	−0.039***	−0.725***
1.281	−2.477	−3.123	−4.225
−0.046	−0.005	−0.009	−0.142
−1.152	−0.206	−0.545	−0.583
0.081**	−0.026	−0.024	−0.525**
2.317	−1.361	−1.691	−2.339
−0.183***	0.057***	0.048***	0.799***
−3.141	4.153	4.102	4.094
−0.181***	0.065***	0.060***	0.907***
−3.311	4.136	4.491	5.361

aggregate measures that may relate to the outcomes across the 31 nations or national regions.[6]

- GDP per capita in purchase price parities (logged to capture percentage change) measures standard of living in 2004 (from Heston, Summers, and Aten, 2006).
- The Gini coefficient of inequality relates to the degree of relative deprivation and comes from data originally compiled by Deininger and Squire (1996) and updated by the World Bank (2009).
- A dummy variable coded 1 for the former Communist nations captures a key source of economic differences in Europe.
- For tobacco control policies, Joossens and Raw (2006) present a scale that combine separate measures—based on data and ratings provided by experts in each of 30 European countries—of price, bans on smoking in public places, public information campaigns, advertising bans, health warnings, and funding for treatment. I use the full scale and also two of its key components—prices and bans on smoking in public places. The full scale ranges from 26 to 74 (with a potential maximum of 100).
- The ban scale measures the extent of smoke-free workplaces, cafes and restaurants, and other public places, with complete and enforced bans receiving high scores and legislated but unenforced bans receiving low scores. The scale ranges from 1 (United Kingdom) to 21 (Ireland).
- The price scale uses data on the price (adjusted for GDP per capita) of Marlboro and the price of cigarettes in the most popular price category. The scale is transformed so that the nation with the most expensive prices gets a score of 30 (United Kingdom) and the nation with the lowest prices gets a score of 7 (Luxembourg).
- For the stage of diffusion, measures of GDP and cigarette consumption in 1950 are not available for many of the nations. An alternative measure, the smoking prevalence of men relative to the smoking prevalence of women in the 2000s, has been used by Gallus et al. (2006). Since adoption of smoking by women lags behind that of men and moves toward parity only in the later stages of diffusion, a ratio close to 1 indicates a later stage of diffusion and a ratio well above 1 indicates an early stage of diffusion. I use two sources for the male and female smoking rates that go into the ratio measure. First, Gallus et al. (2006) report figures on male and female prevalence in the early 2000s from the Tobacco Control Country Profiles that

---

[6] I assign the same values for the aggregate variables to East and West Germany, Great Britain and Northern Ireland, and the Cyprus Republic and Cypriot Turkish Community.

are gathered independently from the Eurobarometer. Second, I use a measure created from the Eurobarometer survey on ever-smoking prevalence at ages 26-64. Although from the same data set, ever-smoking differs from the outcome variable of current smoking and reduces definitional overlap. With either source of prevalence data, the ratio of male to female smoking is an obvious and trivial predictor of the likelihood of smoking among men or women, but it may indicate less obviously how the stage of cigarette diffusion moderates the influence of SES on individual smoking.

To summarize these results briefly, the measures of cigarette diffusion have consistently significant coefficients in the expected direction, but the others do not. The earlier the stage (or the higher the male-to-female ratio), the weaker the effect of education (i.e., the positive effect of an early stage moderates the otherwise negative effect of the SES variables). Conversely, the later the stage (or the lower the male-to-female ratio), the stronger the negative effect of education. Of the 12 interaction coefficients for the diffusion measures, 10 reach significance. Partly consistent with these results are the significant negative effects of GDP for women. The higher income nations, generally those at later stages of diffusion, have stronger female SES disparities in smoking. Otherwise, the Gini coefficient has little influence on the individual coefficients, and ex-Communist nations do not differ from the other nations in the effects of the SES variables.

The results for restrictive tobacco policies show little consistent association. Moreover, the direction of the relationship often is opposite to that expected. The policies are associated with lower smoking for men, but higher smoking for women, and all the significant effects on SES disparities in smoking are negative. That is, restrictive policies are associated with stronger negative effects of SES or with larger rather than smaller disparities. The small number of nations warrants use of simple level-2 models and prevents additional tests of various combinations of variables. Moreover, rigorous tests of the impact of policies require longitudinal data and comparisons of smoking before and after a policy change. Even with these limitations, the results consistently show that the diffusion measures produce the expected effects, whereas the tobacco policy variables do not.

Cutler and Glaeser (2006) offer an alternative explanation based on stronger antitobacco beliefs in the United States compared with Europe. They note that taxes, prices, and regulations fail to explain lower U.S. smoking, as all these tend to be greater in Europe than the United States. However, a higher percentage of survey respondents in the United States than in Europe agree with statements about the harm of smoking for health. To minimize cognitive dissonance bias—smokers rejecting scientific evidence as a way to justify their habit—Cutler and Glaeser examine beliefs among nonsmokers. For this subset of respondents, data from the 1994 General Social Survey show that 94 percent of Americans agreed that smoking causes cancer, while data from the 1994 Eurobarometer show that an average of 90 percent across 14 Western European nations agreed. Cutler and Glaeser interpret this difference as evidence that stronger American beliefs in the harm of smoking reduce prevalence. The stronger beliefs result from concerted efforts of government and health advocacy groups to publicize the facts. Government decentralization, the prominence of specialized interest groups, and the actions of numerous health advocacy groups contribute to the lower smoking in the United States. As Cutler and Glaeser (2006) say, "While greater U.S. entrepreneurship and economic openness led to more smoking during an earlier era (and still leads to more obesity today), it also led to faster changes in beliefs about smoking and ultimately less cigarette consumption."

However, beliefs as well as smoking may be associated with the stage of diffusion; the United States is exceptional in regard to its long history of smoking as well as its antismoking beliefs. In a simple test, I correlate the figures on beliefs and smoking from Cutler and Glaeser (2006, Tables 5-1 and 5-4) and the measures of GDP and cigarette consumption from 1950.[7] With a sample size of 14 nations, the correlation of beliefs with smoking equals –.19, while the correlations of 1950 GDP and cigarette consumption with smoking equal –.01 and –.27, respectively. That consumption 44 years earlier correlates with smoking at least as well as current beliefs highlights the importance of the long-term diffusion process.[8] Moreover, 1950 cigarette consumption has a positive correlation of .20 with beliefs. The truncated sample makes these results only suggestive, but it could be that beliefs change with the stage of the epidemic.

DISCUSSION

The analyses presented in this study, although limited methodologically in many ways, tend to tell a consistent story about national variation in levels, trends, and SES differences of smoking: cigarette smoking is initially adopted by high-SES men, the habit diffuses first to men in other SES groups and later to high-SES women, high-SES men then reject smoking, male and female smoking rates converge, and SES disparities in smoking grow (Mackenbach, 2006). Based on diffusion processes of innovations, class distinction, and imitation and on the balance of costs and

---

[7] The analysis drops Luxembourg because of lack of data on past cigarette use.

[8] Cutler and Glaeser (2006) drop Greece from their analysis because its GDP is so much lower than those of the other nations. Even without Greece, high cigarette consumption in 1950 correlates with both lower smoking and beliefs in 1994.

benefits of smoking for SES groups, the pattern of change seems to be similar across countries. What differs is the timing of the start of the epidemic and diffusion process, with early-starting nations having advanced farther in the process than nations starting later. Thus, smoking spread earlier in English-speaking nations and Belgium and the Netherlands than in Southern European nations. A perspective based on diffusion helps answer several questions about differences across nations.

What caused some countries like the United States to have smoked more heavily in the past and dropped more steeply in recent decades than other nations? These nations started the epidemic earlier. This explanation seems to work better than alternatives focusing on policies, inequality, and beliefs. And why did some nations start earlier? One reason is economic—citizens in high-income nations like the United States could afford to start earlier. Results thus show that high GDP in 1950 relates to the early rise in smoking and to subsequent decline. In Southern Europe, later economic development slowed the start of the epidemic. No doubt cultural factors play a role as well. Events unique to the United States, such as the domestic cultivation of the tobacco plant, the invention of the cigarette rolling machine, and the development of innovative advertising to attract smokers, affected the early start of the epidemic here and in English-speaking trading partners. Thus, the seven nations with highest per capita cigarette consumption in 1950 were Australia, Belgium, Canada, Ireland, New Zealand, the United Kingdom, and the United States. Among the lowest were Austria, Germany, Italy, Portugal, and Spain.

What causes convergence in male and female smoking rates in nations like the United States and Sweden but substantially lower smoking among women than men in Southern Europe? Again, this pattern fits the diffusion argument. In nations at later stages, the drop in smoking among men has occurred more quickly than among later adopting women and has produced some convergence (Schaap et al., 2008). The Southern European nations are in the earlier stages of diffusion, so women are just starting to follow men in the adoption of smoking and the gap remains large. A good predictor of current female smoking is the level of male smoking several decades earlier. Nations with high smoking in 1950 have low male smoking today but relatively high female smoking, while nations with low smoking in 1950 have high male smoking today and low female smoking. If the pattern continues, this too will change. Female smoking in nations at later stages will drop, while female smoking in nations at earlier stages will rise. Several previous studies further suggest that gender equality does little to influence these trends and patterns in female smoking (Pampel, 2001, 2002, 2003).

Why has smoking become much more prevalent among low-SES groups? Common explanations focus on several traits of disadvantaged groups: higher stress, lower health benefits from quitting, orientations toward short-term utility, low efficacy to deal with the difficulties of resisting and quitting, exposure to more advertising, greater opportunities to buy and use cigarettes in poor communities, and lower social and cultural capital. In cross-national comparisons, however, variation in SES effects appears consistent with the diffusion argument. Among nations at later stages of diffusion, early adoption by high-SES groups in the past leads to low current smoking rates and later adoption by low-SES groups leads to higher rates of current smoking—which jointly produce the growing disparities observed in many nations. Among nations at earlier stages of diffusion and among later adopting women, however, the process has proceeded less far and disparities are smaller.

How can government policies speed the process of change toward lower smoking? Government tobacco restrictions are certainly associated with lower prevalence rates; U.S. studies show the benefits of comprehensive antismoking policies (Fiori and Baker, 2009). However, the policies may affect men and high-SES groups most—those already most likely to reject smoking, according to diffusion arguments. For example, despite more than a decade of higher taxes and bans on smoking, SES disparities among native-born whites and blacks in the United States remain just as large today as in 1990 (Pampel, 2009).

In Europe, Finland, Ireland, Italy, Norway, Sweden, and the United Kingdom have the strongest tobacco control policies, and Austria, Denmark, Germany, Greece, Portugal, and Spain, have the weakest. Although Italy is an exception, the former group has consistently lower smoking rates among men than the latter group. However, the Eurobarometer data show little association between restrictive policies and female smoking prevalence or SES disparities in smoking. If anything, tobacco control policies are associated with greater rather than smaller SES disparities. The Eurobarometer data do not allow the kind of test needed to properly evaluate the impact of policies on disparities, but the pattern of results tends to favor the diffusion argument. A study of quit ratios in 18 European countries similarly finds that the least educated smokers benefited no more than highly educated smokers from tobacco control policies (Schaap et al., 2008).

If in the context of cigarette diffusion, policies to raise taxes, ban smoking in public places, and otherwise restrict access to cigarettes all lower the level of smoking but fail to moderate disparities, tobacco reduction efforts may need to more directly target low-SES groups. Such strategies might include worksite-based smoking cessation interventions (Sorensen et al., 2004), education efforts focused more specifically on priority groups with high risks of smoking (Barbeau et al., 2004), and recognition that techniques of behavior change may differ substantially across SES backgrounds (Frohlich and Potvin, 2008). The same kind of policies may help nations at early stages of the epidemic do more to prevent adoption of smoking by women and low-SES groups who have yet to start smoking in large numbers. Such changes might alter the spread of the epidemic and quicken its passage.

More generally, gains to longevity among low-SES groups may help speed the decline in smoking during the diffusion process. As Cutler and Glaeser (2006) argue, the trend toward adoption of smoking with income growth reverses when the health costs of smoking come to exceed the short-term benefits. High-SES groups reach this reversal point soonest, but reductions in mortality from nonsmoking causes among low-SES groups may foster the rejection of smoking.

What are the limitations of the findings? To qualify claims on behalf of the diffusion argument, the evidence is more illustrative than authoritative. The measures of smoking across nations show inconsistencies, the measures of diffusion are imprecise, and the measures of tobacco control policies cover only the more recent years. Furthermore, analyses comparing a relatively small number of nations have weak statistical power. Additional analyses of the Eurobarometer data by age or cohort groups might give additional insights but would still be limited by the cross-sectional design. The evidence suggests promise rather than confirmation of the diffusion theory's predictions of variation in smoking across time, nations, and social groups.

One might object on theoretical grounds as well. The mechanisms underlying the regularities of adoption and rejection of smoking by gender and SES seem vague compared with the concrete influences of higher prices, smoking bans, deprivation, and knowledge of the harm of tobacco. Given inadequacies of the cross-national data and measures available for analysis, the chapter neither specifies nor tests for underlying SES-based mechanisms relevant to smoking, A guide to doing so comes from work on diffusion and fertility decline. Casterline (2001) defines diffusion as change in behavior of some that affects the likelihood of change in behavior among others, and he identifies mechanisms of social influence, social learning, social comparison or emulation, social coercion, and social capital through which diffusion operates. Palloni (2001), after arguing that the diffusion-of-innovation theories fail to identify the decision-making processes that give meaning to the underlying mechanisms, further suggests refinements to make the theories more complete. However, similar theoretical development has not occurred with regard to the spread of smoking.

Two types of data would allow better tests of diffusion arguments and evaluation of the ability of policies to speed the process of change toward smoking reduction. First, at the macro level, over-time survey data on smoking prevalence and national-level changes in policies across nations would allow one to evaluate the effect of policy changes. Without following individuals over time, consecutive cross-sectional data that cover a decade or more and have comparable measures across a large number of nations can better establish causal relations by comparing changes over time as well as differences across nations in policies, diffusion stage, and SES disparities. If the data also identify areas within nations, particularly those with different linguistic, religious, and ethnic compositions, it might give further insight into the social dynamics of diffusion.

Second, more micro-oriented designs can help identify the mechanisms underlying the spread of smoking or smoking cessation. Casterline (2001) identifies the kinds of data needed to test diffusion arguments. The data should be longitudinal, include measures of social exposure to innovations, both informal and formal, and relate perceptions of the attitudes and behaviors of others at time one to outcomes at time two. Some success with this kind of approach comes from the analysis of education-based networks in the Framingham Heart Study by Christakis and Fowler (2008). Studies of teen smoking likewise have focused on the strong influence of peer networks and interpersonal influence on initiation and adoption (see Jacobson et al., 2001, for a review). Comparative studies would likewise benefit from more detailed micro-level measures of diffusion variables.

REFERENCES

Barbeau, E., Krieger, N., and Soobader, M.-J. (2004). Working class matters: Socioeconomic disadvantage, race/ethnicity, gender, and smoking in NHIS 2000. *American Journal of Public Health, 94*(2), 269-278.

Becker, G.S., and Murphy, K.M. (1988). A theory of rational addiction. *Journal of Political Economy, 96*(4), 675-700.

Brandt, A.M. (2007). *The Cigarette Century: The Rise, Fall, and Deadly Persistence of the Product That Defined America.* New York: Basic Books.

Casterline, J.B. (2001). Diffusion processes and fertility transition: Introduction. In National Research Council, *Diffusion Processes and Fertility Transition: Selected Perspectives* (pp. 1-38). Committee on Population, J.B. Casterline (Ed.) Division of Behavioral and Social Sciences and Education. Washington DC: National Academy Press.

Christakis, N.A., and Fowler, J.H. (2008). The collective dynamics of smoking in a large social network. *New England Journal of Medicine, 358*(21), 2249-2258.

Cutler, D.M., and Glaeser, E.L. (2006). *Why Do Europeans Smoke More Than Americans?* National Bureau of Economic Research Working Paper 12124. Available: http://www.nber.org/papers/w12124 [accessed June 2010].

Cutler, D.M., and Lleras-Muney, A. (2008). Education and health: Evaluating theories and evidence. In R.F. Schoeni, J.S. House, G.A. Kaplan, and H. Pollack (Eds.), *Making Americans Healthier: Social and Economic Policy as Health Policy* (pp. 29-60). New York: Russell Sage Foundation.

Davis, R.M., Wakefield, M., Amos, A., and Gupta, P.C. (2007). The hitchhiker's guide to tobacco control: A global assessment of harms, remedies, and controversies. *Annual Review of Public Health, 28,* 171-194.

Deininger, K., and Squire, L. (1996). A new data set measuring income inequality. *World Bank Economic Review, 10*(3), 565-591.

Dube, S.R., Asman, K., Malarcher, A., and Carabollo, R. (2009). Cigarette smoking among adults and trends in smoking cessation—United States, 2008. *Morbidity and Mortality Weekly Report, 58*(44), 1227-1232.

Eriksen, M.P., and Cerak, R.L. (2008). The diffusion and impact of clean indoor air laws. *Annual Review of Public Health, 29,* 171-185.

Fagan, P., King, G., Lawrence, D., Petrucci, S.A., Robinson, R.G., Banks, D., Marable, S., and Grana, R. (2004). Eliminating tobacco-related health disparities: Directions for future research. *American Journal of Public Health, 94*(2), 211-217.

Farrelly, M.C., and Bray, J. (1998). Response to increases in cigarette prices by race/ethnicity, income, and age groups—United States, 1976-1993. *Morbidity and Mortality Weekly Report, 47*(29), 605-609.

Farrelly, M.C., Evans, M.N., and Sfekas, A.E. (1999). The impact of workplace smoking bans: Results from a national survey. *Tobacco Control, 8*(3), 272-277.

Fiori, M.C., and Baker, T.B. (2009). Stealing a march in the 21st century: Accelerating progress in the 100-year war against tobacco addiction in the United States. *American Journal of Public Health, 99*(7), 1170-1175.

Forey, B., Hamling, J., Lee, P., and Wald, N. (Eds.). (2002). *International Smoking Statistics (2nd ed.).* Oxford, England: Oxford University Press.

Forey, B., Hamling, J., Hamling, J., and Lee, P. (2009). *International Smoking Statistics Web Edition.* P.N. Lee Statistics and Computing. Available: http://www.pnlee.co.uk/ISS.htm [accessed June 2010].

Frohlich, K.L., and Potvin, L. (2008). The inequality paradox: The population approach and vulnerable populations. *American Journal of Public Health, 98*(2), 216-221.

Gallus, S., Schiaffino, A., La Vecchia, C., Townsend, J., and Fernandez, E. (2006). Price and cigarette consumption in Europe. *Tobacco Control, 15*(2), 114-119.

Giskes, K., Kunst, A.E., Benach, J., Borrell, C., Costa, G., Dahl, E., Dalstra, J.A.A., Federico, B., Helmert, U., Judge, K., Lahelma, E., Moussa, K., Ostergren, P.O., Platt, S., Prattala, R., Rasmussen, N.K., and Mackenbach. J.P. (2005). Trends in smoking behaviour between 1985 and 2000 in nine European countries by education. *Journal of Epidemiology and Community Health, 59*(5), 395-401.

Heston, A., Summers, R., and Aten, B. (2006). *Penn World Table Version 6.2.* Center for International Comparisons of Production, Income and Prices at the University of Pennsylvania. Available: http://pwt.econ.upenn.edu/php_site/pwt_index.php [accessed June 2010].

Huisman, M., Kunst, A.E., and Mackenbach, J.P. (2005a). Inequalities in the prevalence of smoking in the European Union: Comparing education and income. *Preventive Medicine, 40*(6), 756-764.

Huisman, M., Kunst, A.E., and Mackenbach, J.P. (2005b). Educational inequalities in smoking among men and women aged 16 years and older in 11 European countries. *Tobacco Control, 14*(2), 106-113.

International Data Resource Center. (2006). *Eurobarometer 66.2: Nuclear Energy and Safety and Public Health Issues, October-November 2006.* Interconsortium for Political and Social Research. Available http://www.icpsr.umich.edu/cocoon/IDRC/STUDY/21460.xml [accessed June 2010].

Jacobson, P.D., Lantz, P., Warner, K., Wasserman, J., Pollack, H., and Ahlstrom, A. (2001). *Combating Teen Smoking: Research and Policy Strategies.* Ann Arbor: University of Michigan.

Joossens, L., and Raw, M. (2006). The Tobacco Control Scale: A new scale to measure country activity. *Tobacco Control, 15*(3), 247-253.

Lawlor, D.A., Frankel, S., Shaw, M., Ebrahim, S., and Davey Smith, G. (2003). Smoking and ill health: Does lay epidemiology explain the failure of smoking cessation programs among deprived populations? *American Journal of Public Health, 93*(2), 266-270.

Levy, D.T., Mumford, E.A., and Compton, C. (2006). Tobacco control policies and smoking in a population of low education women, 1992-2002. *Journal of Epidemiology and Community Health, 60*(supplement 2), ii20-ii26.

Link, B.G. (2008). Epidemiological sociology and the social shaping of population health. *Journal of Health and Social Behavior, 49*(4), 367-384.

Lopez, A.D. (1995). The lung cancer epidemic in developed countries. In A.D. Lopez, G. Caselli, and T. Valkonen (Eds.), *Adult Mortality in Developed Countries: From Description to Explanation* (pp. 111-143). Oxford, England: Clarendon.

Lopez, A.D., Collishaw, N.E., and Piha, T. (1994). A descriptive model of the cigarette epidemic in developed countries. *Tobacco Control, 3*(3), 242-247.

Mackay, J., Eriksen, M., and Shafey, O. (2006). *The Tobacco Atlas, 2nd edition*. Geneva, Switzerland: World Health Organization. Available: http://www.cancer.org/docroot/AA/content/AA_2_5_9x_Tobacco_Atlas.asp [accessed June 2010].

Mackenbach, J.P. (2006). *Health Inequalities: Europe in Profile. An Independent, Expert Report Commissioned by the UK Presidency of the EU*. Rotterdam, Germany: Erasmus University Medical Center.

Mendez, D., and Warner, K.E. (2004). Adult cigarette smoking prevalence: Declining as expected (not as desired). *American Journal of Public Health, 94*(2), 251-252.

Moskowitz, J.M., Lin, Z., and Hudes, E.S. (2000). The impact of workplace smoking ordinances in California on smoking cessation. *American Journal of Public Health, 90*(5), 757-761.

Murphy, K.M., and Topel, R.H. (2006). The value of health and longevity. *Journal of Political Economy, 114*(5), 871-904.

Palloni, A. (2001). Diffusion in sociological analysis. In National Research Council, *Diffusion Processes and Fertility Transition: Selected Perspectives* (pp. 66-114). Committee on Population, J.B. Casterline (Ed.). Division of Behavioral and Social Sciences and Education. Washington DC: National Academy Press.

Pampel, F.C. (2001). Cigarette diffusion and sex differences in smoking. *Journal of Health and Social Behavior, 42*(4), 388-404.

Pampel, F.C. (2002). Cigarette use and the narrowing sex differential in mortality. *Population and Development Review, 28*(1), 77-104.

Pampel, F.C. (2003). Declining sex differences in lung cancer mortality in high income nations. *Demography, 40*(1), 45-65.

Pampel, F.C. (2005). Diffusion, cohort change, and social patterns of smoking. *Social Science Research, 34*(1), 117-139.

Pampel, F.C. (2007). National income, inequality, and global patterns of cigarette use. *Social Forces, 86*(2), 455-466.

Pampel, F.C. (2009). The persistence of educational disparities in smoking. *Social Problems, 56*(3), 526-542.

Peto, R., Lopez, A.D., Boreham, J., Thun, M., and Heath, C., Jr. (1994). *Mortality from Smoking in Developed Countries 1950-2000: Indirect Estimates from National Vital Statistics*. Oxford, England: Oxford University Press.

Preston, S.H., and Wang, H. (2006). Sex mortality differences in the United States: The role of cohort smoking patterns. *Demography, 43*(4), 631-646.

Raudenbush, S., Bryk, A.S., Cheong, Y.F., and Congdon, R. (2004). *HLM 6: Hierarchical Linear and Nonlinear Modeling*. Chicago: Scientific Software International.

Rock, V.J., Malarcher, A., Kahende, J.W., Asman, K., Husten, C., and Caraballo, R. (2007). Cigarette smoking among adults—United States, 2006. *Morbidity and Mortality Weekly Report, 56*(44), 1157-1161.

Rogers, E.M. (2003). *Diffusion of Innovations.* New York: Free Press.

Satcher, D., Thompson, T.G., and Kaplan. J.P. (2002). Women and smoking: A report of the surgeon general. *Nicotine and Tobacco Research, 4*(1), 7-20.

Schaap, M.M., Kunst, A.E., Leinsalu, M., Regidor, E., Ekholm, O., Dzurova, D., Helmert, U., Klumbiene, J., Santana, P., and Mackenbach, J.P. (2008). Effect of nationwide tobacco control policies on smoking cessation in high and low educated groups in 18 European countries. *Tobacco Control, 17*(4), 248-255.

Shafey, O., Dolwick, S., and Guindon, G.E. (Eds.). (2003). *Tobacco Control Country Profiles, 003.* Atlanta: American Cancer Society.

Sorenson, G., Barbeau, E., Hunt, M.K., and Emmons, K. (2004). Reducing social disparities in tobacco use: A social contextual model for reducing tobacco use among blue-collar workers. *American Journal of Public Health, 94*(2), 230-239.

Thomas, S., Fayter, D., Misso, K., Ogilvie, D., Petticrew, M., Sowden, A., Whitehead, M., and Worthy, G. (2008). Population tobacco control interventions and their effects on social inequalities in smoking: Systematic review. *Tobacco Control, 17*(4), 230-237.

Townsend, J.L. (1987). Cigarette tax, economic welfare and social class patterns of smoking. *Applied Economics, 19*(3), 355-365.

U.S. Department of Health and Human Services. (2001). *Women and Smoking: A Report of the Surgeon General.* Rockville, MD: Author.

Warner, K.E. (2000). The economics of tobacco control: Myths and realities. *Tobacco Control, 9*(1), 78-89.

Warner, K.E. (2005). Tobacco policy in the United States: Lessons for the obesity epidemic. In D. Mechanic, L.B. Rogut, and D.C. Colby (Eds.), *Policy Challenges in Modern Health Care* (pp. 99-114). New Brunswick, NJ: Rutgers University Press.

Wilkinson, R.G. (1996). *Unhealthy Societies: The Afflictions of Inequality.* London, England: Routledge.

World Bank. (2009). *Measuring Income Inequality Database: Research at the World Bank.* Available: http://go.worldbank.org/UVPO9KSJJ0 [accessed July 2009].

World Health Organization. (1997). *Tobacco or Health: A Global Status Report.* Geneva, Switzerland: Author.

World Health Organization. (2009). *WHO Mortality Database: Tables.* Health Statistics and Health Information Systems. Available: http://www.who.int/healthinfo/morttables/en/index.html [accessed June 2010].

ANNEX 5A

To measure education, the Eurobarometer survey asks respondents at what age they finished school. The responses are coded as (0) still studying, (1) no education and age 13 and under, (2) age 14, (3) age 15, (4) age 16, (5) age 17, (6) age 18, (7) age 19, (8) ages 20-21, (9) ages 22-24, and (10) ages 25 and older. Another variable that equals 0 for those still studying and 1 for all others complements the education variable. Controlling for both variables shows the effect of completed education independent of those still studying.[9] This measure of age of finishing school aims to avoid problems of comparability across diverse education systems that affect measures of formal degrees. However, the age measure may overstate the attainment of those finishing at a later age because of slowness and problems in school rather than advanced degrees.

The measure of occupation uses the EB classification of current or last job in the following categories: (0) no job; (1) farmer or fisherman; (2) unskilled manual, servant; (3) skilled manual; (4) service—hospital, restaurant, police; (5) supervisor; (6) shop owner, craftsman, self-employed; (7) traveling—salesman, driver; (8) work mainly at a desk; (9) middle management—department head, junior manager, teacher, technician; (10) business proprietor, partner or full owner of a company; (11) general management, director, top management; and (12) professional—lawyer, doctor, accountant, architect. The measure treats the categories as a continuous scale, and, given the diverse mix of occupations in some of the categories, the ranking has some arbitrariness. However, the measure relates closely to smoking, and rearranging categories (4 and 7, for example) does little to change the results. Much as for education, a second occupational variable that equals 1 for those with a current or former job and 0 for those never having done any paid work complements the occupation measure.

To measure economic standing, the surveys ask about ownership of goods rather than income. A scale based on the proportion of the following goods owned by the respondent has an alpha reliability of .764: household phone, mobile phone, television, DVD player, music CD player, computer, Internet connection, car, and paying for an apartment or house. Given reporting errors common in usual income measures, goods-based measures do better to predict smoking (Schaap et al., 2008).

Other control variables include age or years since birth treated as a quadratic term to reflect the increase and decrease in smoking prevalence

---

[9]Let D equal the dummy variable for completed education and E equal the age of completing education as a centered variable with a mean of zero. The equation $Y = a + b1*D + b2*E*D$ reduces to $Y = a$ for those still studying. Then b1 represents the average (i.e., when E equals its mean of zero) difference in Y between those still studying and those with completed education, and b2 represents the effect of schooling for those with completed education.

over the life course. Dummy variables code women as 1, and code married, remarried, or currently living with a partner as 1. A measure of residence codes rural area or village as 1, small or middle-sized town as 2, and large town as 3.

6

Can Obesity Account for Cross-National Differences in Life-Expectancy Trends?

Dawn E. Alley, Jennifer Lloyd, and Michelle Shardell

The prevalence of obesity has increased dramatically in the United States since the 1970s across all sex, race, and socioeconomic groups (Flegal et al., 1998, 2002). Because obesity is associated with a variety of chronic conditions, disability, and mortality, this trend raises important concerns about the current and future health of the U.S. population. The purpose of this review is to examine the implications of trends in obesity for trends in life expectancy, in order to determine whether obesity might account for cross-national differences in life-expectancy trends.

Available evidence suggests that this is unlikely, for at least two reasons: (1) the epidemic of obesity is not confined to the United States. Although the prevalence of obesity in U.S. adults is the highest of any country included in this report, other countries are also experiencing rising obesity rates. (2) The association between obesity and mortality is relatively weak, particularly at older ages. The best available estimates of the effect of obesity on life expectancy suggest that it may be a small contributor to differences in life-expectancy trends, but it is not likely to fully account for them.

However, obesity's importance as a determinant of life expectancy is likely to grow with the aging of younger cohorts, and obesity is importantly related to other indicators of population health and quality of life, including disease, disability, and health care costs. Several trends suggest that the effect of obesity on life expectancy will increase in the future, including (1) an increase in abdominal adiposity, reflected by higher waist circumference at a given body mass index (BMI); (2) an increased prevalence of obesity at all ages, particularly younger ages, in which the association between obesity and mortality is stronger; (3) the increasing severity of obesity; and (4) the increasing duration of obesity.

In an effort to be responsive to the question at hand (i.e., Can obesity account for cross-national differences in life-expectancy trends at age 50?), the following review focuses on BMI in older cohorts. First, we examine international trends in obesity and life expectancy. Second, we review the association between obesity and mortality, prioritizing estimates that are generalizable to the U.S. population. Third, we provide estimates of the effect of obesity on life expectancy in the United States. Fourth, we discuss limitations in the use of BMI to predict mortality and the implications of these limitations for cross-national comparisons. Finally, we discuss implications of rising obesity rates for future trends in life expectancy and other population health indicators. Throughout the review, we rely on published results and our own analysis of the National Health and Nutrition Examination Survey (NHANES), a nationally representative repeated cross-sectional survey of U.S. adults that includes both a questionnaire and a physical exam, including height and weight measurement (National Center for Health Statistics, 2009).

INTERNATIONAL TRENDS IN OBESITY AND LIFE EXPECTANCY

The World Health Organization (WHO) defines obesity as a BMI (dividing weight in kg over squared height in meters) of $30 kg/m^2$ or more. Figure 6-1 presents obesity prevalence estimates for adults in 10 countries over time.[1] Among adult men, the United States has the highest obesity prevalence at all observed time points. In approximately 1978 (data collected 1976-1980), the prevalence of obesity among men in the United States was 13 percent. Around the same time, the prevalence varied from a low of 0.8 percent in Japan to a high of 12 percent in Canada. By 2003, the prevalence of obesity among American men had more than doubled, to 32 percent. The most recent estimates from other countries show that 23 percent of British and Canadian men are obese, followed by 19 percent of Australian men, 12 percent of Danish, French, and Spanish men, and 10 percent of Dutch men. Only men in Italy and Japan have an obesity prevalence below 10 percent.

Overall patterns are similar among adult women. Around 1978, the prevalence of obesity among women in the United States was already 17 percent, and it rose to 35 percent in 2003. The prevalence of obesity

---

[1] Age ranges vary. The majority of data sources were designed to be nationally representative (with the exception of data before 1999 in Australia and all data from the Netherlands, which were collected in major cities only). Where surveys spanned multiple years, prevalence estimates are shown based on the midpoint of survey collection.

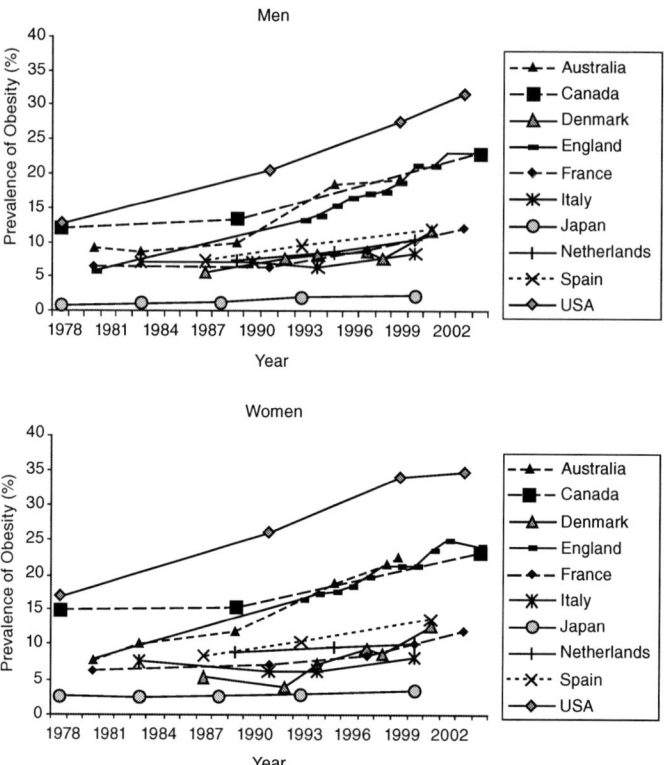

FIGURE 6-1 Trends in adult obesity prevalence by country and sex, 1978-2004.
SOURCES: Data are nationally representative unless otherwise noted. Australia: measured height and weight, ages 25-64 (1980-1989), ages 18+ (1995), ages 25+ (1999-2000), data before 1999 are from urban areas only (Australian Institute of Health and Welfare, 2009); Canada: measured height and weight, ages 20-64 (1978-1989) (Torrance, Hooper, and Reeder, 2002), ages 18+ (2004) (Tjepkema, 2005); Denmark: self-reported height and weight, ages 16+ (Bendixen et al., 2004); England: measured height and weight, ages 16+ (Department of Health, 2009; Rennie and Jebb, 2005); France: self-reported height and weight, ages 20+ (1980-1991) (Maillard et al., 1999), ages 18+ (1997-2003) (Charles, Eschwege, and Basdevant, 2008); Italy: self-reported height and weight, ages 15+ (1983-1994) (Pagano et al., 1997), ages 18+ (1999) (Calza, Decarli, and Ferraroni, 2008); Japan: measured height and weight, ages 20+ (Yoshiike, Kaneda, and Takimoto, 2002; Yoshiike et al., 2002); Netherlands: measured height and weight, ages 20-59, from three cities (International Association for the Study of Obesity, 2009; Seidell, Verschuren, and Kromhout, 1995; Visscher, Kromhout, and Seidell, 2002); Spain: self-reported height and weight, ages 21+ (1987, 1993), ages 17+ (2001) (Martínez, Moreno, and Martínez-González, 2004); United States: measured height and weight, ages 20-74 (1978, 1991, 1999) (Flegal et al., 2002), author analysis of NHANES data, ages 20-74 (2003).

in women is now between 20 and 25 percent in Australia, Canada, and England. Again, only Italy and Japan currently have an obesity prevalence below 10 percent.

Figure 6-2 presents obesity trends among older adults. In 1978, the prevalence of obesity was similar among older men and women in Canada and the United States, with the prevalence of obesity around 13-14 percent in men and 23-24 percent in women. Today, more than 25 percent of older men and 30 percent of older women are obese in Australia, England, and the United States, although the United States now has the highest rate of obesity in both men (35 percent) and women (38 percent) in this age group. Table 6-1 provides recent data from the Survey of Health, Ageing, and Retirement in Europe and the Health and Retirement Study to provide a snapshot of the obesity prevalence measured comparably (based on corrected estimates of self-reported height and weight) in the population ages 50+ in several countries (Michaud, van Soest, and Andreyeva, 2007). The prevalence of obesity among older adults is highest in the United States, followed by older adults in Spain.

Several patterns emerge in this examination of obesity trends across countries. First, the increase in the prevalence of obesity is not confined to the United States, but instead was observed across all 10 countries examined. Nonetheless, obesity levels and trends vary greatly by country. There appears to be a cluster of Anglo-Saxon countries (Australia, Canada, England, and the United States) that have experienced both higher levels and a more rapid rise in the prevalence of obesity. It is notable that the prevalence of obesity in the United States in the late 1970s was already higher than the prevalence in most other countries today. In addition, differences between the United States and other countries are larger when comparing obesity prevalence among adults of all ages than when comparing obesity prevalence among older adults. This suggests that cross-national differences in obesity prevalence are even larger at younger ages, which may be important in determining morbidity and mortality burden in the future.

Figure 6-3 summarizes trends in obesity along with trends in life expectancy at age 50 (see Glei, Meslé, and Vallin, Chapter 2, in this volume). Because of the limited amount of published obesity data on the population over age 50, the slope of the obesity trend was calculated using adult obesity prevalence. The first and last estimates of adult obesity prevalence available for each country between 1978 and 2004 were used to estimate annual change in obesity prevalence.

Among the 10 countries included here, the United States ranked eighth in life expectancy at age 50 for men (28.9 years) in 2004. The United States had the highest prevalence of adult obesity (31.7 percent) and the most rapid rate of obesity change (0.76 percent per year). Men in Australia had the highest life expectancy at age 50 in 2004 (31.0 years), followed by Japan

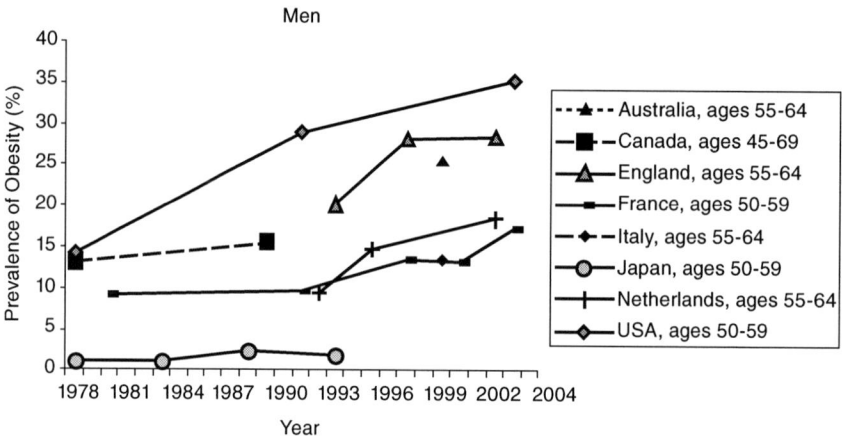

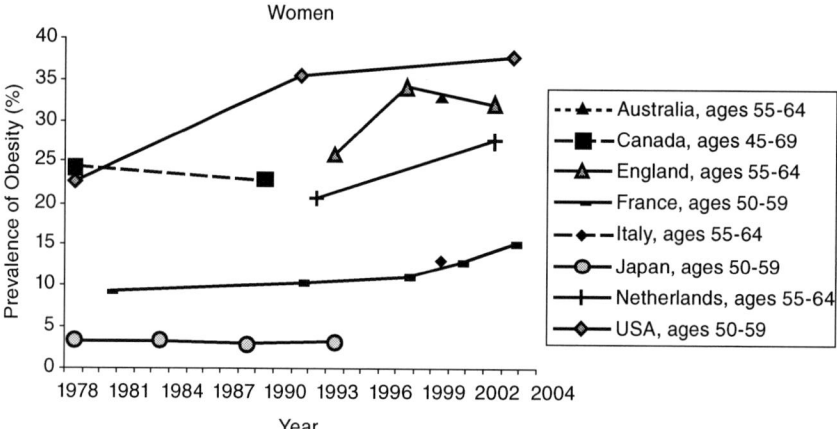

FIGURE 6-2 Trends in obesity prevalence by country and sex: Older adults, 1978-2004.
SOURCES: Data are nationally representative unless otherwise noted. Australia: measured height and weight (Cameron et al., 2003); Canada: self-reported height and weight (Torrance, Hooper, and Reeder, 2002); England: measured height and weight (Rennie and Jebb, 2005); France: self-reported height and weight (Charles, Eschwege, and Basdevant, 2008; Maillard et al., 1999); Italy: self-reported height and weight (Calza et al., 2008); Japan: measured height and weight (Yoshiike, Seino et al., 2002); Netherlands: measured height and weight, from three cities (Schokker et al., 2007); United States: measured height and weight (Flegal et al., 2002) and author analysis of NHANES data.

TABLE 6-1 Prevalence of Obesity Among Adults Ages 50+, by Country and Sex, 2004

	Males (%)	Females (%)
Denmark	17.5	18.2
France	16.2	20.3
Italy	15.6	23.4
Netherlands	15.3	23.2
Spain	20.8	33.6
United States	29.6	36.0

SOURCE: Data from Michaud et al. (2007).

(30.7 years), Italy (30.2 years), and Canada (30.1 years). Among men, there was little correlation between change in obesity prevalence and change in life expectancy after age 50 (r = 0.126). Countries with the longest life expectancy included the two countries with the lowest obesity prevalence (Italy and Japan), as well as two countries with high obesity rates and large increases in obesity (Australia and Canada). Australia and England both experienced increases in life expectancy of more than 5 years across this period at the same time that obesity prevalence increased at a rate of more than 0.5 percent per year.

Among women, there was some evidence of a negative association between change in adult obesity prevalence and changes in life expectancy at age 50 (r = –0.421). Life expectancy at age 50 in 2004 was highest for women in Japan (36.9 years), followed by France (35.5 years), Italy (35.0 years), and Australia and Spain (34.9 years). The United States ranked ninth (32.6 years). While women in the United States had the highest prevalence of adult obesity, Australia had the most rapid increase in obesity (0.76 percent per year). The rate of increase in obesity prevalence exceeded 0.5 percent per year in Australia, Canada, Denmark, England, and the United States. The Netherlands appears to be an outlier, with relatively low increases in both obesity and life expectancy. If we were to exclude the Netherlands from this analysis, the correlation between change in obesity prevalence and change in life expectancy would have been greater.

These comparisons suggest that the correlation between obesity and life expectancy is stronger in women than in men. While prior analysis suggests that associations between obesity and mortality are similar in men and women or that the association is stronger in men (Fontaine et al., 2003; Stevens et al., 1999), this finding is consistent with women's higher prevalence of obesity and recent evidence that women account for more than two-thirds of years of life lost to obesity in the United States (Finkelstein et al., 2010).

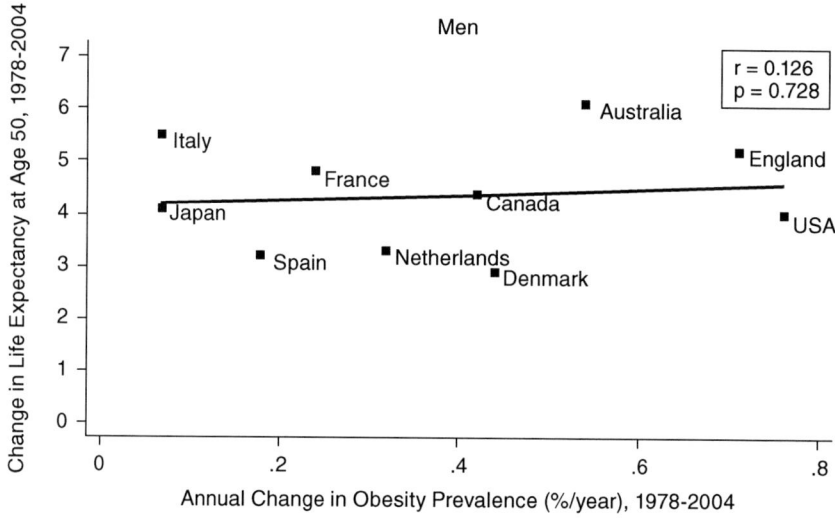

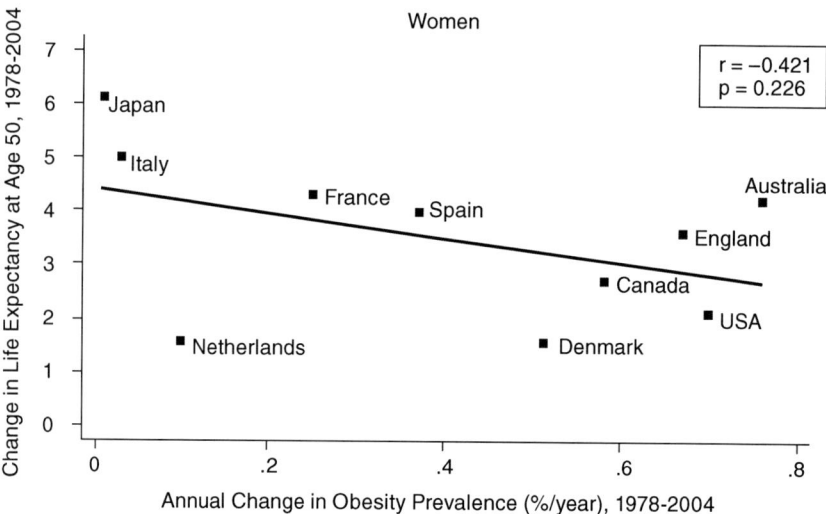

FIGURE 6-3 Trends in life expectancy at age 50 and adult obesity prevalence by country and sex.
SOURCE: Figure 6-1 and Glei, Meslé, and Vallin, Chapter 2, in this volume.

It is difficult to draw substantive conclusions from these ecological comparisons, which cannot determine whether obesity accounts for trends in life expectancy across countries. For example, life expectancy in Australia might have increased even more if the prevalence of obesity had not also been increasing. Many other factors have changed over time in the countries assessed here, and these changes may obscure differences in life expectancy due to obesity. An additional limitation of these comparisons is that they examine contemporaneous changes in obesity and life expectancy. If there is a long latency period between development of obesity and increased mortality risk, we might observe a substantial time lag between increases in the prevalence of obesity and changes in life expectancy.

Nonetheless, these comparisons provide a context for considering the role of obesity in international life expectancy trends. If obesity is slowing life expectancy gains in the United States, it is likely that it is also affecting life expectancy trends in other countries, particularly countries like Australia, Canada, and England, which have also experienced rapid increases in obesity prevalence. Among men, there was little evidence of an association between changes in adult obesity prevalence and changes in life expectancy at age 50, although we did find some evidence of an association among women. This is particularly important, because gains in life expectancy of American women have not kept pace with those of women in most European countries.

ASSOCIATION BETWEEN OBESITY AND MORTALITY

Obesity may affect mortality risk both directly and indirectly. Fat can be thought of as an endocrine organ, secreting hormones and inflammatory proteins that are important risk factors for diabetes and cardiovascular disease (Snijder et al., 2006; Trayhurn and Beattie, 2001). Obesity is also a mediator through which physical activity and diet affect health. Obesity is clearly associated with risk factors for mortality, including high blood pressure, high cholesterol, and diabetes (Must et al., 1999; Prospective Studies Collaboration, 2009). Nonetheless, the association between BMI and mortality remains a topic of significant controversy, in part because it varies greatly by age, race, and cause of death and is confounded by smoking history.

The following review of this association relies on published reports of population-based data from the United States (except where noted). Depending on the population or population subgroup examined, the association between BMI and mortality has been characterized as linear and positive (Ajani et al., 2004; Baik et al., 2000; Gelber et al., 2007), U-shaped (Ajani et al., 2004; Allison et al., 1997; Gelber et al., 2007; Matkin Dolan et al., 2007), J-shaped (Freedman et al., 2006; Manson et al., 1995), nonexistent (Baik et al., 2000; Diehr et al., 1998), or negative (Diehr et al., 1998; Grabowski and Ellis, 2001). Despite this variability, several conclusions can be drawn from the existing literature.

First, at the population level, obesity is associated with a modest increase in all-cause mortality relative to normal weight, and the association between obesity and mortality increases with obesity severity. Results from a recent meta-analysis based on data from 26 studies, including both sexes, several racial and ethnic groups and multiple countries are shown in Figure 6-4 (McGee and Diverse Populations Collaboration, 2005). Among men, obesity was associated with a 20 percent increase in all-cause mortality risk (RR = 1.201, 95% CI: 1.119-1.289) and a 51 percent increased risk of mortality from coronary heart disease (RR = 1.508, 95% CI: 1.362-1.67), but was not significantly associated with cancer mortality (RR = 1.055, 95% CI: 0.978-1.138). Among women, obesity was associated with approximately a 28 percent increased risk of all-cause mortality (RR = 1.275, 95% percent CI:1.183-1.373), a 62 percent increased risk of mortality from coronary heart disease (RR = 1.624, 95% CI: 1.459-1.806), and a 10 percent increased risk of cancer mortality (RR = 1.103, 95% CI: 1.001-1.215).

These associations increase with obesity severity. An analysis of international data from 894,576 participants ages 35 and older found that each 5kg/m^2 increase in BMI is associated with approximately 30 percent higher overall mortality (Prospective Studies Collaboration, 2009). In one large cohort study of adults ages 50-71 at baseline, the excess mortality risk associated with obesity (relative to a BMI of 23.5-24.9) increased from 10 percent (RR = 1.10, 95% CI: 1.06-1.14) among men with Class I obesity (BMI of 30.0-34.9kg/m^2), to 35 percent (RR = 1.35, 95% CI: 1.28-1.42) among those with Class II obesity (BMI: 35.0-39.9), to 83 percent (RR = 1.83, 95% CI: 1.70-1.97) among men with Class III obesity (BMI ≥ 40.0) (Adams et al., 2006). Results were similar among women, with an excess mortality risk ranging from 18 percent (RR = 1.18, 95% CI: 1.12-1.25) among those with Class I obesity to 94 percent (RR = 1.94. 95% CI: 1.79-2.09) among those with Class III obesity.

Although the majority of research on the relationship between BMI and mortality has utilized the WHO cut points to define risk groups, another way to characterize this relationship is to examine the continuous association. In one analysis of a nationally representative cohort study (the NHANES I Epidemiologic Follow-up Study), the BMI associated with minimum mortality ranged from 24.3-27.1 for different race-gender groups (Durazo-Arvizu et al., 1998). The authors determined the range of BMI values over which all-cause mortality risk would increase no more than 20 percent relative to the minimum; this interval was nine BMI units wide and included 70 percent of the U.S. population ages 25-74. Similarly, in an analysis of the association between BMI and mortality using National Health Interview Survey data for adults ages 18-64, there was no difference in mortality observed for participants with BMIs between 20 and 35, which included 85.9 percent of the population (Gronniger, 2006). Taken together, these results suggest that associations between BMI and mortality are small in most adults, increasing rapidly for those with extreme BMI values.

Second, the association between BMI and mortality changes with age. The closest associations between obesity and mortality have been observed

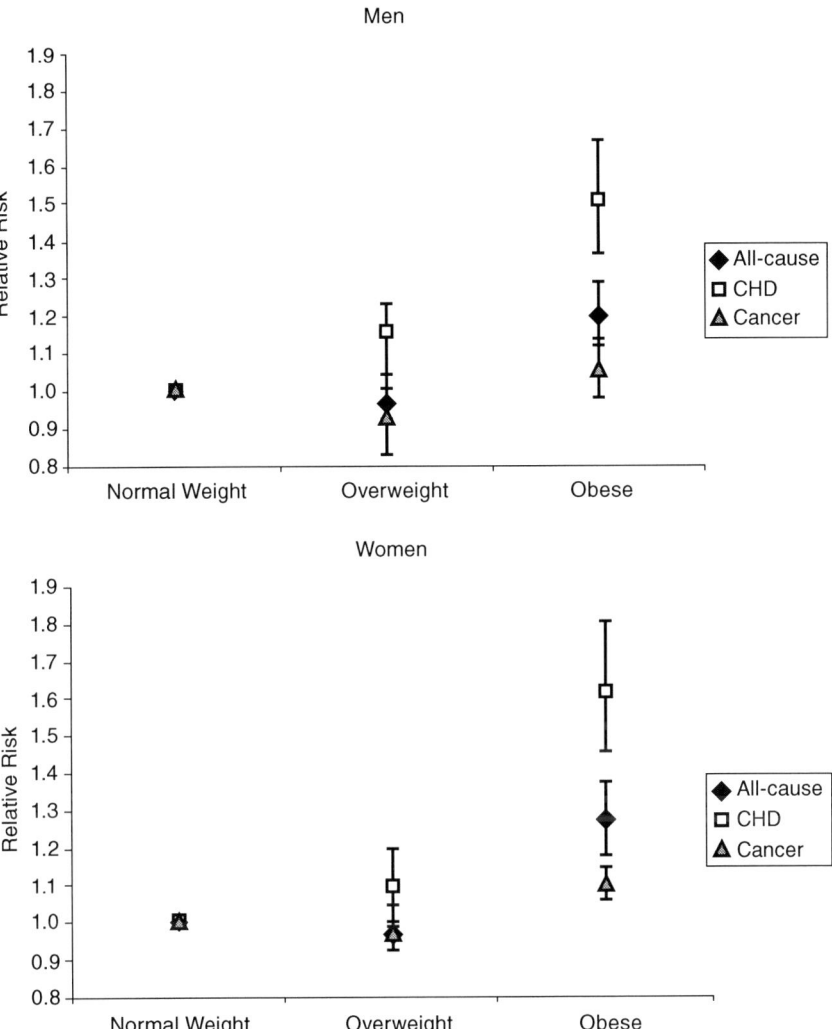

FIGURE 6-4 Association between BMI group and mortality in adults by sex and cause of death.
SOURCE: McGee and Diverse Populations Collaboration (2005); CHD = coronary heart disease; normal weight = body mass index (BMI) 18.5-24.9kg/m^2; overweight = BMI 25.0-29.9kg/m^2; obese = BMI ≥ 30kg/m^2.

for adults under age 50 (Bender et al., 1999; Stevens et al., 1998; Thorpe and Ferraro, 2004). As age increases, the greatest risk of mortality is associated with the most extreme ends of the BMI spectrum: the lowest (underweight) and highest BMI categories (Class II and Class III obesity). Recent reviews of the association between BMI and mortality risk in the elderly have found that obesity is associated with a 10 percent increase in mortality risk (RR = 1.10, 95% CI: 1.06-1.13) (Janssen and Mark, 2007) and that "the overall trends for the relation between BMI and mortality in older adults can be represented as a U-shaped curve, with a large flat bottom and a right curve that starts to rise for BMIs of more than 31 to 32" (Heiat, Vaccarino, and Krumholz, 2001).

Third, smoking confounds the relationship between BMI and mortality. Smoking is associated with both lower weight and higher mortality. Thus, smoking modifies the effect of BMI on mortality, so that obesity appears less harmful among current and former smokers. Excluding ever-smokers from analysis of the BMI-mortality relationship reduces the risk associated with underweight and suggests a stronger, more linear association between BMI and mortality (Adams et al., 2006; Ajani et al., 2004; Calle et al., 1999; Freedman et al., 2006; Manson et al., 1995).

In summary, the association between BMI and mortality is moderate at the population level but stronger in some subgroups, including persons with Class II or III obesity and never-smokers. The following section explores the potential effects of BMI on trends in life expectancy.

OBESITY AND LIFE EXPECTANCY

In order to move from a discussion of mortality risks at an individual level to a discussion of life expectancy at the population level, we must examine the size of the population at increased risk for poor outcomes. Figure 6-5 provides trends in the prevalence of Class II and Class III obesity by sex in the United States. Among men ages 50-59 and 60-69, the prevalence of Class II obesity reached a high of nearly 10 percent in 2003-2006, an increase of 5-6 percent from 1988-1994 and 7-8 percent from 1976-1980. The prevalence of Class III obesity has also increased markedly in men but remains fairly rare, affecting fewer than 5 percent of men ages 50 and older. Among women ages 50-59 and 60-69, the prevalence of Class II obesity reached a high of nearly 11 percent in 2003-2006, an increase of approximately 5 percent since 1976-1980. The prevalence of Class III obesity increased dramatically in women of all age groups, particularly women under age 70, in whom the prevalence of Class III obesity was 3-4 times higher in 2003-2006 than in 1976-1980.

Fontaine and colleagues (2003) estimated the years of life lost (YLL) for different BMI levels, relative to a BMI of 24, using NHANES data (see Figure 6-6). As discussed above, the effect of obesity on mortality, and in this case life expectancy, decreases with age. Among white men, Class I obesity was associated with an average of 0-1 years of life lost, Class II obesity was associated with 1-3 years of life lost, and Class III obesity was associated with 1-7 years of life lost, depending on age. These associations were similar

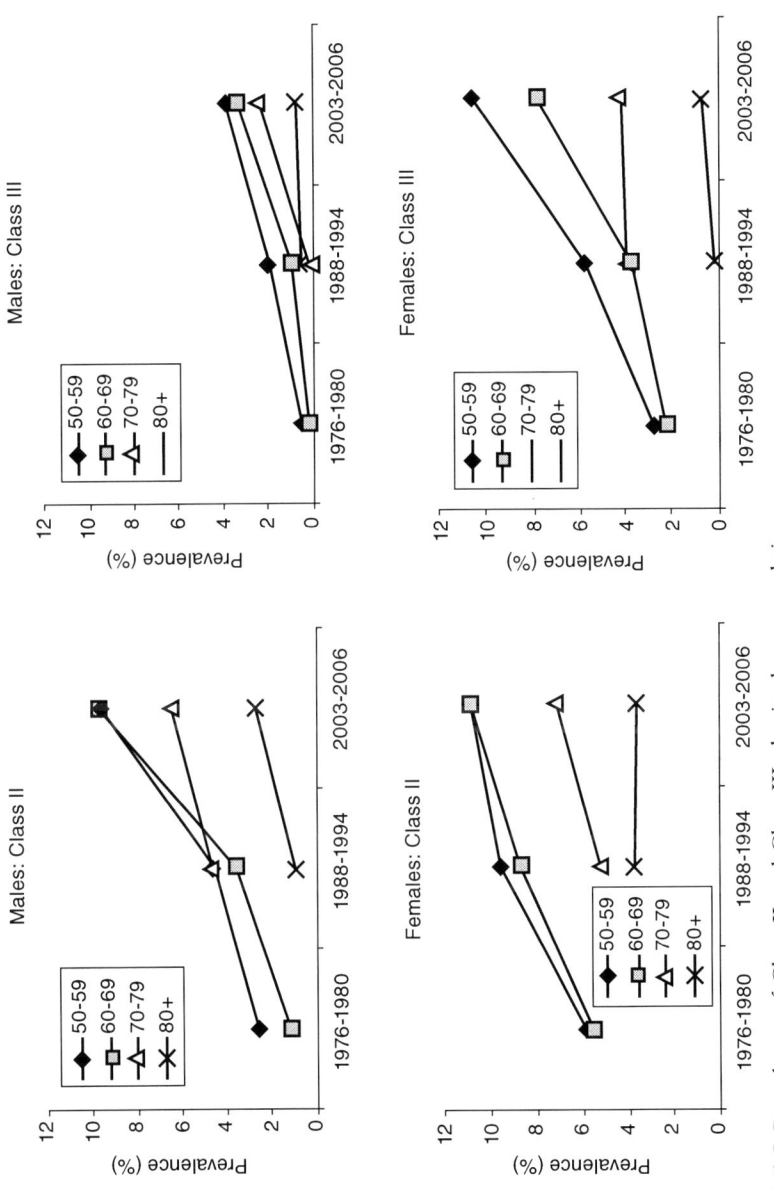

FIGURE 6-5 Prevalence of Class II and Class III obesity by age and time.
SOURCES: Flegal et al. (1998) and author analysis of NHANES data. Class II obesity: BMI = 35.0–39.9kg/m^2; Class III obesity: BMI ≥ 40.0kg/m^2.

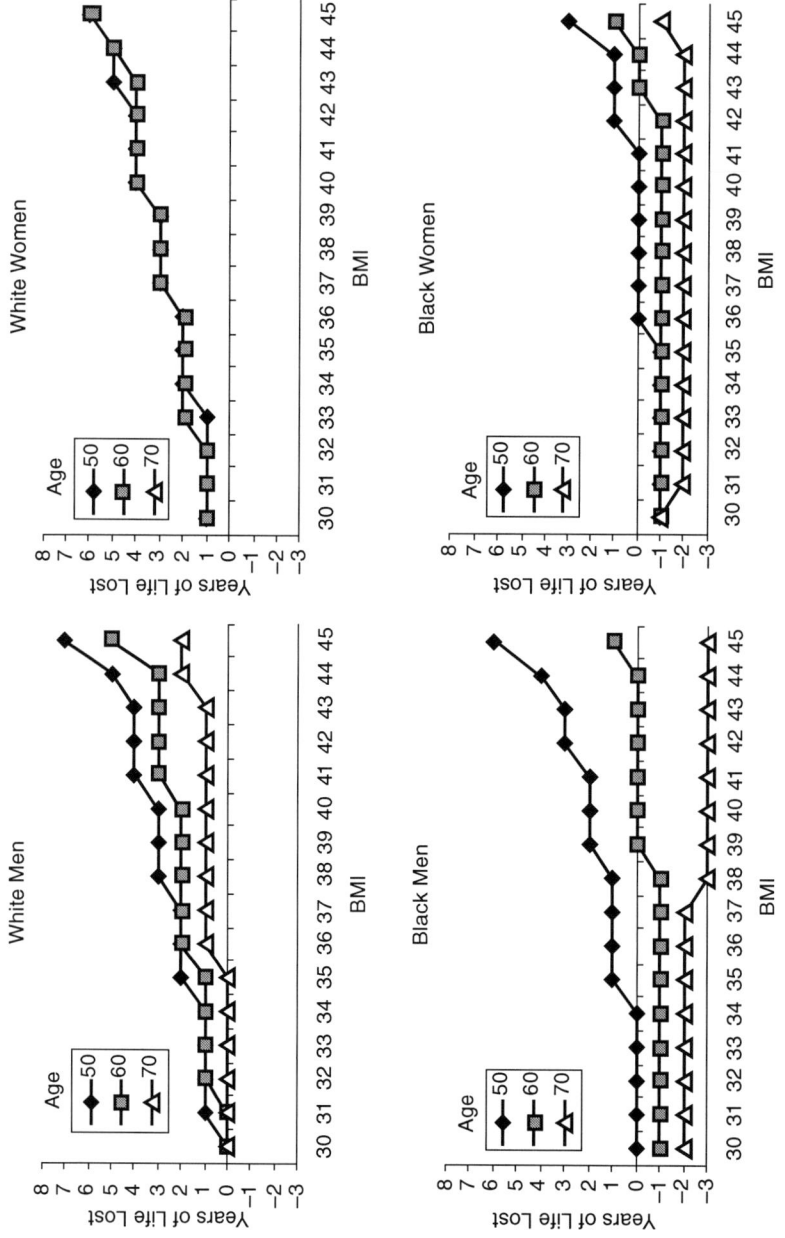

FIGURE 6-6 Years of life lost relative to life expectancy for a BMI of 24, by age, race, and sex.
SOURCE: Fontaine et al. (2003).

in white women (although estimates for women ages 70 and older were not available, because life expectancy for this group exceeded age 85). However, associations differed markedly by race. The negative effects of obesity on life expectancy among black men and women were observed only at younger ages and among those with very high BMIs.

Olshansky and colleagues (2005) estimated the effect of obesity on total life expectancy by estimating the potential gain in life expectancy at birth in 2000 if obesity were eliminated completely among U.S. adults ages 20-85. They found that, without obesity, life expectancy in the United States would be higher by 0.33-0.93 years for white men, 0.30-0.81 years for white women, 0.30-1.08 years for black men, and 0.21-0.73 years for black women. These estimates demonstrate that obesity is clearly a large and important contributor to life expectancy, but they represent an upper bound related to the specific questions in this chapter for two reasons. First, these estimates were based on mortality for ages 20-85. Because the association between obesity and mortality is roughly twice as large from ages 20-49 as it is for ages 50 and above (decreasing even further for those above 65) (Thorpe and Ferraro, 2004), much of this effect was probably due to deaths before age 50. Second, these estimates were based on eliminating obesity entirely in the U.S. population. Effects would be smaller if obesity were simply reduced to the prevalence already present in the U.S. population in the 1970s or to the prevalence observed in other countries today.

In order to estimate the effect of increasing obesity prevalence on trends in life expectancy at age 50 in the United States, we applied Fontaine and colleagues' estimates (Fontaine et al., 2003) of YLL at age 50 to the BMI distribution from NHANES II (1976-1980) and NHANES 2001-2004 (see Annex for details). Results showing the estimated effect of obesity on life expectancy at age 50 are included in Table 6-2. Results are provided for whites only, because estimates for blacks were unstable.

The BMI distribution for white men at age 50 in 1976-1980 is projected to result in a reduction in life expectancy of 0.19 years in this group relative to life expectancy if all obese individuals had a BMI of 24. Because of increases in the prevalence of obesity, the effect of obesity on life expectancy is expected to increase to 0.43 years among men age 50 in 2001-2004. However, as discussed in more detail below, little is known about the lag time necessary for obesity to affect mortality risk, so it is unclear how long it will take to observe these changes at the population level. Nonetheless, these results suggest that obesity growth during this period will slow improvements in life expectancy across these cohorts of white men by approximately 0.24 years. Obesity for white women age 50 in 1976-1980 is projected to result in a reduction of 0.33 years for this group, and this effect is expected to increase to 0.73 years among women age 50 in 2001-2004. Thus, increases

TABLE 6-2 Projected Population-Level Reductions in Life Expectancy at Age 50 (years) due to Obesity, by Age and Sex, 1976-1980 and 2001-2004

	1976-1980 (A)	2001-2004 (B)	Difference (B − A)
White men	0.19	0.43	0.24
White women	0.33	0.73	0.40

NOTE: Relative to a BMI of 24. See Annex for more information.

in obesity prevalence during this period are likely to reduce life-expectancy improvements in white women at age 50 by approximately 0.40 years.

These results are extremely sensitive to the choice of YLL estimates used to generate them. We chose Fontaine and colleagues' estimates for three reasons: (1) estimates are based on measured height and weight, (2) the population used to generate estimates was a representative sample of U.S. adults, and (3) sufficient detail was provided in online appendices to the publication to allow us to generate estimates. Because of a lack of complete data on age- and sex-specific BMI trends in other countries, as well as country-specific estimates of YLL due to excess BMI, we focus this analysis on the association between obesity and life expectancy in the United States. However, it is notable that Fontaine and colleagues' estimates are lower than those from a recent large-scale collaborative analysis of 57 prospective studies. The Prospective Studies Collaboration (2009) found that life expectancy at age 35 was reduced by 2-4 years among participants who reached a BMI of 30-35 by midlife and by 8-10 years among participants who reached a BMI of 40-45 by midlife, compared with Fontaine and colleagues' estimates of a loss of approximately 1 year of life in whites with a BMI of 30-35 and 3-7 years in whites with a BMI of 40-45. More generally, estimates of YLL have varied widely across studies (for an excellent review and comparison, see Finkelstein et al., 2010). Estimates of projected reductions in life expectancy due to obesity are directly proportional to the estimate of YLL used to generate them, allowing the reader to calculate alternative scenarios. For example, if all sex- and BMI-specific YLLs were uniformly twice as high as those estimated by Fontaine and colleagues, the projected reduction in life expectancy would be twice as high.

These data suggest that increasing obesity prevalence is likely to slow life-expectancy growth in the United States. However, it is unknown to what extent these changes have already begun to manifest themselves in the countries examined in this chapter. As noted above, all of the comparison countries included in this report also experienced significant increases in obesity during this time period. It is unlikely that the small increases in obesity occurring before 1980 explain current life-expectancy trends in the

United States or differences between trends in the United States and other countries. Between 1980 and 2004, life expectancy at age 50 in U.S. men grew by 4.0 years, while it grew by 6.1 years in Australia. In that same period, life expectancy at age 50 in U.S. women grew by 2.1 years, while it grew by 6.1 years in Japan. Based on available estimates, obesity may be a contributor to these trends, but it is unlikely to explain them. Nonetheless, the large increase in obesity prevalence in the United States since the late 1970s is likely to have important implications for life expectancy in the coming decades.

LIMITATIONS IN MEASUREMENT OF EFFECTS OF OBESITY ON MORTALITY

The purpose of this review is to summarize literature on obesity and mortality in order to determine whether obesity might account for cross-national differences in life-expectancy trends. We have attempted to address this question using the extensive published literature on the association between BMI and mortality. However, three important limitations of existing research may affect our conclusions: (1) confounding due to chronic disease, (2) lack of data on body composition, and (3) limited understanding of the natural history of obesity's effect on mortality.

First, we are likely to underestimate the effect of BMI on mortality at older ages due to chronic disease. Although obesity is associated with increased incidence of chronic diseases, including diabetes and cardiovascular disease, many of these chronic conditions are also associated with both involuntary weight loss and increased mortality. Thus, BMI appears to have an attenuated or negative association with mortality among those with existing illness. In this group, mortality risk is particularly high at low BMIs and generally flat at higher BMIs. For example, in a review of the association between BMI and mortality among patients with coronary artery disease, patients with a low BMI had the highest total mortality risk (RR = 1.37, 95% CI: 1.32-1.43), overweight patients had the lowest risk (RR = 0.87, 95% CI: 0.81-0.94), and risk among obese patients was not significantly different from normal weight patients (RR = 0.93, 95% CI: 0.85-1.03 for Class I, RR = 1.10, 95% CI: 0.87-1.41 for Class II/III) (Romero-Corral et al., 2006).

A variety of approaches have been used to attempt to generate estimates of the effect of obesity on mortality unconfounded by chronic disease. One common approach is to exclude deaths occurring within 5 years of weight measurement. However, exclusion of early deaths does not substantially change estimated associations between BMI and mortality (Allison et al., 1999). Another approach is to restrict analyses to healthy individuals, excluding persons with preexisting chronic diseases. This approach results in a stronger, more linear association between BMI and mortality, but it potentially excludes the majority of older persons (Adams et al., 2006; Calle et al., 1999). A final approach is to use a measure of BMI obtained earlier in life, before disease-related weight loss is likely to have begun. Available literature demonstrates that midlife BMI is more closely associated than current BMI with mortality in old age. For example, Figure 6-7 provides estimates of the adjusted relative risk of mortality by BMI group based on current BMI and recalled BMI at age 50 (Adams et al., 2006). For both men and women, using BMI at age 50 reduces the relative risk associated with underweight relative to using current BMI. In addition, when BMI groups are based on BMI at age 50, every BMI category above 26.5 was associated with significant increases in mortality risk. Thus, using an indicator of weight earlier in life may help avoid confounding in the association between BMI and mortality due to unintentional weight loss associated with chronic conditions.

Second, BMI has important limitations as a measure of adiposity (fatness), especially in older persons. BMI is a widely used measure because it provides an indicator of weight uncorrelated with height that is easy to measure and associated with health outcomes. However, BMI does not distinguish between muscle and fat and provides no information about the distribution of body fat, which may be important. Visceral fat, or intra-abdominal fat in the organ cavity, appears to be particularly harmful to health (Bergman et al., 2006; Snijder et al., 2006). Body composition measurement is difficult to implement in population-based surveys, because commonly used methods including computed tomography (CT) and dual energy x-ray absorptiometry (DXA) require equipment that is not transportable in the field. However, simple measures of anthropometry can provide useful indicators of body composition and fat distribution. In particular, waist circumference, an indicator of abdominal adiposity, may provide a useful indicator of mortality risk (Baik et al., 2000; Koster et al., 2008; Visscher et al., 2001).

Issues of body composition may be particularly important in cross-national comparisons. If Americans at a given BMI have a higher body fat or higher waist circumference relative to other populations, then comparisons based on BMI would underestimate the effect of obesity trends on cross-national differences in life expectancy. However, data on cross-national differences in body composition are limited (see Figure 6-8). As we would expect given higher BMIs in the United States, American adults have a higher waist circumference relative to European adults, especially in women. More importantly, waist circumference has been increasing in the United States even more than would be expected given concurrent BMI trends (Elobeid et al., 2007). This suggests that the obesity epidemic is resulting not only in changes in body size, but also in changes in body fat distribution, a trend that has also been identified in the Netherlands (Visscher and Seidell, 2004).

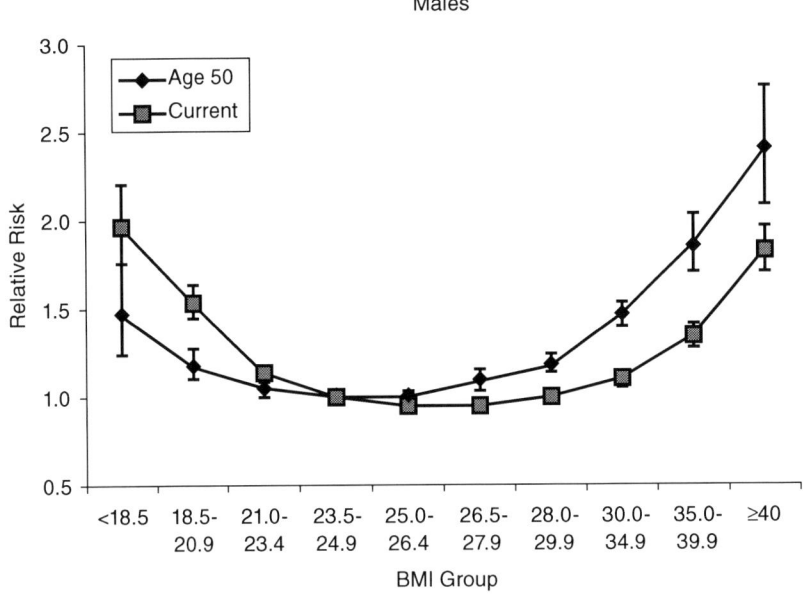

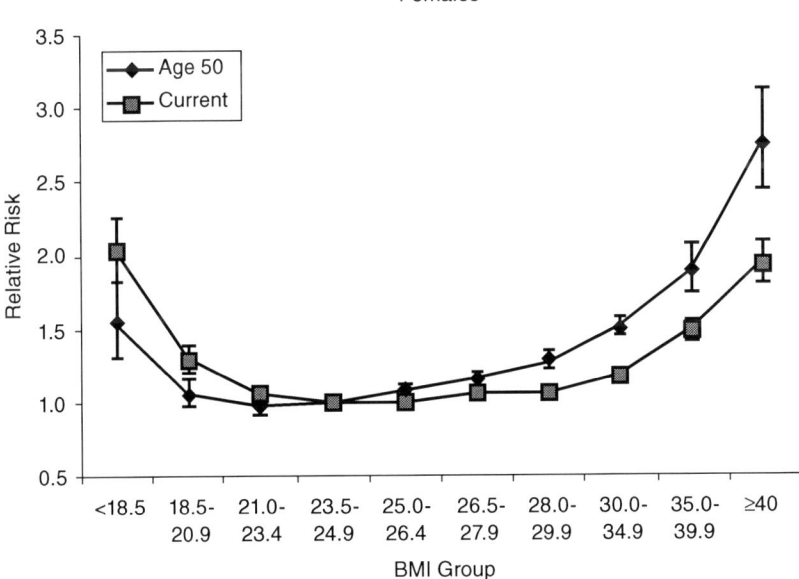

FIGURE 6-7 Association between BMI and mortality by sex, based on current BMI (ages 50-71) and BMI at age 50.
SOURCE: Adams et al. (2006).

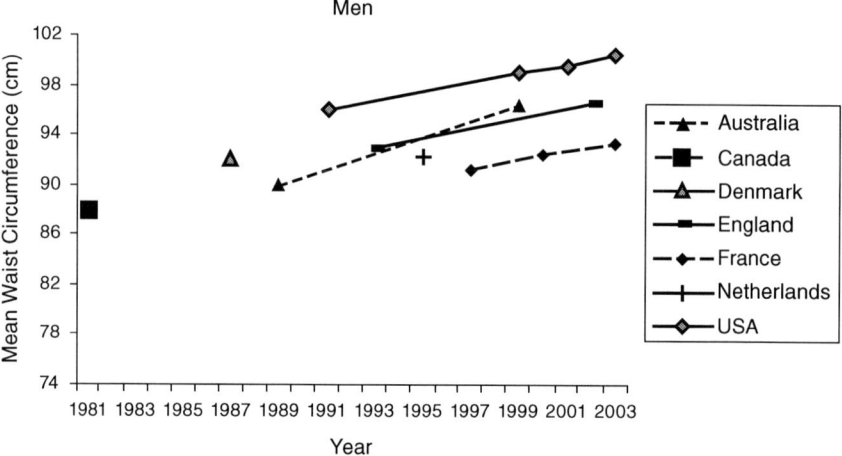

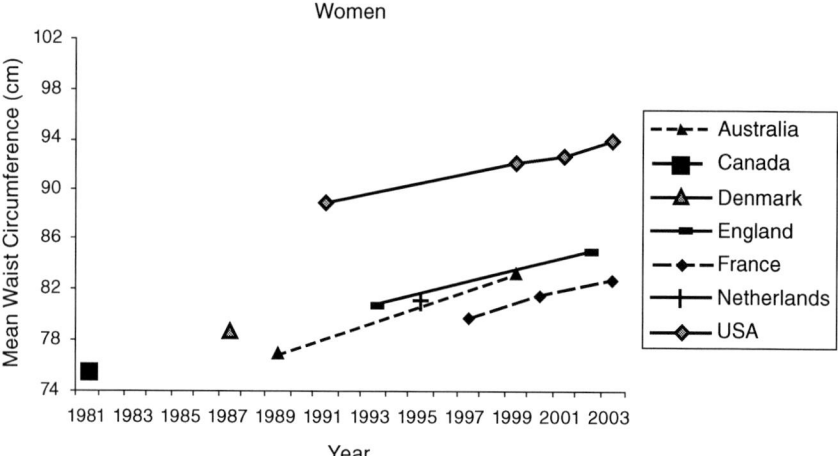

FIGURE 6-8 Trends in mean waist circumference by country and sex, 1981-2003.
SOURCES: Data are nationally representative unless otherwise noted. Australia: measured waist circumference, sample representative of Australian capital cities, ages 20-69 (1989) (Welborn, Dhaliwal, and Bennett, 2003), nationally representative ages 25+ (1999) (Snijder et al., 2004); Canada: measured waist circumference, ages 20-69 (1981) (Katzmarzyk, Craig, and Bouchard, 2002); Denmark: measured waist circumference, ages 35-65 (Heitmann, Frederiksen, and Lissner, 2004); France: self-reported waist circumference, ages 18+ (Charles, Eschwege, and Basdevant, 2008); England: measured waist circumference, ages 18-64 (Wardle and Boniface, 2007); Netherlands: measured waist circumference, representing three towns, ages 20-59 (Visscher and Seidell, 2004); United States: measured waist circumference, ages 20+ (Li et al., 2007).

Few studies have directly compared body composition across countries at a given BMI, but a recent comparison of body shape between American and British adults showed that body composition differs between them (Wells et al., 2007). American men have greater waist circumference compared with British men, even after adjusting for hip or thigh girth. American women had smaller waist circumference than British women after adjusting for hip or thigh girth, possibly related to greater total body size. These results suggest that it is important to consider body composition in cross-national comparisons in the health consequences of obesity.

A final limitation in our analysis of the association between obesity and mortality is that very little is known about how long it will take for us to observe the full effect of the increasing obesity prevalence on health outcomes at the population level. Many researchers have suggested that current increases in obesity-related chronic conditions represent the tip of the iceberg and the real impact of obesity will not be realized until cohorts with high levels of obesity at younger ages begin to age into disease and disability (Kumanyika, 2001; Sturm, Ringel, and Andreyeva, 2004). However, little is known about the lag time necessary for obesity to affect mortality risk. Clearly, the growth in childhood obesity is likely to result in an increased risk of obesity-related diseases in future cohorts of adults. Increased duration of obesity is associated with increased risk of diabetes (Wannamethee and Shaper, 1999), suggesting a potential lag between development of obesity and development of diabetes. However, there is little evidence of a lag time for obesity-related cancer development (Polendak, 2003), and research suggests that cardiovascular disease risk factors respond quickly to moderate weight loss (Klein et al., 2004). Thus, it is difficult to predict the extent to which the rise in obesity prevalence since the 1970s has already resulted in changes in life expectancy or has yet to exert its most important effects.

It is unclear how our assessment of the role of obesity as a contributor to cross-national differences in life expectancy would be different if obesity were defined based on waist circumference, weight at midlife, or different lag times between changes in obesity and changes in mortality—or all three. However, it is likely that available data using current BMI underestimate the association between obesity and mortality. Future work incorporating waist circumference and weight history data collected comparably across countries could help address these issues.

OBESITY AND MORTALITY IN THE FUTURE

Obesity's effect on life expectancy in future cohorts will depend on at least two factors: (1) changes in the prevalence of obesity at different ages and (2) changing associations between obesity and health outcomes. Rising rates of obesity at younger ages have two important implications for mortality. First, because the association between obesity and mortality is higher at younger ages, a rising prevalence of obesity at these ages is likely to have a greater effect on population life expectancy. Second, because more recent cohorts have an earlier average age of obesity onset (and recovery from obesity is rare), future cohorts will experience a longer duration of obesity (Leveille, Wee, and Iezzoni, 2005; Reynolds and Himes, 2007). Figure 6-9 provides the likelihood of obesity for three birth cohorts: by age 40, more than 30 percent of women in the 1969 cohort were projected to be obese, compared with only 6 percent in the 1919 cohort (Reynolds and Himes, 2007). In this relatively short time period, the duration of obesity appears to be increasing dramatically across cohorts. Few studies have examined

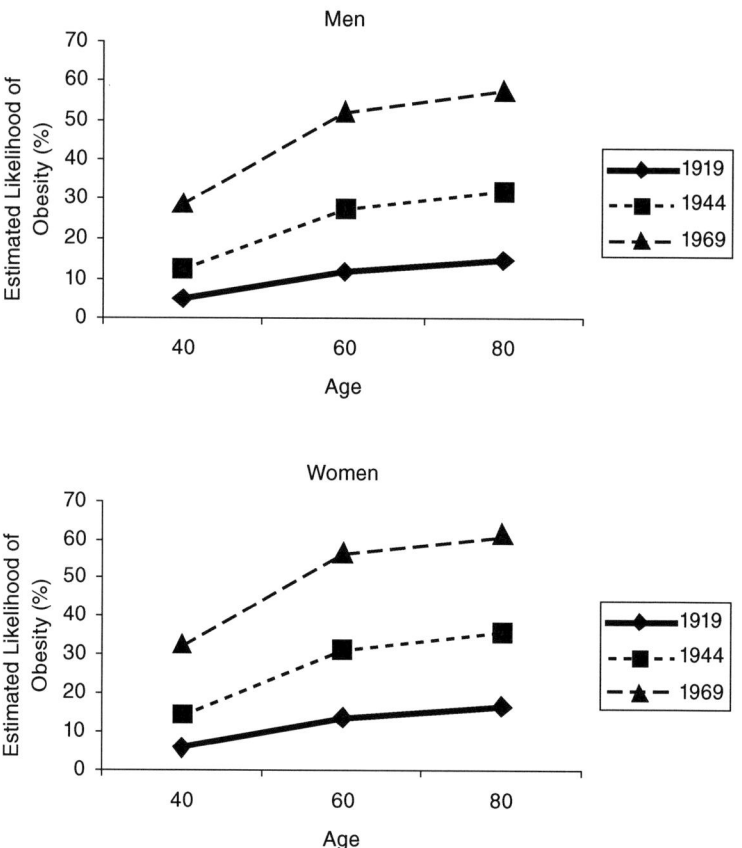

FIGURE 6-9 Estimated likelihood of obesity by age in successive birth cohorts.
SOURCE: Reynolds and Himes (2007); likelihood of obesity adjusted for age, race, ethnicity, and education.

the association between obesity duration and mortality, but a longer duration of obesity is clearly associated with increased risk of diabetes and disability (Stenholm et al., 2007; Wannamethee and Shaper, 1999). Given the increased prevalence of obesity at all ages, the strong association between obesity at younger ages and mortality, the increasing severity of obesity, and the increasing duration of obesity, it is likely that the effect of obesity on life expectancy will increase in the future.

However, there is some indication that the association between obesity and mortality, particularly cardiovascular mortality, may be decreasing over time (Flegal et al., 2005, 2007) possibly due to advances in treatment of cardiovascular risk factors (Gregg et al., 2005). This finding has not been replicated in other studies (Calle, Teras, and Thun, 2005), making predictions about the future effects of obesity on life expectancy controversial. Given rapidly rising rates of obesity at younger ages, it is likely that obesity will have a negative effect on advances in life expectancy in the future, but the magnitude of this effect is difficult to predict.

OBESITY AND OTHER HEALTH OUTCOMES

Even if obesity does not account for cross-national differences in life expectancy, rising obesity rates have important population health implications. For a variety of reasons, obesity is more closely associated with chronic conditions and disability than with mortality in old age. Thus, increases in obesity prevalence have important effects on the population burden of morbidity. As BMI increases, disability risk increases more than mortality risk (Al Snih et al., 2007; Lang et al., 2008). For example, Al Snih and colleagues (2007) found that disability risk increases above a BMI of approximately 24, while mortality risk did not begin to increase until a BMI of 27 in adults ages 65 and older. Furthermore, the slope of the BMI-disability relationship is steeper than that of the BMI-mortality relationship. This leads to a reduction in active life expectancy among the obese, even when total life expectancy is not affected (Reynolds, Saito, and Crimmins, 2005).

Similarly, obesity is associated with incidence of many chronic diseases and, as noted above, is not clearly associated with mortality in persons with chronic disease. Recent research has highlighted an "obesity paradox" in many chronic diseases associated with unintentional weight loss, particularly congestive heart failure, chronic kidney disease, and chronic obstructive pulmonary disease. This paradox refers to a combination of higher disease incidence in obese persons and lower mortality. The combination of earlier disease onset and lower mortality leads to a reduced healthy life expectancy and longer life expectancy with morbidity among these patients (Curtis et al., 2005; Kalantar-Zadeh et al., 2004, 2005; Landbo et al., 1999). A complete discussion of the possible mechanisms underlying obesity's differing associations with morbidity and mortality is beyond the scope of this chapter (Ferrucci and Alley, 2007). However, it is important to note that obesity may importantly contribute to cross-national differences in morbidity. Obesity is also associated with excess annual health care costs of $70 to $100 billion in the United States, further emphasizing the importance of obesity as a major public health issue (Allison, Zannolli, and Narayan, 1999; Wolf and Colditz, 1998).

CONCLUSION

At an individual level, obesity is associated with excess mortality risk, particularly among younger persons and those with severe obesity. Although the rise in obesity prevalence is likely to slow life-expectancy growth in the United States in the future, it is unlikely to account for current cross-national differences in life expectancy. Because obesity is becoming both more common and more severe at younger ages, its contribution to life expectancy is likely to grow. Furthermore, obesity remains a critical population health concern because of its effects on disease, disability, and health care costs.

ACKNOWLEDGMENTS

Support for this research was provided by National Institute on Aging grant no. T32 AG000262 and National Institute of Child Health and Human Development grant no. K12 HC043489 and by the Organized Research Center on Aging at the University of Maryland, Baltimore.

REFERENCES

Adams, K.F., Schatzkin, A., Harris, T.B., Kipnis, V., Mouw, T., Ballard-Barbash, R., et al. (2006). Overweight, obesity, and mortality in a large prospective cohort of persons 50 to 71 years old. *New England Journal of Medicine, 355*, 763-778.

Ajani, U.A., Lotufo, P.A., Gaziano, J.M., Lee, I.M., Spelsberg, A., Buring, J.E., et al. (2004). Body mass index and mortality among U.S. male physicians. *Annals of Epidemiology, 14*, 731-739.

Al Snih, S., Ottenbacher, K.J., Markides, K.S., Kuo, Y., Eschbach, K., and Goodwin, J.S. (2007). The effect of obesity on disability versus mortality in older Americans. *Archives of Internal Medicine, 167*, 774-780.

Allison, D.B., Gallagher, D., Heo, F., and Heymsfield, S. (1997). Body mass index and all-cause mortality among people ages 70 and older: The Longitudinal Study of Aging. *International Journal of Obesity, 21*, 424-431.

Allison, D.B., Zannolli, R., and Narayan, K.M. (1999). The direct health care costs of obesity in the United States. *American Journal of Public Health, 89*, 1194-1199.

Allison, D.B., Faith, M.S., Heo, M., Townsend-Butterworth, D., and Williamson, D.F. (1999). Meta-analysis of the effect of excluding early deaths on the estimated relationship between body mass index and mortality. *Obesity Research, 7*, 417-419.

Australian Institute of Health and Welfare. (2009). *AIHW Analysis of the 1980, 1983 and 1989 Risk Factor Prevalence Surveys, 1995 National Nutrition Survey and 1999-2000 Australian Diabetes, Obesity and Lifestyle (AusDiab) Study.* Available: http://www.aihw. gov.au/dataonline/riskfactors/index.cfm [accessed June 2009].

Baik, I., Ascherio, A., Rimm, E.B., Giovannucci, E., Spiegelman, D., Stampfer, M.J., et al. (2000). Adiposity and mortality in men. *American Journal of Epidemiology, 152,* 264-271.

Bender, R., Jockel, K., Trautner, C., Spraul, M., and Berger, M. (1999). Effect of age on excess mortality in obesity. *Journal of the American Medical Association, 281,* 1498-1504.

Bendixen, H., Holst, C., Sorensen, T.I.A., Raben, A., Bartels, E.M., and Astrup, A. (2004). Major increase in prevalence of overweight and obesity between 1987 and 2001 among Danish adults. *Obesity, 12,* 1464-1472.

Bergman, R.N., Kim, S.P., Catalono, K.J., Hsu, I.R., Chiu, J.D., Kabir, M., et al. (2006). Why visceral fat is bad: Mechanisms of the metabolic syndrome. *Obesity, 14,* 16S-19S.

Calle, E., Thun, M., Petrelli, J., Rodriguez, C., and Heath, C.J. (1999). Body-mass index and mortality in a prospective cohort of U.S. adults. *New England Journal of Medicine, 341,* 1097-1105.

Calle, E., Teras, L., and Thun, M. (2005). Obesity and mortality. *New England Journal of Medicine, 353,* 2197-2199.

Calza, S., Decarli, A., and Ferraroni, M. (2008). Obesity and prevalence of chronic diseases in the 1999-2000 Italian National Health Survey. *BMC Public Health, 8,* 140.

Cameron, A.J., Welborn, T.A., Zimmet, P.Z., Dunstan, D.W., Owen, N., Salmon, J., et al. (2003). Overweight and obesity in Australia: The 1999-2000 Australian Diabetes, Obesity and Lifestyle Study (AusDiab). *Medical Journal of Australia, 178,* 427-432.

Charles, M.-A., Eschwege, E., and Basdevant, A. (2008). Monitoring the obesity epidemic in France: The ObEpi surveys 1997-2006. *Obesity, 16,* 2182-2186.

Curtis, J., Selter, J., Wang, Y., Rathore, S., Jovin, I., Jadbabaie, F., et al. (2005). The obesity paradox: Body mass index and outcomes in patients with heart failure. *Archives of Internal Medicine, 165,* 55-61.

Department of Health (United Kingdom). (2009). *Health Survey for England.* Available: http://www.heartstats.org [accessed June 2009].

Diehr, P., Bild, D., Harris, T., Duxbury, A., Siscovick, D., and Rossi, M. (1998). Body mass index and mortality in nonsmoking older adults: The Cardiovascular Health Study. *American Journal of Public Health, 88,* 623-629.

Durazo-Arvizu, R., McGee, D., Cooper, R., Liao, Y., and Luke, A. (1998). Mortality and optimal body mass index in a sample of the U.S. population. *American Journal of Epidemiology, 147,* 739-749.

Elobeid, M.A., Desmond, R.A., Thomas, O., Keith, S.W., and Allison, D.B. (2007). Waist circumference values are increasing beyond those expected from BMI increases. *Obesity, 15,* 2380-2383.

Ferrucci, L., and Alley, D. (2007). Obesity, disability, and mortality: A puzzling link. *Archives of Internal Medicine, 167,* 750-751.

Finkelstein, E.A., Brown, D.S., Wrage, L.A., Allaire, B.T., and Hoerger, T.J. (2010). Individual and aggregate years-of-life-lost associated with overweight and obesity. *Obesity, 18,* 333-339.

Flegal, K.M., Carroll, M.D., Kuczmarski, R.J., and Johnson, C.L. (1998). Overweight and obesity in the United States: Prevalence and trends, 1960-1994. *International Journal of Obesity, 22,* 39-47.

Flegal, K.M., Carroll, M.D., Ogden, C.L., and Johnson, C.L. (2002). Prevalence and trends in obesity among U.S. adults, 1999-2000. *Journal of the American Medical Association, 288,* 1723-1727.

Flegal, K.M., Graubard, B.I., Williamson, D.F., and Gail, M.H. (2005). Excess deaths associated with underweight, overweight, and obesity. *Journal of the American Medical Association, 293,* 1861-1867.

Flegal, K.M., Graubard, B.I., Williamson, D.F., and Gail, M.H. (2007). Cause-specific excess deaths associated with underweight, overweight, and obesity. *Journal of the American Medical Association, 298,* 2028-2037.

Fontaine, K., Redden, D., Wang, C., Westfall, A., and Allison, D. (2003). Years of life lost due to obesity. *Journal of the American Medical Association, 289,* 187-193.

Freedman, D.M., Ron, E., Ballard-Barbash, R., Doody, M.M., and Linet, M.S. (2006). Body mass index and all-cause mortality in a nationwide U.S. cohort. *International Journal of Obesity, 30,* 822-829.

Gelber, R.P., Kurth, T., Manson, J.E., Buring, J.E., and Gaziano, J.M. (2007). Body mass index and mortality in men: Evaluating the shape of the association. *International Journal of Obesity, 31,* 1240-1247.

Grabowski, D., and Ellis, J. (2001). High body mass index does not predict mortality in older people: Analysis of the Longitudinal Study of Aging. *Journal of the American Geriatrics Society, 49,* 968-979.

Gregg, E., Cheng, Y., Cadwell, B., Imperatore, G., Williams, D., Flegal, K., et al. (2005). Secular trends in cardiovascular disease risk factors according to body mass index in U.S. adults. *Journal of the American Medical Association, 293,* 1868-1874.

Gronniger, J.T. (2006). A semiparametric analysis of the relationship of body mass index to mortality. *American Journal of Public Health, 96,* 173-178.

Heiat, A., Vaccarino, V., and Krumholz, H.M. (2001). An evidence-based assessment of federal guidelines for overweight and obesity as they apply to elderly persons. *Archives of Internal Medicine, 161,* 1194-1203.

Heitmann, B.L., Frederiksen, P., and Lissner, L. (2004). Hip circumference and cardiovascular morbidity and mortality in men and women. *Obesity Research, 12,* 482-487.

International Association for the Study of Obesity. (2009). *Global Prevalence of Adult Obesity.* Available: http://www.iotf.org/database/documents/GlobalPrevalenceofAdultObesityJune2009updateonweb.pdf [accessed June 2009].

Janssen, I., and Mark, A.E. (2007). Elevated body mass index and mortality risk in the elderly. *Obesity Reviews, 8,* 41-59.

Kalantar-Zadeh, K., Block, G., Horwich, T., and Fonarow, G. (2004). Reverse epidemiology of conventional cardiovascular risk factors in patients with chronic heart failure. *Journal of the American College of Cardiology, 43,* 1439-1444.

Kalantar-Zadeh, K., Kopple, J.D., Kilpatrick, R.D., McAllister, C.J., Shinaberger, C.S., Gjertson, D.W., et al. (2005). Association of morbid obesity and weight change over time with cardiovascular survival in a hemodialysis population. *American Journal of Kidney Disease, 46,* 489-500.

Katzmarzyk, P.T., Craig, C.L., and Bouchard, C. (2002). Adiposity, adipose tissues distribution and mortality rates in the Canada Fitness Survey follow-up study. *International Journal of Obesity, 26,* 1054-1059.

Klein, S., Burke, L.E., Bray, G.A., Blair, S., Allison, D.B., Pi-Sunyer, X., et al. (2004). Clinical implications of obesity with specific focus on cardiovascular disease: A statement for professionals from the American Heart Association Council on Nutrition, Physical Activity, and Metabolism: Endorsed by the American College of Cardiology Foundation. *Circulation, 110,* 2952-2967.

Koster, A., Leitzmann, M.F., Schatzkin, A., Mouw, T., Adams, K.F., van Eijk, J.T.M., et al. (2008). Waist circumference and mortality. *American Journal of Epidemiology, 167,* 1465-1475.

Kumanyika, S.K. (2001). Minisymposium on obesity: Overview and some strategic considerations. *Annual Review of Public Health, 22,* 293-308.

Landbo, C., Prescott, E., Lange, P., Vestbo, J., and Almdal, T.P. (1999). Prognostic value of nutritional status in chronic obstructive pulmonary disease. *American Journal of Respiratory and Clinical Care Medicine, 160,* 1856-1861.

Lang, I.A., Llewellyn, D.J., Alexander, K., and Melzer, D. (2008). Obesity, physical function, and mortality in older adults. *Journal of the American Geriatrics Society, 56,* 1474-1478.

Leveille, S.G., Wee, C.C., and Iezzoni, L.I. (2005). Trends in obesity and arthritis among baby boomers and their predecessors, 1971-2002. *American Journal of Public Health, 95,* 1607-1613.

Li, C., Ford, E.S., McGuire, L.C., and Mokdad, A.H. (2007). Increasing trends in waist circumference and abdominal obesity among U.S. adults. *Obesity, 15,* 216-216.

Maillard, G., Charles, M.-A., Thibult, N., Forhan, A., Sermet, C., Basdevant, A., et al. (1999). Trends in the prevalence of obesity in the French adult population between 1980 and 1991. *International Journal of Obesity, 23,* 389-394.

Manson, J., Willett, W., Stampfer, M., Colditz, G., Hunter, D., Hankinson, S., et al. (1995). Body weight and mortality among women. *New England Journal of Medicine, 333,* 677-685.

Martínez, J.A., Moreno, B., and Martínez-González, M.A. (2004). Prevalence of obesity in Spain. *Obesity Reviews, 5,* 171-172.

Matkin Dolan, C., Kraemer, H., Browner, W., Ensrud, K., and Kelsey, J. (2007). Associations between body composition, anthropometry, and mortality in women aged 65 years and older. *American Journal of Public Health, 97,* 913-918.

McGee, D.L., and Diverse Populations Collaboration. (2005). Body mass index and mortality: A meta-analysis based on person-level data from twenty-six observational studies. *Annals of Epidemiology, 15,* 87-97.

Michaud, P., van Soest, A.H.O., and Andreyeva, T. (2007). Cross-country variation in obesity patterns among older Americans and Europeans. *Forum for Health Economics and Policy, 10.*

Must, A., Spadano, J., Coakley, E.H., Field, A.E., Colditz, G., and Dietz, W.H. (1999). The disease burden associated with overweight and obesity. *Journal of the American Medical Association, 282,* 1523-1529.

National Center for Health Statistics. (2009). *National Health and Nutrition Examination Survey.* Available: http://www.cdc.gov/nchs/nhanes.htm [accessed June 2009].

Olshansky, S., Passaro, D., Hershow, R., Layden, J., Carnes, B., Brody, J., et al. (2005). A potential decline in life expectancy in the United States in the 21st century. *New England Journal of Medicine, 352,* 1138-1145.

Pagano, R., La Vecchia, C., Decarli, A., Negri, E., and Franceschi, S. (1997). Trends in overweight and obesity among Italian adults, 1983 through 1994. *American Journal of Public Health, 87,* 1869-1870.

Polendak, A.P. (2003). Trends in incidence rates for obesity-associated cancers in the U.S. *Cancer Detection and Prevention, 27,* 415-421.

Prospective Studies Collaboration. (2009). Body-mass index and cause-specific mortality in 900,000 adults: Collaborative analyses of 57 prospective studies. *Lancet, 373,* 1083-1096.

Rennie, K.L., and Jebb, S.A. (2005). Prevalence of obesity in Great Britain. *Obesity Reviews, 6,* 11-12.

Reynolds, S.L., and Himes, C.L. (2007). Cohort differences in adult obesity in the United States: 1982-2002. *Journal of Aging and Health, 19,* 831-850.

Reynolds, S.L., Saito, Y., and Crimmins, E.M. (2005). The impact of obesity on active life expectancy in older American men and women. *Gerontologist, 45,* 438-444.

Romero-Corral, A., Montori, V., Somers, V., Korinek, J., Thomas, R., Allison, T., et al. (2006). Association of bodyweight with total mortality and with cardiovascular events in coronary artery disease: A systematic review of cohort studies. *Lancet, 368,* 666-678.

Schokker, D.F., Visscher, T.L.S., Nooyens, A.C.J., van Baak, M.A., and Seidell, J.C. (2007). Prevalence of overweight and obesity in the Netherlands. *Obesity Reviews, 8,* 101-107.

Seidell, J.C., Verschuren, W.M., and Kromhout, D. (1995). Prevalence and trends of obesity in the Netherlands 1987-1991. *International Journal of Obesity and Related Metabolic Disorders, 19,* 924-927.

Snijder, M.B., Zimmet, P.Z., Visser, M., Dekker, J.M., Seidell, J.C., and Shaw, J.E. (2004). Independent and opposite associations of waist and hip circumferences with diabetes, hypertension and dyslipidemia: The AusDiab Study. *International Journal of Obesity and Related Metabolic Disorders, 28,* 402-409.

Snijder, M.B., van Dam, R.M., Visser, M., and Seidell, J.C. (2006). What aspects of body fat are particularly hazardous and how do we measure them? *International Journal of Epidemiology, 35,* 83-92.

Stenholm, S., Rantanen, T., Alanen, E., Reunanen, A., Sainio, P., and Koskinen, S. (2007). Obesity history as a predictor of walking limitation at old age. *Obesity, 15,* 929-938.

Stevens, J., Cai, J., Pamuk, E.R., Williamson, D.F., Thun, M., and Wood, J.L. (1998). The effect of age on the association between body-mass index and mortality. *New England Journal of Medicine, 338,* 1-7.

Stevens, J., Cai, J., Thun, M.J., Williamson, D.F., and Wood, J.L. (1999). Consequences of the use of different measures of effect to determine the impact of age on the association between obesity and mortality. *American Journal of Epidemiology, 150,* 399-407.

Sturm, R., Ringel, J., and Andreyeva, T. (2004). Increasing obesity rates and disability trends. *Health Affairs, 23,* 199-205.

Thorpe, R., and Ferraro, K. (2004). Aging, obesity, and mortality: Misplaced concern about obese older people? *Research on Aging, 26,* 108-129.

Tjepkema, M. (2005). *Measured Obesity. Adult Obesity in Canada: Measured Height and Weight.* Ottawa: Statistics Canada.

Torrance, G.M., Hooper, M.D., and Reeder, B.A. (2002). Trends in overweight and obesity among adults in Canada (1970-1992): Evidence from national surveys using measured height and weight. *International Journal of Obesity, 26,* 797-804.

Trayhurn, P., and Beattie, J.H. (2001). Physiological role of adipose tissue: White adipose tissue as an endocrine and secretory organ. *Proceedings of the Nutrition Society, 60,* 329-339.

Visscher, T.L.S., and Seidell, J.C. (2004). Time trends (1993-1997) and seasonal variation in body mass index and waist circumference in the Netherlands. *International Journal of Obesity and Related Metabolic Disorders, 28,* 1309-1316.

Visscher, T.L.S., Seidell, J.C., Molarius, A., van der Kuip, D., Hofman, A., and Witteman, J.C.M. (2001). A comparison of body mass index, waist-hip ratio and waist circumference as predictors of all-cause mortality among the elderly: The Rotterdam Study. *International Journal of Obesity, 25,* 1730-1735.

Visscher, T.L.S., Kromhout, D., and Seidell, J.C. (2002). Long-term and recent time trends in the prevalence of obesity among Dutch men and women. *International Journal of Obesity, 26,* 1218-1224.

Wannamethee, S., and Shaper, A. (1999). Weight change and duration of overweight and obesity in the incidence of type 2 diabetes. *Diabetes Care, 22,* 1266-1272.

Wardle, J., and Boniface, D. (2007). Changes in the distributions of body mass index and waist circumference in English adults, 1993/1994 to 2002/2003. *International Journal of Obesity, 32,* 527-532.

Welborn, T.A., Dhaliwal, S.S., and Bennett, S.A. (2003). Waist-hip ratio is the dominant risk factor predicting cardiovascular death in Australia. *Medical Journal of Australia, 179*, 580-585.

Wells, J.C.K., Cole, T.J., Bruner, D., and Treleaven, P. (2007). Body shape in American and British adults: Between-country and inter-ethnic comparisons. *International Journal of Obesity, 32*, 152-159.

Wolf, A., and Colditz, G. (1998). Current estimates on the economic cost of obesity in the United States. *Obesity Research, 6*, 97-106.

Yoshiike, N., Kaneda, F., and Takimoto, H. (2002). Epidemiology of obesity and public health strategies for its control in Japan. *Asia Pacific Journal of Clinical Nutrition, 11*, S727-S731.

Yoshiike, N., Seino, F., Tajima, S., Arai, Y., Kawano, M., Furuhata, T., et al. (2002). Twenty-year changes in the prevalence of overweight in Japanese adults: The National Nutrition Survey 1976-95. *Obesity Reviews, 3*, 183-190.

ANNEX 6A

We first estimated the proportion at each BMI at approximately age 50 for both sexes using data from NHANES II (1976-1980) and NHANES (2001-2004). In order to generate a relatively smooth BMI distribution, we estimated the BMI distribution for the population ages 48-52 at each BMI in both surveys.

We then used the following formula to calculate the effect of obesity on life expectancy:

$$RLE = \sum_b p_{BMI=b} * E[YLL \mid BMI = b]$$

where:

RLE = expected reduction in life expectancy (years) at age 50
$p_{BMI=b}$ = proportion of population with BMI = b (range 30-45+) at ages 48-52
$E[YLL \mid BMI = b]$ = expected years of life lost given BMI = b, from Fontaine et al. (2003).

A BMI of 24 was defined as the reference category. Therefore, $E[YLL \mid BMI = 24]$ was defined to be 0, and $E[YLL \mid BMI = b]$ is interpreted as expected YLL at age 50, comparing those with BMI b with those with BMI 24.

This approach assumes that age-specific mortality and the association between BMI and mortality were constant.

7

The Contribution of Physical Activity to Divergent Trends in Longevity

Andrew Steptoe and Anna Wikman

Physical activity is fundamental to the maintenance of physical health, mobility, independent living, and the quality of life of older people. Sustained physical activity in the elderly is likely to minimize health and social care costs, reduce the risk of falls and fractures, and enhance cognition and positive well-being either directly or indirectly, through promoting social participation. The extent to which differences in physical activity contribute to variations in health and life expectancy across countries is poorly understood.

One reason is that there are limits to the validity of the standard questionnaire measures of physical activity used in studies of older people. These measures can be somewhat insensitive to variations in light and moderate activity, and there may be differences in interpretation of activity intensity items. In addition, there may be incomplete recall among older participants, particularly with respect to the timing and duration of activities across days of the week. Objective assessments using accelerometers or pedometers are being used more frequently, but they have yet to be applied to nationally representative samples in comparative studies. These factors conspire against definite conclusions at this point in time concerning the contribution of physical activity to differences in longevity across countries. There are, however, pointers toward the relevance of physical activity to cross-country variations in health and well-being.

The purpose of this chapter is to review the current evidence concerning physical activity and highlight issues for future research. We begin with a brief overview of the benefits of physical activity at older ages for physical and mental health and cognitive functioning. The scientific literature is large, so we draw on two recent comprehensive reports that have reviewed this work, namely the 2008 report of the Physical Activity Guidelines Advisory Committee (2008) and the position stand on physical activity for older adults from the American College of Sports Medicine (Chodzko-Zajko et al., 2009). A particular difficulty of studying the health benefits of physical activity at older ages is establishing an incontrovertible level of proof. Intervention studies with disease outcomes are rare, so much of the evidence is based on observational studies or short-term interventions with intermediate health endpoints. Nevertheless, the weight of the data indicates that physical activity is associated both with an enhanced life span and good health and functioning at older ages.

Any discussion of the contribution of physical activity to divergent trends in longevity across countries depends on accurate assessment. The second section of the chapter therefore addresses the strengths and limitations of self-report and objective measures and suggests ways in which self-report assessments might be improved. Third, we review the current literature concerning physical activity levels in developed countries in relation to longevity. A key issue in these cross-country comparisons is whether countries should be judged in terms of the proportion of their population attaining recommended levels of physical activity, or the proportion that is sedentary and does no activity at all. Population rates of physical activity and sedentary behavior do not have a simple reciprocal relationship, and country rankings vary depending on which measure is used. While monitoring adherence to physical activity guidelines is valuable for public health promotion, many of the adverse effects of being inactive are likely to occur at the lower end of the activity/inactivity distribution. The timing of important relationships is also poorly understood. Is it the current level of physical activity or sedentary behavior among older adults that is important, or the levels of activity that were present in the country when these individuals were in middle age?

BENEFITS OF PHYSICAL ACTIVITY AT OLDER AGES

Regular physical activity is thought to be among the most important lifestyle factors for the maintenance of health and prevention of premature disease and mortality. Across developed regions of the world, inactivity ranks alongside tobacco, alcohol, and adiposity as a leading cause of reduced healthy life expectancy (Ezzati et al., 2003). An analysis of the Nurses' Health Study estimated that the population attributable risk (PAR) for physical inactivity was 16.5 percent of deaths from any cause, 27.7 percent of cardiovascular deaths, and 9.3 percent of cancer deaths (van Dam et al., 2008). In the INTERHEART study of myocardial infarction in 52 countries, the PAR for inactivity was 12.2 percent across all regions of the world and was as strong as 24-38 percent in Western Europe and North America (Yusuf et al., 2004). Globally, the World Health Organization recently estimated that inactivity is responsible for around 5.5 percent of deaths (World Health Organization, 2009). Many types of physical activity appear to be protective, including leisure-time physical activity, walking, and active commuting (Hamer and Chida, 2008; Landi et al., 2008; Manson et al., 2002). Physical activity is also relevant to the secondary prevention of physical disease and is a major component of most programs of cardiac or respiratory rehabilitation.

Physical inactivity contributes to many specific health and function problems in old age. Table 7-1 outlines some of the positive health benefits of regular physical activity for older adults. For example, physical activity is a key component of many programs to reduce risk of falls through improving strength, balance, and confidence. Falls are an important cause of morbidity in older populations; more than a third of people age 65 and over fall every year, and many falls result in fractures, soft tissue injury, or head injury (Tinetti, 2003). A recent longitudinal population study in Australia showed that physical activity was associated with a substantially reduced risk of falls over a 3-5 year period, independent of age, education,

TABLE 7-1 Health Benefits of Regular Physical Activity for Older Adults

How Physical Activity Can Improve Physical Functioning	How Physical Activity Can Improve Mental Functioning	How Physical Activity Can Be Beneficial at Older Ages in General
• Improves cardiorespiratory fitness • Improves glucose metabolism and insulin sensitivity • Reduces blood pressure • Improves lipid profiles • Reduces levels of inflammatory markers • Induces growth factors • Improves balance • Improves strength, flexibility and joint mobility (range of motion) • Reduces decline in bone density • Helps maintain a healthy weight	• Enhances emotional well-being • Provides relaxation and helps lower stress levels • Helps maintain cognitive function and alertness • Helps reduce depression • Enhances perceptions of coping ability • Improves sleep	• Helps maintain independence • Improves quality of life • Increases energy • Helps maintain social connectedness

body weight, eyesight problems, chronic conditions, and other covariates (Heesch, Byles, and Brown, 2008).

The Physical Activity Guidelines Advisory Committee concluded that there is a dose-response relationship with fracture risk, so greater physical activity results in greater risk reduction. The MacArthur Studies of Successful Aging have demonstrated that deterioration in objectively defined physical functioning over a 2.5-year period was attenuated in more physically active individuals, both with and without chronic health problems (Seeman and Chen, 2002). Another longitudinal study found that regular activity was associated with reduced risk of the development of impairments in activities of daily living in both normal and overweight participants, independent of covariates (Bruce, Fries, and Hubert, 2008), and favorable effects on physical function appear to be maintained into very old age (Yates et al., 2008).

Physical activity is also associated with improved prognosis of chronic obstructive lung disease, in particular improvements in health-related quality of life and functional exercise capacity (Langer et al., 2009). The effects of regular physical activity on the biological systems noted in Table 7-1 have been observed both in observational and intervention trials (Kelley and Kelley, 2006, 2007). Physical activity also appears to help maintain cognitive function in old age (Hamer and Chida, 2009), as well as promoting emotional well-being and quality of life (Martin et al., 2009; Steptoe, 2006).

Most longitudinal observational studies do not begin with populations that are completely free of subclinical or early-stage illness or risk factors. Exercise in middle and old age is more common among people who have been active in their early lives (Chakravarty et al., 2008). This makes it difficult to be confident whether physical activity really precedes illness, or whether early presymptomatic illness or risk factors lead to reduced physical activity. Nonetheless, some studies have shown that changes in levels of physical activity in middle-aged and older people are associated with changes in risk factors, functional independence, and mortality (Byberg et al., 2001, 2009; Stessman et al., 2009).

Table 7-2 summarizes the conclusions drawn by the 2008 Physical Activity Guidelines Advisory Committee about the role of physical activity in major diseases that contribute to longevity in developed countries. The evidence is strong in most cases for an inverse relationship between regular physical activity and reduced risk of cardiovascular and metabolic diseases, with graded effects in many cases. The associations with cancer vary by the site of malignancy, with the strongest evidence for colorectal and breast cancer. Potentially, therefore, it is plausible that physical activity is a modifiable risk factor for diseases of old age that could contribute to international variations in longevity.

TABLE 7-2 Physical Activity and Major Health Conditions of Older Age

Health Condition	Committee Conclusion	Reviews and Meta-analyses
Cardiovascular disease	A strong inverse relationship between habitual physical activity and coronary heart disease and cardiovascular disease morbidity and mortality. Sedentary behavior is an independent risk factor for middle-aged and older men and women, with those reporting moderate activity having a 20 percent lower risk and those reporting higher activity having approximately a 30 percent lower risk than least active persons. Physical activity is also protective for stroke.	Sofi et al. (2008); Wendel-Vos et al. (2004)
Metabolic syndrome	There is an inverse dose-response association between level of activity and risk of metabolic syndrome. Many studies indicate that a goal of 150 minutes per week of moderate intensity activity is desirable.	Orozco et al. (2008)
Type 2 diabetes	Randomized controlled trials and observational studies indicate that 150 minutes per week of moderate intensity physical activity will help prevent type 2 diabetes.	Orozco et al. (2008)
Cancers	People who carry out aerobic physical activity for about 3 to 4 hours per week at moderate or greater intensity have an average 30 percent reduction in colon cancer risk and a 20 to 40 percent lower risk of breast cancer, compared with sedentary individuals. Compared with sedentary people, available epidemiological data suggest that active people show reductions of approximately 20, 30, and 20 percent in risk of lung, endometrial, and ovarian cancers, respectively.	Friedenreich and Cust (2008); Wolin et al. (2009)
Cognitive function/ dementia	Prospective cohort studies support the conclusion that physical activity delays the incidence of dementia and the onset of age-related cognitive decline.	Hamer and Chida (2009)

SOURCE: Adapted from 2008 Physical Activity Guidelines Advisory Committee.

RECOMMENDED LEVELS OF ACTIVITY IN OLDER ADULTS

There are some variations in government and authoritative agency recommendations about the levels of physical activity that should be achieved, and older adults may have physical problems that limit their capacity to attain high levels of activity. The U.S. 2008 physical activity guidelines for older adults are summarized in Box 7-1 (U.S. Department of Health and Human Services, 2008). The first guideline—that people should carry out any activity rather than none, since even modest exercise is better than none

> **BOX 7-1**
> **2008 Physical Activity Guidelines for Older Adults**
>
> - All adults should avoid inactivity. Some physical activity is better than none, and adults who participate in any amount of physical activity gain some health benefits.
> - For substantial health benefits, adults should do at least 150 minutes (2 hours and 30 minutes) a week of moderate-intensity, or 75 minutes (1 hour and 15 minutes) a week of vigorous-intensity aerobic physical activity, or an equivalent combination of moderate- and vigorous-intensity aerobic activity. Aerobic activity should be performed in episodes of at least 10 minutes, and, preferably, it should be spread throughout the week.
> - For additional and more extensive health benefits, adults should increase their aerobic physical activity to 300 minutes (5 hours) a week of moderate-intensity, or 150 minutes a week of vigorous-intensity aerobic physical activity, or an equivalent combination of moderate- and vigorous-intensity activity. Additional health benefits are gained by engaging in physical activity beyond this amount.
> - Adults should also do muscle-strengthening activities that are of moderate or high intensity and involve all major muscle groups on 2 or more days a week, as these activities provide additional health benefits.
> - When older adults cannot do 150 minutes of moderate-intensity aerobic activity a week because of chronic conditions, they should be as physically active as their abilities and conditions allow.
> - Older adults should do exercises that maintain or improve balance if they are at risk of falling.
> - Older adults should determine their level of effort for physical activity relative to their level of fitness.
> - Older adults with chronic conditions should understand whether and how their conditions affect their ability to do regular physical activity safely.
>
> SOURCE: Adapted from the 2008 Physical Activity Guidelines for Americans.

at all—is potentially relevant to international trends, since health problems associated with physical activity are likely to be most prominent among the sedentary population, not those who are moderately versus highly active.

The current recommendation is for 150 minutes per week of aerobic activity of moderate intensity in episodes of at least 10 minutes. This is equivalent to around 20 minutes per day, ideally spread throughout the week. Muscle-strengthening activity is also recommended, with older adults being advised to carry out exercises that help maintain balance. The proportion of the population that fulfills these criteria in the United States and Western Europe is not as high as is desirable, as detailed later in this chapter. But there are two immediate implications of the guidelines that are relevant to the theme of this chapter. First, providing a complete assessment of the different activity components in population studies is difficult. While it may be possible to gauge the amount of aerobic activity, measures of muscle-strengthening activities and balance exercises are less well developed, and it is not clear whether the different elements can be integrated into a single score of physical activity. Second, the guidelines use the terms *moderate-intensity* and *vigorous-intensity* activity. These are open to interpretation, and there may be variation among individuals and among countries in how different types of activity are perceived.

MEASUREMENT OF PHYSICAL ACTIVITY

The issue of accurate measurement is of course fundamental to analyses of the contribution of physical activity to divergent trends in longevity. Most population studies are based on self-report of physical activity. A number of standardized measures have been developed, such as the Paffenbarger Physical Activity Questionnaire and the Minnesota Leisure Time Physical Activity Questionnaire. Questionnaires designed specifically for older men and women have also been devised, including the Yale Physical Activity Survey for Older Adults, the Physical Activity Scale for the Elderly (PASE), and the Community Health Activity Model Program for Seniors (CHAMPS) scale. Cross-national studies need to take account of the different forms of activity in different cultures: bicycling for transport is very common in the Netherlands, gardening is popular in the United Kingdom, and some countries show wide seasonal variations in activity because of their climates. Instruments have therefore been developed specifically for international comparison work, such as the International Physical Activity Questionnaire (IPAQ) and the European Prospective Investigation into Cancer (EPIC) measure. The applied research measurement resource of the National Cancer Institute lists the details of more than 100 physical activity questionnaires, together with many validation studies (see http://appliedresearch.cancer.gov/tools/paq/reflist.html [accessed June 8, 2010]). Nevertheless, there are limitations to the accuracy of all self-report measures (Shephard, 2003), and agreement with gold standard measures, such as doubly labeled water (a measure of metabolic rate based on the speed of elimination of heavy isotopes), is modest (Westerterp, 2009).

Some of the limitations of self-report measures are common to all ages, but there are particular problems in older adults, and these are exacerbated in cross-national studies (see Table 7-3). Responses to questionnaires may not be accurate because of incomplete recall and impaired cognitive ability; in older age groups, many activities are of light or moderate intensity and occur as part of everyday life, so they may be missed. Questionnaires typically provide crude summary indices of physical activity, so they may provide little information about the pattern of activity across the day and

TABLE 7-3 Adherence to Physical Activity Recommendations

Proportion (standard error) based on objective assessment of activity

Age	Men % (SE)	Women % (SE)	Total % (SE)
16-19	7.1 (1.0)	4.1 (1.0)	5.6 (0.8)
20-59	3.8 (0.4)	3.2 (0.3)	3.5 (0.3)
60+	2.5 (0.4)	2.3 (0.5)	2.4 (0.4)

SOURCE: Adapted from NHANES 2003-2004 (Troiano et al., 2008).

through the week. Much of older people's activity is not done in designated exercise periods, so the frequency of activity is less easy to gauge than in younger groups. Some questionnaires suffer from floor effects, are based only on the assessment of designated leisure-time activities rather than all types of activity, or do not even include the low-intensity activities that are common in the older population (Shephard, 2003). In addition, disability can have an influence on the interpretation of items concerning activity intensity, with disabled individuals rating particular activities as more intense than nondisabled people (Rikli, 2000). This means that comparisons between people with very different levels of physical function and frailty groups may be compromised. Finally, there may be important cultural differences across countries in what constitutes exercise, vigorous exercise in particular.

Objective measurement of physical activity is therefore desirable. Several types of measure are available, including doubly labeled water and heart rate monitoring, but the most useful objective method for population studies is motion sensing using accelerometers (Westerterp, 2009). Accelerometers are robust, lightweight devices that can be worn for several days without discomfort. Because the information is time-stamped, patterns of activity through the day can be determined. Useful information about the amount of time people spend inactive or at relatively low levels of activity can also be obtained. Pedometers are also an option, particularly for older people for whom walking is a primary mode of activity. Pedometers are simple to use, inexpensive, and very practical for older age samples. Recordings correlate well with accelerometers, but they do not capture the intensity of activity or the pattern of activity over time (Harris et al., 2009b). There are also specific devices, such as the activPAL™ physical activity logger, that are designed specifically for monitoring leg activity (Busse, van Deursen, and Wiles, 2009).

The importance of the pattern of activity over the day is illustrated in Figure 7-1, which compares activity counts averaged over 7 days recorded from 163 community-dwelling older men and women in England (age 76

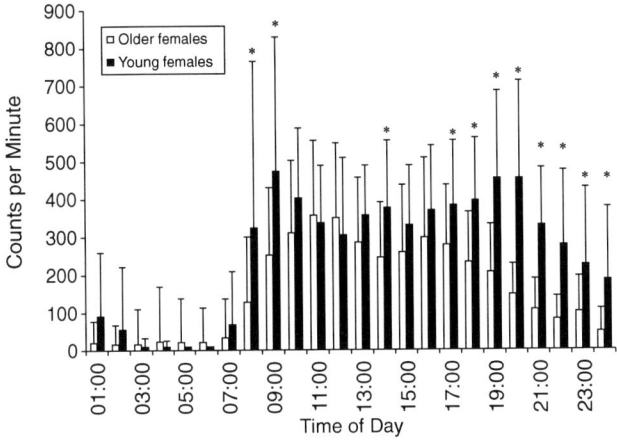

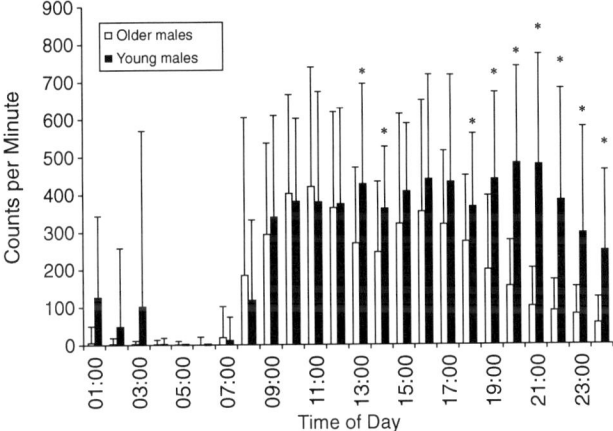

FIGURE 7-1 Weekday hourly mean accelerometer counts per minute for older and younger women (upper panel) and men (lower panel).
NOTE: The asterisks indicate significant age differences.
SOURCE: Davis and Fox (2007). Permission to reprint obtained from Springer-Verlag 2006, and M.G. Davis and K.R. Fox. Exercise, Nutrition, and Health Sciences, School of Applied and Community Health, Centre for Sport, Exercise & Health, University of Bristol, Tyndall Avenue, Bristol, BS8 1TP, UK.

on average) with 45 young adults age 27 (Davis and Fox, 2007). Distinct patterns of activity are apparent, with comparable activity in the morning in the older group, but markedly less activity in older than younger participants in the evening. Overall counts were around one-third lower in the older group, which also engaged in much less high-intensity activity.

There are particular issues in using accelerometers with older people that should not be ignored. They do not, of course, provide information about the type of activity being carried out. Changes in body composition and declines in basal metabolic rate mean that algorithms designed to convert accelerometer counts into units of energy expenditure need to be interpreted with caution. The assessment of people with chronic physical disability may be problematic, with different positioning of devices around the waist or wrist being necessary. Finally, accelerometers are relatively expensive and labor-intensive to analyze, so they may not prove the ultimate solution to general survey work unless these practical and economic issues are resolved. An iterative process involving conjoint assessment of objective and self-report measures may help improve subjective measures.

Two other approaches to measuring physical activity are relevant in studies of older populations. The first is the assessment of cardiorespiratory fitness. Fitness can be measured through a number of standard protocols using treadmills, step tests, and bicycle ergometers (American College of Sports Medicine, 2005). Cardiorespiratory fitness is moderately correlated with activity questionnaire measures, although the two are not interchangeable and may have independent effects on health (Chase et al., 2009; Wei et al., 2000). Second, measuring walking speed can provide a simple yet useful method of measuring health-relevant physical activity capacity in the elderly. One recent study demonstrated that slow walking speed over 6 meters in older people was strongly associated with an increased risk of cardiovascular mortality (Dumurgier et al., 2009); those with a walking speed in the lower third of the distribution had about a threefold increased risk of cardiovascular death, but no increased risk of mortality from cancer or other causes of death. In an analysis of apparently healthy older participants in the Whitehall II cohort, we demonstrated that speed on a very short (8 ft) walk was associated with greater subclinical coronary atherosclerosis (Hamer et al., in press).

DISCREPANCIES BETWEEN SELF-REPORT AND OBJECTIVE MEASURES

Ratings on self-report measures of physical activity are moderately correlated with objective measures using accelerometers and pedometers (Friedenreich et al., 2006; Hagstromer, Oja, and Sjöström, 2006). Studies of older adults have shown correlations of .34 to .49 for accelerometers and .36 to .56 for pedometers (Harris et al., 2009b; Stel et al., 2004; Washburn and Ficker, 1999). Of greater concern are discrepancies in the absolute levels of physical activity reported, since these are relevant both for public policy and for understanding associations with longevity.

The largest representative study to date is the National Health and

Nutrition Examination Survey (NHANES) 2003-2004, which involved collection of 7 days of accelerometry from 7,176 individuals (Troiano et al., 2008). Data for 4 or more days were obtained from 4,867 participants. There was a marked decline in activity counts with age, falling from mean counts per minute of 423.6 and 327.2 for men and women ages 20-29, to 256.7 and 251.2 for men and women ages 60-69. The proportion of individuals of different ages whose activity attained the recommended levels is detailed in Table 7-3. The criterion was 30 or more minutes of moderate or vigorous activity at least 5 days per week, a somewhat less stringent threshold than that shown in Box 7-1, since activity in this analysis did not have to be accumulated in bouts of at least 10 minutes. Nevertheless, it is apparent that the proportion of individuals in the population who are adherent is very small, even among adolescents, and only about 1 in 40 for participants age 60 and older.

The proportion of the population apparently complying with national recommendations is much smaller with objective than self-report measures. Figures from the Behavioral Risk Factor Surveillance System (see http://www.cdc.gov/brfss/ [accessed June 8, 2010]) indicate that, in 2005, 48.8 percent of adults in the United States reported 30 or more minutes of moderate physical activity on 5 or more days of the week, or vigorous activity of at least 20 minutes duration on 3 or more days. According to the Healthy People 2010 Database (see http://wonder.cdc.gov/data2010/ [accessed June 8, 2010]), only 14 percent of people ages 65-74 fulfill criteria for being sufficiently active.

The NHANES findings are reproduced elsewhere. A smaller accelerometer study of men and women age 65 or older in the United Kingdom showed that only 2.5 percent achieved the recommended amount of 150 minutes per week in bouts of at least 10 minutes (Harris et al., 2009a). A Swedish population study across a wider age range (ages 18-69) found that 57 percent accumulated at least 30 minutes daily, although if these had to be obtained through bouts of 10 minutes or more, the proportion fell to 1 percent (Hagstromer, Oja, and Sjöström, 2007). Equally worrying from the public health perspective is the high incidence of sedentary behavior, as defined by low activity counts on accelerometers. Analysis of the NHANES 2003-2004 data indicates that individuals aged 60-69 years spent an average 8.41 hours (more than 60 percent of their time) per day in sedentary behavior (Matthews et al., 2008). Interestingly, this is somewhat higher than the average of 7.52 hours per day recorded for Swedish men and women ages 65-79, although the sample was small (Hagstromer, Oja, and Sjöström, 2007).

The data collected using objective measures therefore shows marked differences from self-report in terms of the amount of activity achieved and very poor adherence to national recommendations. One possible explanation is that people overestimate their physical activity and misclassify their activities as involving more energy expenditure than they actually do. Sedentary behavior is often defined in self-report studies in terms of the amount of time spent in inactive pursuits, such as watching TV or using a computer; the accelerometer studies indicate that such measures capture only a small proportion of the time spent without moving in a typical day. It is also possible that accelerometers fail to assess some types of activity accurately, leading to underestimation. Accelerometers are taken off when people are swimming, and they are relatively poor at monitoring such activities as cycling. Important though these activities are, they probably contribute a modest amount to overall physical activity in population studies. In addition, static activities involving complex movements may be underestimated using accelerometers (Matthews, 2005). Another issue that is being actively investigated is whether the cut points used to define sufficient objective activity in these accelerometer studies are correct for the general population.

It should also be pointed out that the guidelines for physical activity have been based predominantly on self-report measures in the population. If these do overestimate actual activity, yet are derived from evidence that these self-report levels are protective, it is possible that, in reality, a lower amount of activity is required for health benefit. Nonetheless, there is clearly scope for improving self-report measures. One useful avenue may be to develop physical activity vignettes that could be used to anchor self-report measures. Vignette questions could describe the activity of a hypothetical person and then ask the respondent to evaluate the exercise of that person. Such a method could help identify systematic variations in the interpretation of activity levels by age or disability level.

INTERNATIONAL DIFFERENCES IN PHYSICAL ACTIVITY

Estimation of the contribution of physical activity to cross-national differences in longevity has to be based on robust estimates of activity in different countries. The previous sections of this chapter indicate that international comparisons are difficult to make. There are no cross-national studies using objective measures, and a key priority for future research is a comparison of objectively assessed activity in representative samples of older adults from different countries, using the same study and measurement protocol. Although there are numerous self-report studies across the developed world, comparisons are difficult to make with different self-report measures, since a common metric is not present. The most reliable comparisons are therefore in cross-national studies in which the same measure has been used on similar sectors of the population in each nation. Another consideration is deciding what aggregate measure of activity is most relevant for longevity; the options include the average levels of physical activity in the population, the proportion who are active above a defined threshold, the levels of sedentary behavior, or (for older people) such indicators as the amount of time spent walking.

Table 7-4 summarizes data from a number of international studies of moderate or vigorous self-reported physical activity. The studies vary in the criterion adopted for assessing moderate or vigorous activity, as well as in the age range tested and sample size. European countries are overrepresented in these studies compared with developed countries in the Americas, Asia, and Australasia, partly because many investigations were focused primarily on the European Union. However, the International Prevalence Study (IPS) of physical activity used the IPAQ to assess activity across 20 countries (Bauman et al., 2009). The IPAQ measures the frequency, duration, and intensity of activity over the last 7 days. Respondents are asked to include all physical activity at work, during transportation, at home, and during leisure time. The criterion presented in the table is the proportion

TABLE 7-4 Ranking of Levels of Moderate or Intense Physical Activity Across Countries

Study	IPS	Eurobarometer	EPIC	EU Study
Age	40-65	≥ 15	50-64	≥ 15
Year	2002-2004	2002	1992-2000	1997
Sample size	52,746	15,000	236,386	15,239
Activity	Moderate/intense activity %	Sufficient activity (IPAQ, %)	Total recreational (hr/week)	MET/h/wk (median %)
Country	Czech R (88.0)	NL (44.2)	NL (19.38)	Sweden (24.0)
Ranking	New Zealand (86.5)	Germany (40.2)	United Kingdom (14.34)	NL (21.0)
	Canada (83.0)	Greece (37.0)	Germany (13.17)	Denmark (19.5)
	United States (82.5)	Denmark (34.1)	Spain (11.82)	United Kingdom (16.0)
	Australia (81.5)	Finland (32.5)	Greece (11.08)	Germany (12.7)
	Sweden (73.0)	United Kingdom (38.7)	Denmark (10.29)	France (10.0)
	Norway (71.0)	Ireland (29.0)	Italy (8.35)	Italy (8.0)
	Spain (70.5)	Italy (25.8)	Sweden (5.86)	Spain (8.0)
	Belgium (51.5)	Spain (25.2)		Greece (8.0)
		Belgium (25.0)		
		France (24.1)		
		Sweden (22.9)		

NOTE: NL = the Netherlands.
SOURCES: Adapted from IPS = International Prevalence Study (Bauman et al., 2009). Eurobarometer Study (Sjöström et al., 2006). EPIC = European Prospective Investigation into Cancer and Nutrition (Haftenberger et al., 2002). Data from the largest center in each country is included. European Union study (Martinez-Gonzalez et al., 2001).

who carried out either moderate activity, measured as 3 days of vigorous activity of at least 20 minutes per day, 5 days of moderate-intensity activity or walking of ≥ 30 minutes per day, or 5 days of combinations that achieve ≥ 600 MET-minutes (metabolic equivalent of task) per week; or high activity, measured as 3 days of vigorous activity that accumulated at least 1,500 MET-minutes per week or ≥ 5 days of any combination achieving at least 3,000 MET-minutes per week. The proportion of respondents ages 40-65 attaining this criterion ranged from more than 85 percent in the Czech Republic and New Zealand to 51.5 percent in Belgium. The IPAQ was also used in the Eurobarometer study in 2002 with a broadly comparable threshold, although in this case a wider age range was included (Sjöström et al., 2006). This again identified low prevalence estimates in Belgium, as well as in France and Sweden.

Physical activity was assessed as part of the EPIC study in a large sample of men and women ages 50-64 (Haftenberger et al., 2002). A short validated questionnaire was administered, and Table 7-4 shows results for total recreational activity for the largest center included in each country. The highest levels were recorded in the Netherlands, the United Kingdom, and Germany, whereas Sweden again ranked low, along with Italy. Finally, an earlier European Union study showed a different profile of responses, with citizens of Northern European countries being more active than those from southern countries like Greece and Spain (Martinez-Gonzalez et al., 2001).

Discussion of the factors driving cross-national differences in physical activity is beyond the scope of this chapter. But issues that are relevant might include variations in cultural factors and attitudes to outdoor pursuits, climate, infrastructure for active commuting, habits (such as the frequent use of bicycles in the Netherlands), exercise facilities, availability of green spaces, and physical activity promotion practices.

CROSS-NATIONAL DIFFERENCES IN
PHYSICAL ACTIVITY AND HEALTH

It is apparent from this brief summary of cross-national studies of physical activity that analyses of the contributions of physical activity to differences in longevity can be made only very tentatively. Since the ranking of countries in terms of physical activity is at best moderately consistent across studies, analyses of relationships with health outcomes must be carried out cautiously. In the analyses described in this section, we decided to use data from the Health and Retirement Study (HRS) in the United States, the Survey of Health, Ageing and Retirement in Europe (SHARE), and the English Longitudinal Study of Ageing (ELSA). The reason is that all three employed a similar measure of physical activity in a large population sample of men and women age 50 or older. We analyzed data from Wave 2 of SHARE (2004-2007) from 14 European countries (see http://www.share-project.org/ [accessed June 8, 2010]), Wave 2 of ELSA (see http://www.ifs.org.uk/elsa/ [accessed June 8, 2010]), and the 2004 HRS (see http://hrsonline.isr.umich. edu/ [accessed June 8, 2010]). Participants were asked about the frequency of vigorous physical activity (cycling, digging, running or jogging, swimming, etc.), moderate activities (dancing, gardening, walking at a moderate pace, etc.), and lightly energetic activities (home repairs, laundry, vacuuming) over the past week.

Figure 7-2 summarizes the proportion of respondents in each country who were vigorously or moderately active at least once a week. Values range from a high of 83.2 percent in Sweden to a low of 56 percent in Poland, with the United States (69.3 percent) and England (74.7 percent) appearing in the middle of the distribution. A second measure was derived to assess inactivity. This was the proportion of individuals who had not been vigorously or moderately active at all over the past week (responses of "hardly ever or never"). Broadly, the profile of countries is the reciprocal of that for vigorous or moderate activity (see Figure 7-3), albeit with exceptions.

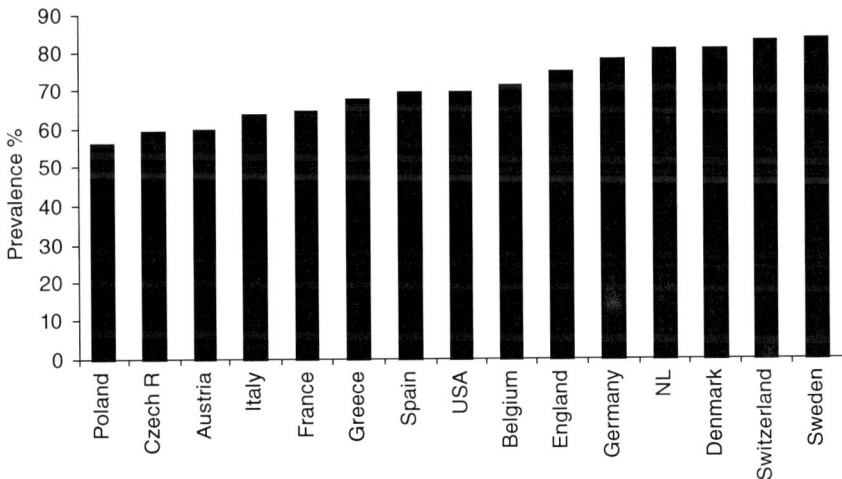

FIGURE 7-2 Proportion of adults age 50 or older who report being moderately or vigorously physically active at least once per week.
NOTE: NL = the Netherlands.
SOURCES: Analyses conducted by the authors based on microdata from Survey of Health, Ageing and Retirement in Europe (SHARE) (see http://www.share-project. org/ [accessed June 22, 2010]) Wave 2, English Longitudinal Study of Ageing (ELSA) (see http://www.ifs.org.uk/elsa/ [accessed June 22, 2010]) Wave 2, and Health and Retirement Study 2004 (see http://hrsonline.isr.umich.edu/ [accessed June 2010]).

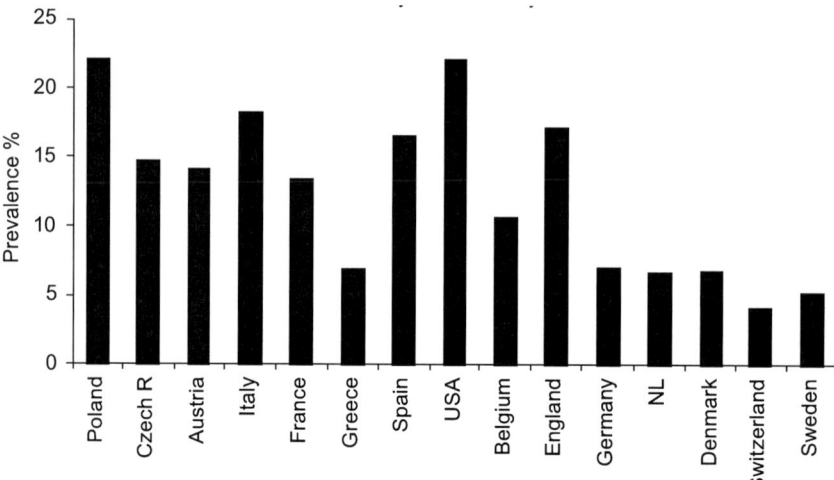

FIGURE 7-3 Proportion of adults age 50 or older who report no moderate or vigorous physical activity.
NOTE: NL = the Netherlands.
SOURCES: Analyses conducted by the authors based on microdata from Survey of Health, Ageing and Retirement in Europe (SHARE) (see http://www.share-project.org/ [accessed June 2010]) Wave 2, English Longitudinal Study of Ageing (ELSA) (see http://www.ifs.org.uk/elsa/ [accessed June 2010]) Wave 2, and Health and Retirement Study 2004 (see http://hrsonline.isr.umich.edu/ [accessed June 2010]).

It is notable that the United States had the highest proportion of inactive respondents (22 percent, matching Poland) and that a relatively large number were also inactive in England (17.1 percent).

In the first set of analyses, we regressed physical activity measures onto the proportion of respondents in each country who rated their own health as only fair or poor, rather than excellent, very good, or good. Significant effects were observed for both men and women, not only for the proportion of individuals who were vigorously or moderately active at least once a week, but also for the proportion who were inactive. Figure 7-4 summarizes results averaged across men and women. In the top panel, it is evident that countries with a higher proportion of individuals who are physically active have a lower prevalence of fair or poor self-rated health ($\beta = -0.866$, 95% C.I. -1.399 to -0.333, $p = 0.004$). Conversely, a high prevalence of inactivity is positively associated with fair or poor self-rated health ($\beta = 1.223$, C.I. 0.400 to 2.046, $p = 0.007$). It should be emphasized that this relationship may not be causal; it could be that poor self-rated health due to physical illness, disability, or mental health problems influences ability or willingness to undertake exercise, or that a third factor affects both self-rated health and physical activity.

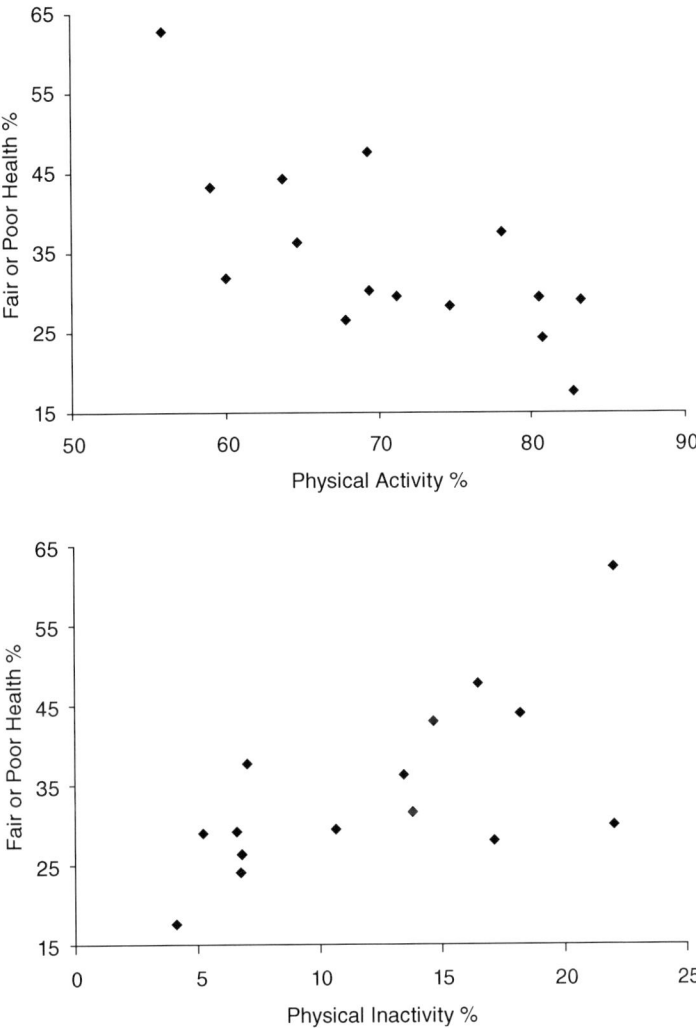

FIGURE 7-4 Scatterplot of the association between fair or poor self-rated health and the proportion of respondents in each country who are vigorously or moderately active at least once a week (upper panel), and the proportion who are inactive (lower panel).
NOTE: Each point represents one country.
SOURCES: Analyses conducted by the authors based on microdata from Survey of Health, Ageing and Retirement in Europe (SHARE) (see http://www.share-project.org/ [accessed June 2010]) Wave 2, English Longitudinal Study of Ageing (ELSA) (see http://www.ifs.org.uk/elsa/ [accessed June 2010]) Wave 2, and Health and Retirement Study 2004 (see http://hrsonline.isr.umich.edu/ [accessed June 2010]).

In addition to analyzing self-rated health, we also assessed associations between reported levels of diabetes and physical activity across countries. Diabetes was selected because of evidence that self-report levels correspond closely with objectively defined diabetes in older adults, at least in England (Pierce et al., 2009). An interesting association between inactivity and the prevalence of diabetes across countries emerged from these analyses ($\beta = 0.320$, C.I. 0.065 to 0.574, $p = 0.018$). As can be seen in Figure 7-5, countries in which a higher proportion of respondents were inactive also had a higher prevalence of diabetes. It should, however, be noted that the prevalence of undetected diabetes may vary across countries and that the impact of these variations on the relationship found in the figure is difficult to estimate.

The measures of both activity and health were derived from the same data sets in these analyses, so their generalizability is uncertain. In order to provide some external validation, a final set of analyses was carried out in which the aggregate estimates of physical activity and inactivity from HRS, ELSA, and SHARE were regressed onto life expectancy at age 50

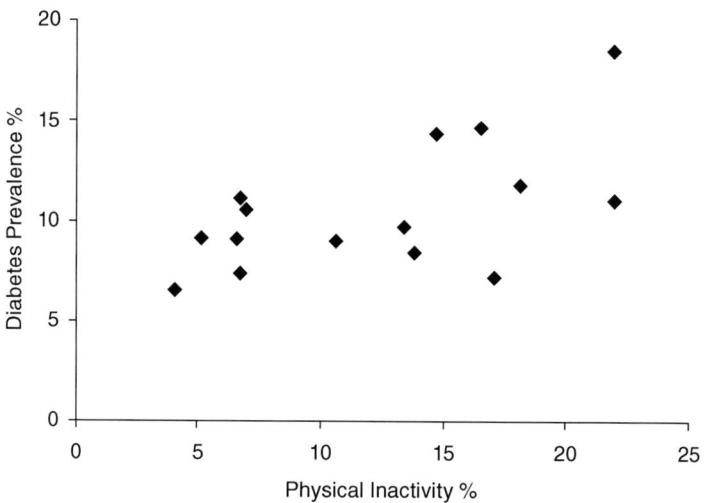

FIGURE 7-5 Scatterplot of the association between self-reported diabetes and the proportion of respondents in each country who are inactive.
NOTE: Each point represents one country.
SOURCES: Analyses conducted by the authors based on microdata from Survey of Health, Ageing and Retirement in Europe (SHARE) (see http://www.share-project.org/ [accessed June 22, 2010]) Wave 2, English Longitudinal Study of Ageing (ELSA) (see http://www.ifs.org.uk/elsa/ [accessed June 2010]) Wave 2, and Health and Retirement Study 2004 (see http://hrsonline.isr.umich.edu/ [accessed June 2010]).

(2004 figures) extracted from the Human Mortality Database (http://www.mortality.org/ [accessed June 8, 2010]). A significant association was observed for life expectancy in men and the proportion reporting vigorous or moderate activity (β = 0.12, 95% C.I. 0.015 to 0.226, p = 0.029), and this is plotted in Figure 7-6. Countries with a higher proportion of vigorously or moderately active men age 50 or older had a greater life expectancy at age 50. The association was strongly influenced by results from the Czech Republic, which had the lowest life expectancy and relatively low prevalence of physically active men. When this country was removed from the analysis, the effect was no longer significant (p = 0.079) although still positive. As can be seen from Figure 7-6, there are also anomalies, such as one country (Denmark) with high activity and relatively low life expectancy, and another (Italy) with low reported activity and high life expectancy. These are bivariate analyses that do not control for other factors, such as smoking or body mass, that might coaggregate with low physical activity. But bearing in mind the likely imprecision of the measure of physical activity, the association is interesting. There was no significant relationship between physical activity

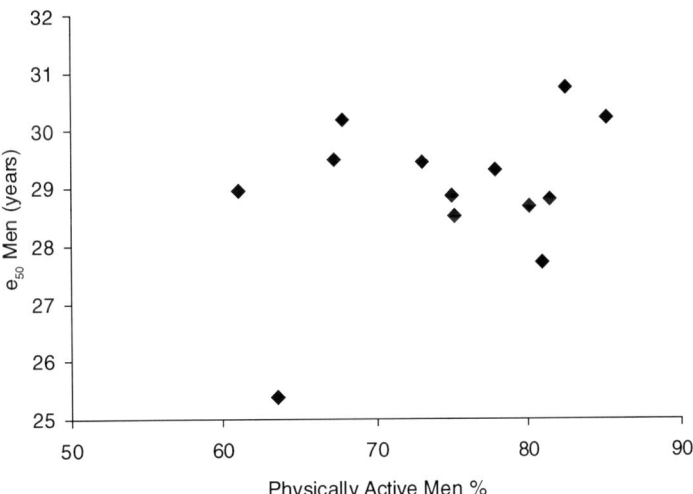

FIGURE 7-6 Scatterplot of the association between life expectancy at age 50 (2004 estimates) in men and the proportion of respondents in each country who are vigorously or moderately active at least once a week.
NOTE: Each point represents one country.
SOURCES: Analyses conducted by the authors based on microdata from Survey of Health, Ageing and Retirement in Europe (SHARE) (see http://www.share-project.org/ [accessed June 2010]) Wave 2, English Longitudinal Study of Ageing (ELSA) (see http://www.ifs.org.uk/elsa/ [accessed June 2010]) Wave 2, and Health and Retirement Study 2004 (see http://hrsonline.isr.umich.edu/ [accessed June 2010]).

and life expectancy among women. The reasons are not clear but could be related to different causes of death or to differences in the suitability of the physical activity measures for men and women.

CONCLUSIONS

The results of the analyses described in the previous section are consistent with the notion that physical activity contributes to cross-national variations in health, but provide only very preliminary evidence. First, the assessments of physical activity were self-reports, and, as argued earlier, these measures are limited. Second, the data from HRS, ELSA, and SHARE are cross-sectional and cannot be interpreted causally; poor self-rated health or the presence of diabetes or other physical or mental health problems may reduce people's activity levels, rather than activity contributing to these health states. Third, the analyses were bivariate and did not control for health behaviors or other factors that may cluster with activity and contribute to morbidity. Fourth, the time course of possible effects of regular physical activity on health outcomes was not considered, and it would be very interesting to track trends in activity over time in relation to changes in longevity. Nonetheless, what these analyses do suggest is that the associations observed among individuals in physical activity and health are reproduced at the ecological level across countries. It is plausible, therefore, that variations in physical activity and in sedentary behavior make a contribution to divergent trends in longevity across nations. Cross-national comparisons of objectively measured physical activity will greatly advance knowledge in this area, as will more sophisticated multivariate analyses of time trends in the activity of people in different countries.

ACKNOWLEDGMENTS

Andrew Steptoe is supported by the British Heart Foundation. We are grateful to Mark Hamer for his comments on earlier drafts of this chapter.

REFERENCES

American College of Sports Medicine. (2005). *ACSM's Guidelines for Exercise Testing and Prescription, (7th ed.)*. New York: Lippincott Williams and Wilkins.

Bauman, A., Bull, F., Chey, T., Craig, C.L., Ainsworth, B.E., Sallis, J.F., Bowles, H.R., Hagstromer, M., Sjöström, M., and Pratt, M. (2009). The International Prevalence Study on Physical Activity: Results from 20 countries. *Journal of Behavioral Nutrition and Physical Activity*, 6, 21.

Bruce, B., Fries, J.F., and Hubert, H. (2008). Regular vigorous physical activity and disability development in healthy overweight and normal-weight seniors: a 13-year study. *American Journal of Public Health*, 98, 1294-1299.

Busse, M.E., van Deursen, R.W., and Wiles, C.M. (2009). Real-life step and activity measurement: Reliability and validity. *Journal of Medical Engineering & Technology, 33*, 33-41.

Byberg, L., Zethelius, B., McKeigue, P.M., and Lithell, H.O. (2001). Changes in physical activity are associated with changes in metabolic cardiovascular risk factors. *Diabetologia, 44*, 2134-2139.

Byberg, L., Melhus, H., Gedeborg, R., Sundstrom, J., Ahlbom, A., Zethelius, B., Berglund, L.G., Wolk, A., and Michaelsson, K. (2009). Total mortality after changes in leisure time physical activity in 50-year-old men: 35-year follow-up of population-based cohort. *British Journal of Sports Medicine, 43*, 482.

Chakravarty, E.F., Hubert, H.B., Lingala, V.B., and Fries, J.F. (2008). Reduced disability and mortality among aging runners: A 21-year longitudinal study. *Archives of Internal Medicine, 168*, 1638-1646.

Chase, N.L., Sui, X., Lee, D.C., and Blair, S.N. (2009). The association of cardiorespiratory fitness and physical activity with incidence of hypertension in men. *American Journal of Hypertension, 22*, 417-424.

Chodzko-Zajko, W.J., Proctor, D.N., Fiatarone Singh, M.A., Minson, C.T., Nigg, C.R., Salem, G.J., and Skinner, J.S. (2009). American College of Sports Medicine position stand: Exercise and physical activity for older adults. *Medicine and Science in Sports and Exercise, 41*, 1510-1530.

Davis, M.G., and Fox, K.R. (2007). Physical activity patterns assessed by accelerometry in older people. *European Journal of Applied Physiology, 100*, 581-589.

Dumurgier, J., Elbaz, A., Ducimetière, P., Tavernier, B., Alpèrovitch, A., and Tzourio, C. (2009). Slow walking speed and cardiovascular death in well functioning older adults: Prospective cohort study. *British Medical Journal, 339*, b4460.

English Longitudinal Study of Ageing. (2010). *English Longitudinal Study of Ageing (ELSA) Wave 2*. Available http://www.ifs.org.uk/elsa/ [accessed June 2010].

Ezzati, M., Hoorn, S.V., Rodgers, A., Lopez, A.D., Mathers, C.D., and Murray, C.J. (2003). Estimates of global and regional potential health gains from reducing multiple major risk factors. *Lancet, 362*, 271-280.

Friedenreich, C.M., and Cust, A.E. (2008). Physical activity and breast cancer risk: Impact of timing, type and dose of activity and population subgroup effects. *British Journal of Sports Medicine, 42*, 636-647.

Friedenreich, C.M., Courneya, K.S., Neilson, H.K., Matthews, C.E., Willis, G., Irwin, M., Troiano, R., and Ballard-Barbash, R. (2006). Reliability and validity of the Past Year Total Physical Activity Questionnaire. *American Journal of Epidemiology, 163*, 959-970.

Haftenberger, M., Schuit, A.J., Tormo, M.J., Boeing, H., Wareham, N., Bueno-de-Mesquita, H.B., Kumle, M., Hjartaker, A., Chirlaque, M.D., Ardanaz, E., Andren, C., Lindahl, B., Peeters, P.H., Allen, N.E., Overvad, K., Tjonneland, A., Clavel-Chapelon, F., Linseisen, J., Bergmann, M.M., Trichopoulou, A., Lagiou, P., Salvini, S., Panico, S., Riboli, E., Ferrari, P., and Slimani, N. (2002). Physical activity of subjects aged 50-64 years involved in the European Prospective Investigation into Cancer and Nutrition (EPIC). *Public Health Nutrition, 5*, 1163-1176.

Hagstromer, M., Oja, P., and Sjöström, M. (2006). The International Physical Activity Questionnaire (IPAQ): A study of concurrent and construct validity. *Public Health Nutrition, 9*, 755-762.

Hagstromer, M., Oja, P., and Sjöström, M. (2007). Physical activity and inactivity in an adult population assessed by accelerometry. *Medicine and Science in Sports and Exercise, 39*, 1502-1508.

Hamer, M., and Chida, Y. (2008). Active commuting and cardiovascular risk: A meta-analytic review. *Preventive Medicine, 46*, 9-13.

Hamer, M., and Chida, Y. (2009). Physical activity and risk of neurodegenerative disease: A systematic review of prospective evidence. *Psychological Medicine, 39*, 3-11.

Hamer, M., Kivimaki, M., Yerramasu, A., Lahiri, A., Deanfield, J.E., Marmot, M.G., and Steptoe, A. (in press). Walking speed and subclinical atherosclerosis in healthy older adults: The Whitehall II Study. Submitted to *Heart*.

Harris, T.J., Owen, C.G., Victor, C.R., Adams, R., and Cook, D.G. (2009a). What factors are associated with physical activity in older people, assessed objectively by accelerometry? *British Journal of Sports Medicine, 43*, 442-450.

Harris, T.J., Owen, C.G., Victor, C.R., Adams, R., Ekelund, U., and Cook, D.G. (2009b). A comparison of questionnaire, accelerometer, and pedometer: Measures in older people. *Medicine and Science in Sports and Exercise, 41*, 1392-1402.

Health and Retirement Study. (2004). *Health and Retirement Study (HRS)*. Available: http://hrsonline.isr.umich.edu/ [accessed June 2010].

Heesch, K.C., Byles, J.E., and Brown, W.J. (2008). Prospective association between physical activity and falls in community-dwelling older women. *Journal of Epidemiology and Community Health, 62*, 421-426.

Kelley, G.A., and Kelley, K.S. (2006). Effects of aerobic exercise on C-reactive protein, body composition, and maximum oxygen consumption in adults: A meta-analysis of randomized controlled trials. *Metabolism, 55*, 1500-1507.

Kelley, G.A., and Kelley, K.S. (2007). Effects of aerobic exercise on lipids and lipoproteins in adults with type 2 diabetes: A meta-analysis of randomized-controlled trials. *Public Health, 121*, 643-655.

Landi, F., Russo, A., Cesari, M., Pahor, M., Liperoti, R., Danese, P., Bernabei, R., and Onder, G. (2008). Walking one hour or more per day prevented mortality among older persons: Results from ilSIRENTE study. *Preventive Medicine, 47*(4), 422-426.

Langer, D., Hendriks, E.J.M., Burtin, C., Probst, V., van der Schans, C.P., Paterson, W.J., Verhoef-de Wijk, M.C.E., Straver, R.V.M., Klaassen, M., Troosters, T., Decramer, M., Ninane, V., Delguste, P., Muris, J., Gosselink, R. (2009). A clinical practice guideline for physiotherapists treating patients with chronic obstructive pulmonary disease based on a systematic review of available evidence. *Clinical Rehabilitation, 23*, 445-462.

Manson, J.E., Greenland, P., LaCroix, A.Z., Stefanick, M.L., Mouton, C.P., Oberman, A., Perri, M.G., Sheps, D.S., Pettinger, M.B., and Siscovick, D.S. (2002). Walking compared with vigorous exercise for the prevention of cardiovascular events in women. *New England Journal of Medicine, 347*, 716-725.

Martin, C.K., Church, T.S., Thompson, A.M., Earnest, C.P., and Blair, S.N. (2009). Exercise dose and quality of life: A randomized controlled trial. *Archives of Internal Medicine, 169*, 269-278.

Martinez-Gonzalez, M.A., Varo, J.J., Santos, J.L., De Irala, J., Gibney, M., Kearney, J., and Martinez, J.A. (2001). Prevalence of physical activity during leisure time in the European Union. *Medicine and Science in Sports and Exercise, 33*, 1142-1146.

Matthews, C.E. (2005). Calibration of accelerometer output for adults. *Medicine and Science in Sports and Exercise, 37*, S512-S522.

Matthews, C.E., Chen, K.Y., Freedson, P.S., Buchowski, M.S., Beech, B.M., Pate, R.R., and Troiano, R.P. (2008). Amount of time spent in sedentary behaviors in the United States, 2003-2004. *American Journal of Epidemiology, 167*, 875-881.

Orozco, L.J., Buchleitner, A.M., Gimenez-Perez, G., Roque, I.F.M., Richter, B., and Mauricio, D. (2008). Exercise or exercise and diet for preventing type 2 diabetes mellitus. *Cochrane Database of Systematic Reviews*, CD003054.

Physical Activity Guidelines Advisory Committee. (2008). *Physical Activity Guidelines Advisory Committee Report, 2008*. Washington, DC: U.S. Department of Health and Human Services.

Pierce, M.B., Zaninotto, P., Steel, N., and Mindell, J. (2009). Undiagnosed diabetes: Data from the English Longitudinal Study of Ageing. *Diabetic Medicine, 26*, 679-685.

Rikli, R.E. (2000). Reliability, validity, and methodological issues in assessing physical activity in older adults. *Research Quarterly for Exercise & Sport, 71*, S89-S96.

Seeman, T., and Chen, X. (2002). Risk and protective factors for physical functioning in older adults with and without chronic conditions: MacArthur Studies of Successful Aging. *Journals of Gerontology Series B: Psychological Sciences and Social Sciences, 57*, S135-S144.

Shephard, R.J. (2003). Limits to the measurement of habitual physical activity by questionnaires. *British Journal of Sports Medicine, 37*, 197-206.

Sjöström, M., Oja, P., Hagstromer, M., Smith, B.J., and Bauman, A. (2006). Health-enhancing physical activity across European Union countries: The Eurobarometer study. *Journal of Public Health, 14*, 291-300.

Sofi, F., Capalbo, A., Cesari, F., Abbate, R., and Gensini, G.F. (2008). Physical activity during leisure time and primary prevention of coronary heart disease: An updated meta-analysis of cohort studies. *European Journal of Cardiovascular Prevention & Rehabilitation, 15*, 247-257.

Stel, V.S., Smit, J.H., Pluijm, S.M., Visser, M., Deeg, D.J., and Lips, P. (2004). Comparison of the LASA Physical Activity Questionnaire with a 7-day diary and pedometer. *Journal of Clinical Epidemiology, 57*, 252-258.

Steptoe, A. (2006). Depression and physical activity. In A. Steptoe (Ed.), *Depression and Physical Illness* (pp. 348-368). Cambridge: Cambridge University Press.

Stessman, J., Hammerman-Rozenberg, R., Cohen, A., Ein-Mor, E., and Jacobs, J.M. (2009). Physical activity, function, and longevity among the very old. *Archives of Internal Medicine, 169*, 1476-1483.

Survey of Health, Ageing and Retirement in Europe. (2010). *SHARE—Survey of Health, Ageing and Retirement in Europe.* Available: http://www.share-project.org/ [accessed June 2010].

Tinetti, M.E. (2003). Clinical practice. preventing falls in elderly persons. *New England Journal of Medicine, 348*, 42-49.

Troiano, R.P., Berrigan, D., Dodd, K.W., Masse, L.C., Tilert, T., and McDowell, M. (2008). Physical activity in the United States measured by accelerometer. *Medicine and Science in Sports and Exercise, 40*, 181-188.

U.S. Department of Health and Human Services. (2008). *2008 Physical Activity Guidelines for Americans.* Washington, DC: Author. Available: http://www.health.gov/paguidelines [accessed June 2010].

van Dam, R.M., Li, T., Spiegelman, D., Franco, O.H., and Hu, F.B. (2008). Combined impact of lifestyle factors on mortality: Prospective cohort study in US women. *British Medical Journal, 337*, a1440.

Washburn, R.A., and Ficker, J.L. (1999). Physical Activity Scale for the Elderly (PASE): The relationship with activity measured by a portable accelerometer. *Journal of Sports Medicine and Physical Fitness, 39*, 336-340.

Wei, M., Gibbons, L.W., Kampert, J.B., Nichaman, M.Z., and Blair, S.N. (2000). Low cardiorespiratory fitness and physical inactivity as predictors of mortality in men with type 2 diabetes. *Annals of Internal Medicine, 132*, 605-611.

Wendel-Vos, G.C., Schuit, A.J., Feskens, E.J., Boshuizen, H.C., Verschuren, W.M., Saris, W.H., and Kromhout, D. (2004). Physical activity and stroke: A meta-analysis of observational data. *International Journal of Epidemiology, 33*, 787-798.

Westerterp, K.R. (2009). Assessment of physical activity: A critical appraisal. *European Journal of Applied Physiology, 105*, 823-828.

Wolin, K.Y., Yan, Y., Colditz, G.A., and Lee, I.M. (2009). Physical activity and colon cancer prevention: A meta-analysis. *British Journal of Cancer, 100*, 611-616.

World Health Organization. (2009). *Global Health Risks: Mortality and Burden of Disease Attributable to Selected Major Risks.* Geneva, Switzerland: Author.

Yates, L.B., Djousse, L., Kurth, T., Buring, J.E., and Gaziano, J.M. (2008). Exceptional longevity in men: Modifiable factors associated with survival and function to age 90 years. *Archives of Internal Medicine, 168,* 284-290.

Yusuf, S., Hawken, S., Ounpuu, S., Dans, T., Avezum, A., Lanas, F., McQueen, M., Budaj, A., Pais, P., Varigos, J., and Lisheng, L. (2004). Effect of potentially modifiable risk factors associated with myocardial infarction in 52 countries (the INTERHEART study): Case-control study. *Lancet, 364,* 937-952.

8

Do Cross-Country Variations in Social Integration and Social Interactions Explain Differences in Life Expectancy in Industrialized Countries?

*James Banks, Lisa Berkman, and James P. Smith
with Mauricio Avendano and Maria Glymour*

INTRODUCTION

Variations in life expectancy among industrialized countries have been attributed to differences in patterns of health behavior, health care, socioeconomic conditions, and variations in social and economic policies. In this chapter, we explore whether variations in morbidity, mortality, and life expectancy are related to variations in the extent to which countries have different levels of social integration or social support. Extensive research suggests that aspects of social networks and social integration may be associated with mortality in a number of countries (Berkman and Syme, 1979; Berkman et al., 2004; Blazer, 1982; Fuhrer and Stansfeld, 2002; Fuhrer et al., 1999; House, Robbins, and Metzner, 1982; Kaplan et al., 1988; Khang and Kim, 2005; Orth-Gomer and Johnson, 1987; Orth-Gomer, Rosengren, and Wilhelmsen, 1993; Orth-Gomer, Unden, and Edwards, 1988; Orth-Gomer et al., 1998; Penninx et al., 1998; Sugisawa, Liang, and Liu, 1994; Welin et al., 1985). But in no studies have we been able to compare either risks or distributions of comparably defined social networks across countries, nor have we been able to understand if variations in social networks and social participation might explain cross-country variations in population health.

We explore these issues from several perspectives. Ideally, we want to assess the variability in distributions of social networks and support in many countries. We would also like to identify whether risks associated with social isolation and various health outcomes are the same in each country. For social networks and support to "explain" cross-country differences in life expectancy, at least one of two conditions must be met. First, a different fraction of the population needs to be exposed to risk factors across countries. Second, the health risk—"toxicity"—associated with risk factors might differ between countries. For common risk factors, even small differences in toxicity may have large population health effects. Differences in toxicity could occur if population differences in exacerbating or compensatory factors influence the risk of disease. For example, if countries had public policies protecting citizens against deleterious health effects of extreme poverty, we might not see health effects manifest themselves there, even though poverty was present. Third, we would hope to assess in a single model whether social integration and support can account for cross-country differences in life expectancy. In this chapter we examine the first two but do not have adequate data to test the third in a compelling way, except for a comparison of England and the United States.

The lack of truly harmonized individual-level data across countries on relevant exposures and health outcomes over time limits our ability to examine this question. To overcome this limitation, we start by comparing associations between social integration and social support in the United States and England, using data from the Health and Retirement Survey (HRS) and the English Longitudinal Study of Ageing (ELSA). Although not identical, these surveys have very comparable measurements of social networks and social support, as well as comparable data on health conditions and associated risks. We then consider ways in which related psychosocial conditions tapping dimensions of stress may explain observed health variations between the United States and England. We examine these questions for a variety of self-reported outcomes and measured biomarkers of disease. In addition, we use the mortality follow-up in HRS and ELSA to examine impacts of social networks and interactions on all-cause mortality.

Since differences in life expectancy between the United States and England are relatively small, we then examine how 28 industrialized countries vary on several dimensions of social networks and support. In these analyses, we draw on recent data from the Gallup World Poll for Japan and a number of European and North American countries. We present data on the distribution of dimensions of social integration explored in our HRS/ELSA comparisons. Although the items are not fully identical, they provide us with a general overview of variations in these dimensions in a wider set of countries. We conclude with suggestions for carrying this work forward by exploring whether variability in social networks is related to a country's level of health and well-being.

The chapter is divided into four sections. First, we compare morbidity and health risks in England and the United States by social networks and support, using cross-sectional data from HRS and ELSA. Second, we briefly report on whether other psychosocial stressors often related to social networks may help explain cross-country differences. Third, we examine mortality risks associated with these social networks in ELSA and HRS. In the last section, we use data from Gallup to examine the extent to which countries vary on domains related to social networks, social integration, and support.

We were unable to explore whether social networks actually explain diverging trends in life expectancy because we do not have data on long-term trends in these conditions across countries. However, this is a first attempt at addressing this question by exploring whether such conditions are able to explain variations in health outcomes contemporaneously and whether variations are large enough in and of themselves to be able to explain diverging trends. We conclude with a summary of our findings and a discussion of strengths and weaknesses of the work as well as ideas for how to extend work in this area.

SOCIAL NETWORKS, SUPPORT, AND HEALTH IN THE UNITED STATES AND ENGLAND

In this section we provide a descriptive portrait of social networks and social support of older residents in the United States and England and examine their association with health outcomes. We concentrate on the United States and England because the most comparable, comprehensive data on social networks and social support are available for them. A recent study (Banks et al., 2006) documented large health differences between England and the United States, and it is possible that social network and social support differences may explain the U.S. disadvantage in health.

Data

For the United States, our research is based on the Health and Retirement Survey, a nationally representative survey that now includes more than 20,000 people over age 50 in the United States (Juster and Suzman, 1995). HRS began in 1991, and new cohorts have been subsequently added to maintain population representation of this age segment. Respondents are reinterviewed biannually.

For England, we use the English Longitudinal Survey of Ageing, which contains around 12,000 respondents recruited from 3 separate years of the Health Survey for England (HSE) providing representative samples of the English population age 50 and over (Marmot et al., 2002). The health data were supplemented by social and economic data collected in the first ELSA wave, fielded in 2002. Like HRS, the initial baseline sample was of the noninstitutionized population, and follow-ups (including of those subsequently moving into institutions) are conducted every 2 years. However, since the ELSA study is still a younger study, in the sense that the baseline is more recent, it will presumably be less representative of the entire population age 50 and over (including those in institutions).

For our analysis we selected key health and social network and support constructs in which strong a priori measurement comparability existed. The 2004 waves of ELSA and HRS were used for analysis, since this was the year in which HRS first contained social network and social support variables directly comparable to those collected in ELSA.

Measures of Chronic Conditions, Biomarkers of Disease Risk, and Health Behaviors

Both surveys collect data on individual self-reports of diseases in the form "Did a doctor ever tell you that you had ___?" In addition, both studies have biomarkers of diabetes risk (HbA1c) and have assessed blood pressure. These two biomarkers permit us to assess diabetes and hypertension status more reliably. The specific diseases analyzed include diabetes (assessed by either self-report of diabetes or HbA1c over 6.5 percent), hypertension (assessed by measured systolic blood pressure ≥ 140 or diastolic blood pressure ≥ 90 or self-report of hypertensive medication), self-reported heart disease, pulmonary function (using a clinical assessment of peak flow), and obesity (body mass index, BMI, ≥ 30).

Lung function in HRS was measured using peak flow (averaged over 3 measures), and in ELSA it was measured with forced expiratory volume (FEV). To account for this difference, we show parameter estimates for each social indicator as a percentage of the average for the reference group. These measures operate similarly with this transformation, as the effect estimated for smoking on lung function is similar in both HRS and ELSA. The two surveys also collect several health-related behaviors in common, including smoking (currently and ever smoked), alcohol consumption (heavy drinking defined as drinking on more than 4 days per week in HRS and twice a day or more/daily or almost daily in ELSA). While other risk factors may be important, we used only these comparably measured variables in our multivariate models.

Measures of Social Networks, Social Support, and Negative Interactions

Measures of the size of social networks and various forms of social participation and quality of social support available to individuals were measured in both surveys using almost identical questionnaires. One key advantage of using these two surveys is that their comparable questions cover many key domains of the social network. Questions were asked in several domains about relationships with children, partners, close family members, and friends. In addition, the surveys included questions about voluntary activities. With regard to children, in addition to the number of children, respondents were asked about the frequency of their interactions with their children on a 4-point scale (a lot, some, a little, not at all). We coded these scores numerically from 0 to 3.

Three questions address elements of positive interaction: (1) do your children really understand the way you feel about things, (2) can you rely on them if you have a serious problem, and (3) can you open up to them if you need to talk about your worries. The other three address negative interactions: (1) how much do your children criticize you, (2) how much do they let you down when you are counting on them, and (3) how much do they get on your nerves. We separated these into two components—positive support and negative interactions—and summed the numerical scores. The total scores for both positive support and negative support vary between 0 and 9. So that high scores on positive and negative interactions mean the same thing, the top score of 9 for negative interactions implies no negative interactions.

HRS and ELSA respondents were asked (not counting those children living with you) about the frequency of contact with children on three dimensions: (1) meeting (arranged and chance meetings), (2) speaking on the phone, and (3) writing an email. The scale for each dimension consists of six possible categories: (1) three or more times a week, (2) once or twice a week, (3) once or twice a month, (4) every few months, (5) once or twice a year, and (6) less than once a year or never. Finally, respondents were asked with how many children they have a close relationship. Our measure does not distinguish between individuals without children and individuals with children who are not close or not in contact, since our measure is intended to capture contact, which would be zero in both cases. However, to assess whether differences between childless individuals and those with children are influencing our results, we also estimated our models for the sample of those with children only. The results were broadly unaffected, with one exception: the social estimated interaction effects were slightly weaker, suggesting that some of the identification of these effects was coming from differences between the childless and those with children. However, since all substantive conclusions of our analysis were unaffected (indeed, if the interaction effects are weaker, our conclusions are strengthened) we do not present this analysis in the tables of results.

Respondents were also asked the same set of questions about positive and negative interactions, frequency of contact, and the number of close relationships they have with other immediate family members, defined as siblings, parents, cousins, or grandchildren. Friends are also a potentially important component of any support network. HRS and ELSA ask the same set of questions (positive and negative interactions), frequency of contact, and number of friends. Scales for positive and negative interactions and frequency of contact are scored in the same way as for children: scores were translated into a scale that ranges from 0 to 9. In the data in these analyses we have summed the total of either positive or negative social interactions across children, friends, and relatives. High scores represent high levels of positive interaction or low levels of negative interactions (in both cases, "high" is the more optimal interaction).

Questions about social participation in voluntary and civic organizations and religious attendance were also asked. In HRS, the item about voluntary activity was framed in terms of frequency of participation, whereas in ELSA it was asked as the number of organizations the participant belonged to. Ties with religious organizations were assessed by attendance. Finally, we developed a summary index of social integration that summed network domains related to children, partner, friends, and relatives and volunteer and religious activities into a single score. This index has six dimensions: (1) married/partnered, (2) frequency of visits with children, (3) frequency of visits with family, (4) frequency of visits with friends, (5) participation in voluntary organizations, and (6) religious attendance. The score could range from 0 to 16, with 0 reflecting no tie and 3 in each domain reflecting high levels of contact. Religious attendance, however, was scored 0 or 1 due to limitations in the availability of more nuanced measures in the ELSA questionnaire (in the HRS-only analysis of mortality, we were able to distinguish between those attending religious services regularly and those attending periodically, and this distinction did prove to be important).

COMPARISONS BETWEEN ENGLAND AND THE UNITED STATES

There are several ways of characterizing social networks, including the existence, number, and type of key people in the network and the nature of interactions taking place, both positive and negative. Although we examined each social network domain individually, in this section we provide tables or figures on summary measures related only to the social network index, the summary measure, and positive and negative social interactions. We describe social networks in England and the United States for spouses, children, other immediate family members, and friends.

Distribution of Social Networks

We begin with a description of an aggregate index of social networks in the two countries. While there are some differences in how older men and women maintain contact with friends, family, and larger civic, religious, and voluntary organizations, the overall distribution of social networks is virtually identical in the two countries.

Figures 8-1A and 8-1B show the distribution of scores for our overall

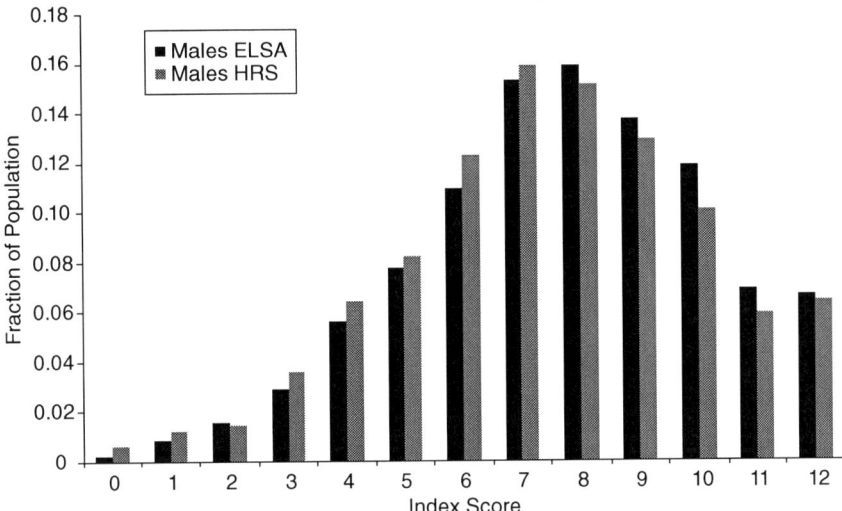

FIGURE 8-1A Distribution of scores of the index of social networks in England and the United States among men.
SOURCES: Authors' calculations from the Health and Retirement Survey (2004) and the English Longitudinal Study of Ageing (2004) microdata.

index of social networks for men and women in HRS and ELSA. For both men and women, the largest numbers of people scored in the mid-range, between 6 and 9, and this concentration of scores is almost identical in England and the United States. Women tended to be slightly more isolated than men, but even among U.S. women (the most isolated), only around 5 percent of older women scored 2 or lower on the summary index.

Some differences in the frequency of contact of specific ties are of some note, but these differences are unlikely to be sufficiently large to explain cross-country variations in health or life expectancy. The prevalence of those with partners, children, other family members, and friends are listed in Table 8-1. Overall, the percentages of those with children are almost identical in the two countries, but there are some cohort differences. Among men and women age 75 and over (those born before 1930), U.S. men and women were more likely to have children than their English counterparts, reflecting greater fertility in the United States among those cohorts. In addition, U.S. men, particularly those ages 65+, were more likely to be living with a partner. Among more recent cohorts (those born in 1940 or later), English men and women were more likely to have children than their U.S. counterparts.

There are conflicting data on closeness of contact and relationship with children in the two countries. For all birth cohorts ages 50+, English

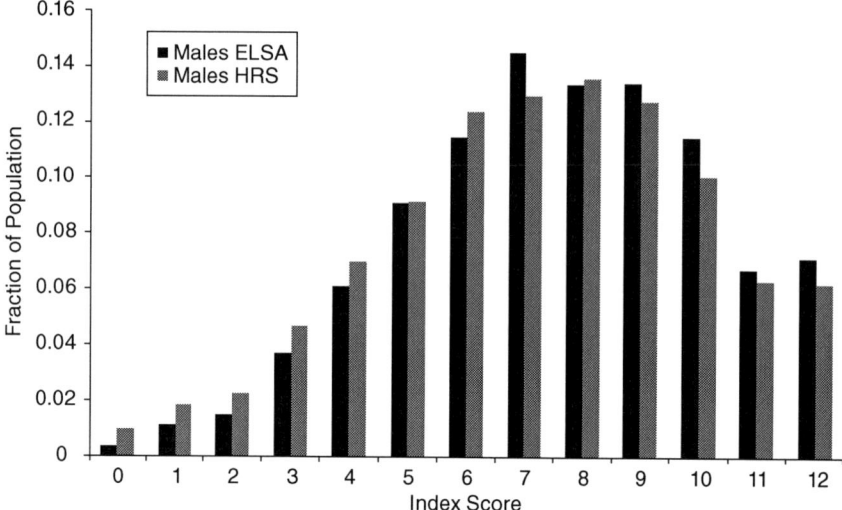

FIGURE 8-1B Distribution of scores of index of social networks in England and the United States among women.
SOURCES: Authors' calculations from the Health and Retirement Study (2004) and the English Longitudinal Study of Ageing (2004) microdata.

TABLE 8-1 Distributions of Social Networks in England and the United States

Age Group	England	USA	England Male	England Female	USA Male	USA Female
Percentage with Spouse/Partner						
50-64	81.3	76.0	85.0	78.7	83.0	71.2
65-74	70.0	75.7	79.9	60.8	85.8	67.8
75 plus	47.6	55.1	65.8	32.1	77.1	39.0
Total	71.9	72.2	79.6	63.4	83.0	64.4
Percentage with Children						
50-64	87.2	85.5	84.5	89.4	83.3	87.0
65-74	86.9	90.1	86.5	87.3	88.9	91.0
75 plus	81.0	83.2	82.3	80.1	85.2	81.8
Total	85.9	86.7	84.7	86.9	85.8	87.5
Percentage with Friends						
50-64	94.0	89.4	93.0	94.8	88.9	89.8
65-74	90.0	90.3	87.7	91.9	88.9	91.3
75 plus	85.1	88.3	81.7	87.5	85.6	90.3
Total	91.2	85.9	89.5	92.6	88.3	90.4

SOURCES: Authors' calculations from the Health and Retirement Study (2004) and the English Longitudinal Study of Ageing (2004) microdata.

men and women with children were more likely to see them at least once a month: 67 percent of English women said that they met with their children at least once a month compared with 62 percent of U.S. women. Comparable numbers for English men and U.S. men are 62 and 56 percent, respectively. These differences may not be surprising, given the relative size of the two countries and much lower mobility among the English compared with Americans. However, one-third of Americans in this age range stated that they are close to three or more of their children compared with a quarter of the English.

Distributions and means of positive interactions with children, friends, and relatives are shown in Figure 8-2A for women and men, and the distribution of negative interactions in Figure 8-2B. There are some differences between the two countries. U.S. men and women reported somewhat lower levels of both positive and negative interactions with children, but there is a clear preretirement and postretirement distinction to this pattern. Preretirement positive interactions with children were worse for Americans, presumably representing a conflict with work. But in postretirement (i.e., after age 65), the pattern switches, and Americans had greater levels of positive interactions with their children. Americans tended to lag behind the English, in that they experienced more negative interactions with children at all these ages. With other family members, however, Americans tended to experience both greater positive interactions and greater absence of negative interactions than their English counterparts. Interestingly, there were no cross-country differences in distributions of positive and negative interactions with friends.

Relationship Between Social Networks, Positive and Negative Interactions, and Five Health Outcomes

Previous evidence suggests that U.S. men and women have higher prevalence of many chronic diseases than their English counterparts (Banks et al., 2006). Table 8-2 shows means of selected health measures in ELSA and HRS, which confirm that Americans had worse health than the English, both using self-reports and biomarkers of disease. Our aim here is twofold: to assess whether associations between social networks and support and morbidity and health risks are similar between countries and to examine whether differences in prevalence of these risk factors can account for observed cross-country variations in health between the United States and England.

Since in most cases distributions of social relations were very similar, our goal was to see if risks or benefits of social relations varied more or less in one country or the other. The weakness of cross-sectional analyses is that it is impossible to determine which condition is shaping the other. In the case

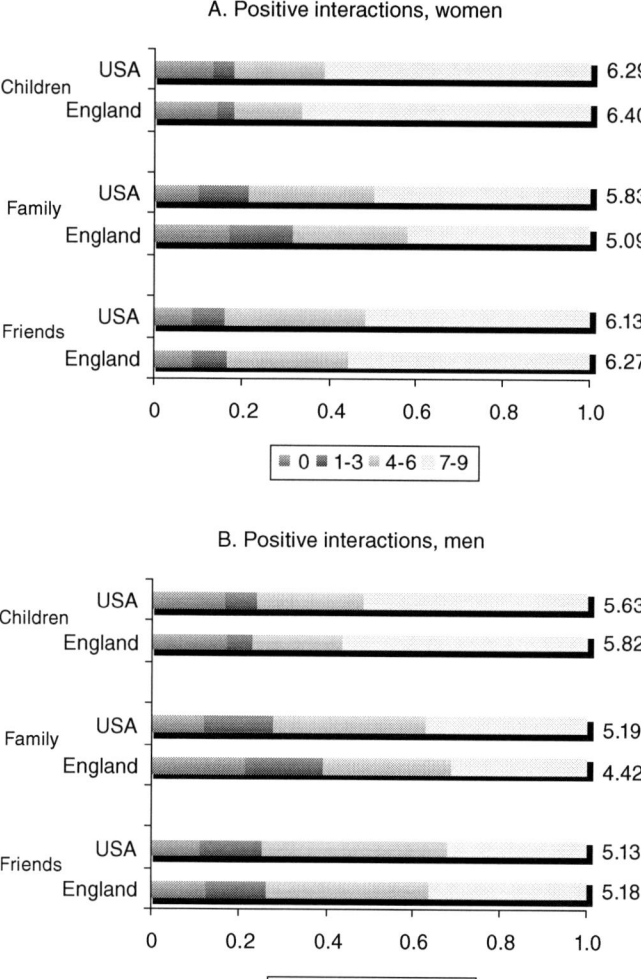

FIGURE 8-2A The distribution of positive interactions with children, family, and friends.
SOURCES: Authors' calculations from the Health and Retirement Study (2004) and the English Longitudinal Study of Ageing (2004) microdata.

of social relations and chronic morbidity, it is very likely that the relations are bidirectional, with strong social ties and support influencing health in a positive way and poor health itself placing stresses on social ties and making interactions difficult. Still, acute illnesses tend to elicit greater expressions of social support, and the provision of care for an ill or disabled family member often requires frequent contact. These processes may create a spurious as-

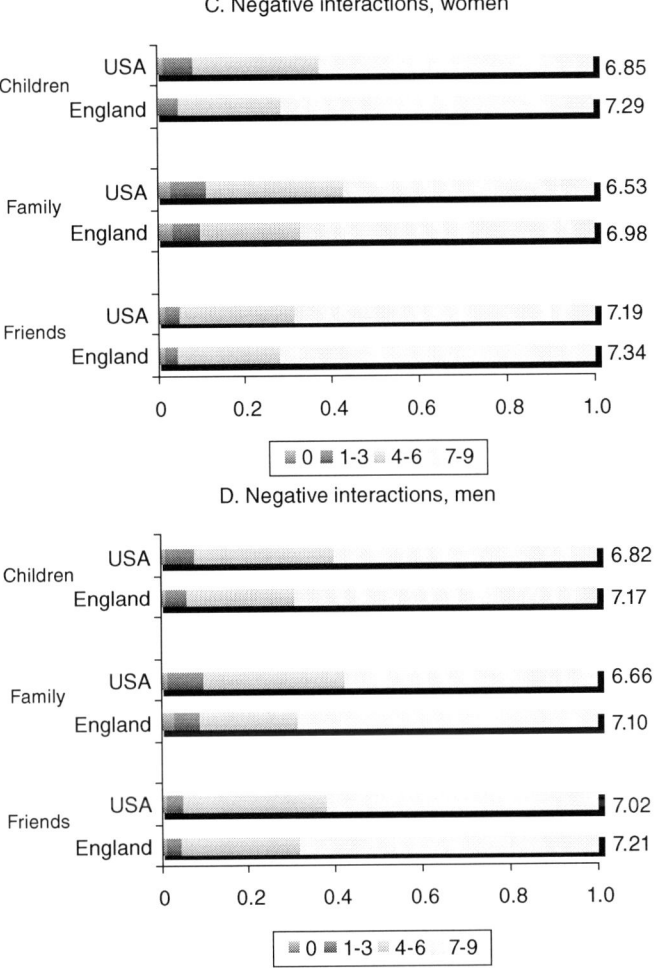

FIGURE 8-2B The distribution of negative interactions with children, family, and friends.
SOURCES: Authors' calculations from the Health and Retirement Study (2004) and the English Longitudinal Study of Ageing (2004) microdata.

sociation between support and poor health in cross-sectional analyses. We conducted cross-sectional analyses on each subdomain of social ties (with children, family, friends, and partners and social and religious activities) as well as associations with interactions with children, friends, and relatives. In this section, we present cross-sectional associations between summary measures of social ties, negative interactions, and partnership in relation

TABLE 8-2 Means of Selected Health Outcomes Among Men and Women in HRS (United States) and ELSA (England)

Variable	HRS		ELSA	
	Mean	STD	Mean	STD
Diabetes	0.20	0.40	0.07	0.26
Hypertension	0.57	0.50	0.44	0.50
Heart	0.23	0.42	0.16	0.36
HbA1c > 6.5%	0.22	0.42	0.09	0.28
SBP ≥ 140 or DBP ≥ 90 or on medication	0.69	0.46	0.60	0.49
Obesity	0.38	0.49	0.29	0.45
Peak flow	341.26	129.40	371.80	143.04
BMI	29.07	5.49	27.89	4.79

NOTES: BMI = body mass index, DBP = diastolic blood pressure, ELSA = English Longitudinal Study of Ageing, HRS = Health and Retirement Survey, SBP = systolic blood pressure.
SOURCES: Authors' calculations from the Health and Retirement Study (2004) and the English Longitudinal Study of Ageing (2004) microdata.

to five health outcomes: hypertension, diabetes, heart disease, obesity, and pulmonary function assessed from a measure of peak flow.

Figures 8-3A and 8-3B show the odds ratios for men and women, respectively, between the social network index and the prevalence of obesity, hypertension, diabetes, and self-reported heart disease. Figure 8-3C shows the association with pulmonary function and the network index for women and men. In these figures, we indicate a statistically significant estimate by an asterisk.

The social network index is not associated with any health outcomes for men with one exception: men with high levels of ties reported somewhat higher levels of heart disease in the United States. Among women in England and the United States, high levels of ties were related to lower health risks, with the exception of obesity. U.S. women with more ties had higher obesity. The social network index is significantly and positively associated with lung function among women in the United States but in not in other groups.

Figures 8-4A, 8-4B, and 8-4C show the relationship between partnership status and the same five health conditions. For both U.S. and English men, having a partner was associated with better lung function. Among English men, having a partner was also associated with lower odds of having hypertension. No other conditions were associated with partnership status among men. Among U.S. women, partnership was associated with lower prevalence of obesity, hypertension, and diabetes. Among English women, partnership was associated only with a lower prevalence of hypertension.

Negative interactions were more strongly related to prevalent health conditions than positive interactions, suggesting the importance of incorporating these measures into further research. Among both English and U.S.

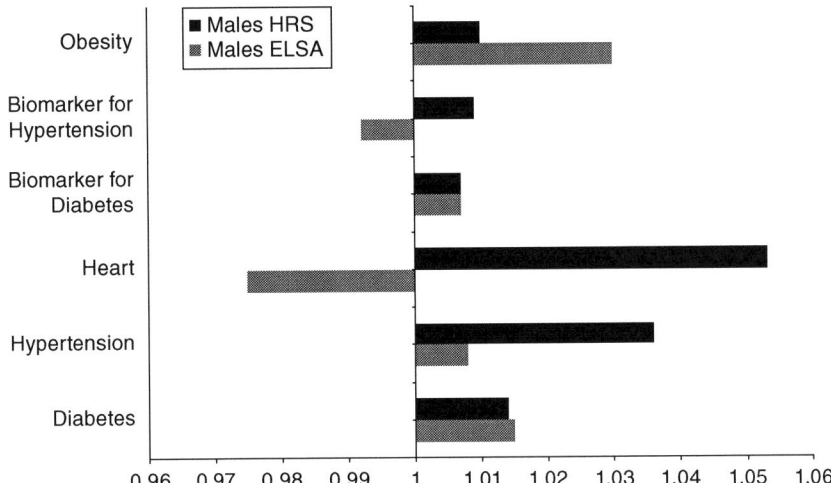

FIGURE 8-3A Odds ratios of disease prevalence for a one-point increase in the social network index for men.
SOURCES: Authors' calculations from the Health and Retirement Study (2004) and the English Longitudinal Study of Ageing (2004) microdata.

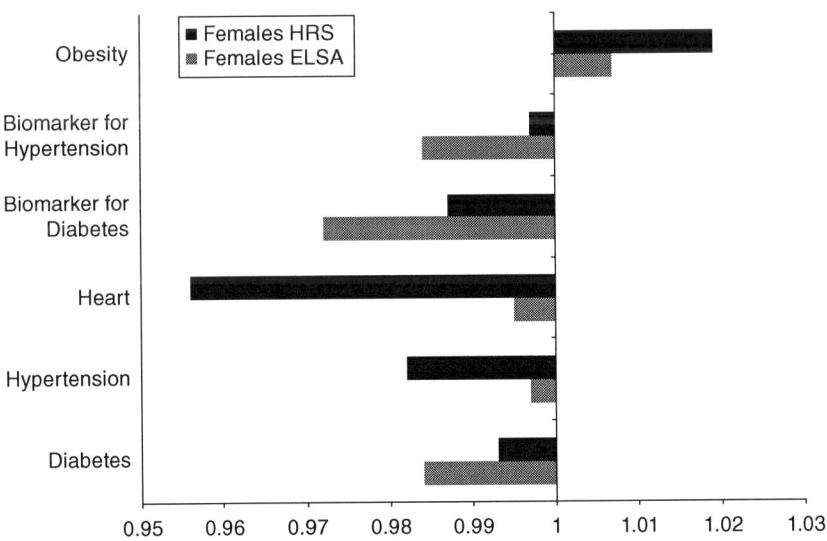

FIGURE 8-3B Odds ratios of disease prevalence for a one-point increase in the social network index for women.
SOURCES: Authors' calculations from the Health and Retirement Study (2004) and the English Longitudinal Study of Ageing (2004) microdata.

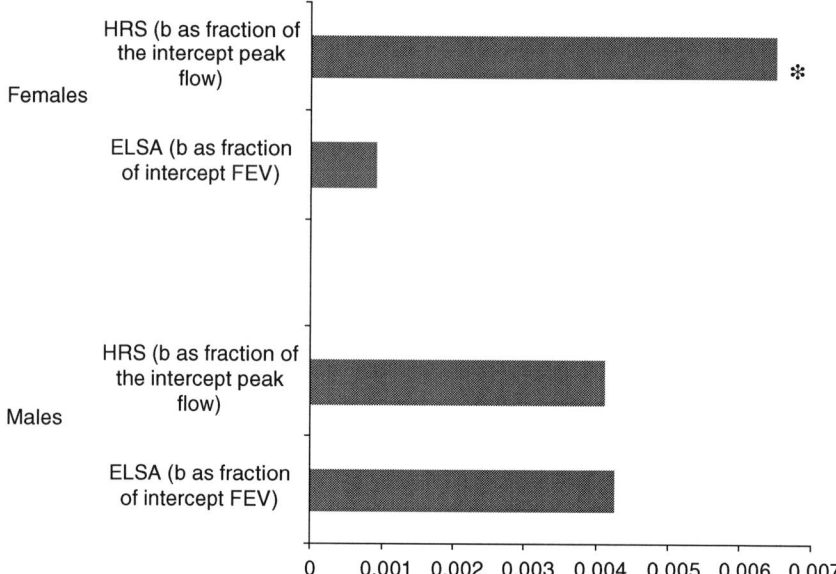

FIGURE 8-3C Association between pulmonary function and the network index for men and women.
NOTES: Statistical significance is indicated by an asterisk, FEV = forced expiratory volume.
SOURCES: Authors' calculations from the Health and Retirement Study (2004) and the English Longitudinal Study of Ageing (2004) microdata.

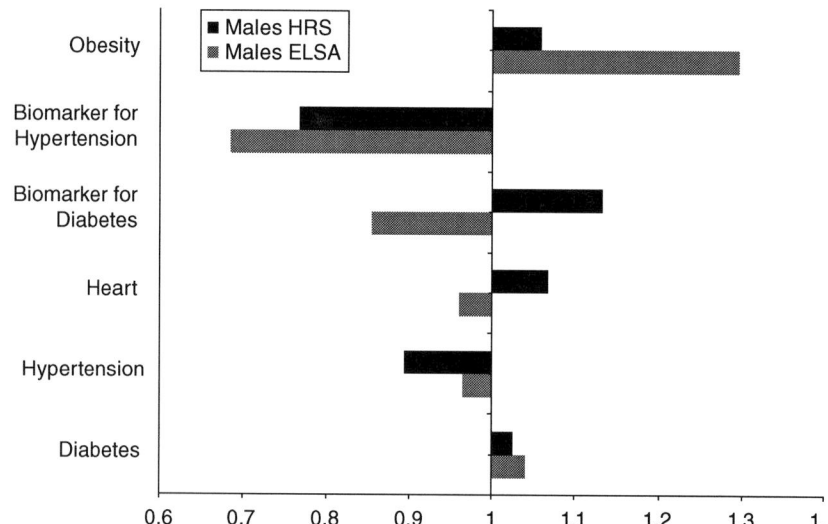

FIGURE 8-4A Odds ratios of disease prevalence by partnership status for men.
SOURCES: Authors' calculations from the Health and Retirement Study (2004) and the English Longitudinal Study of Ageing (2004) microdata.

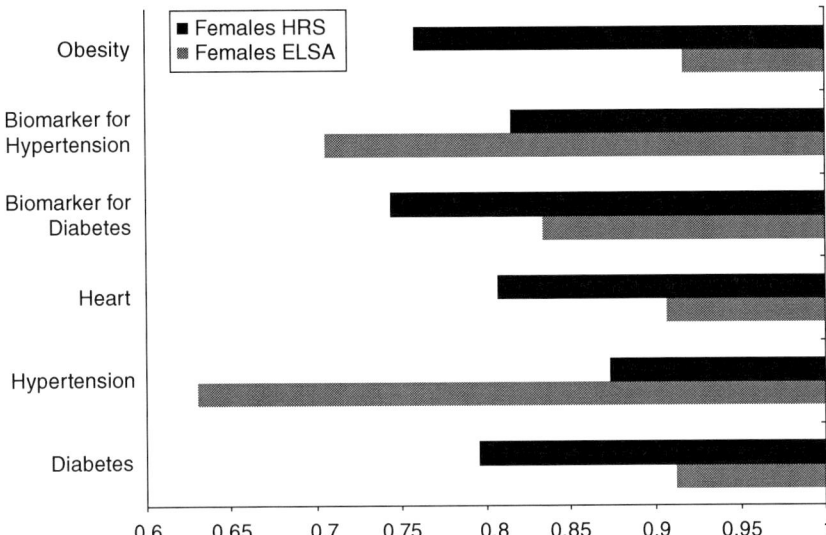

FIGURE 8-4B Odds ratios of disease prevalence by partnership status for women.
SOURCES: Authors' calculations from the Health and Retirement Study (2004) and the English Longitudinal Study of Ageing (2004) microdata.

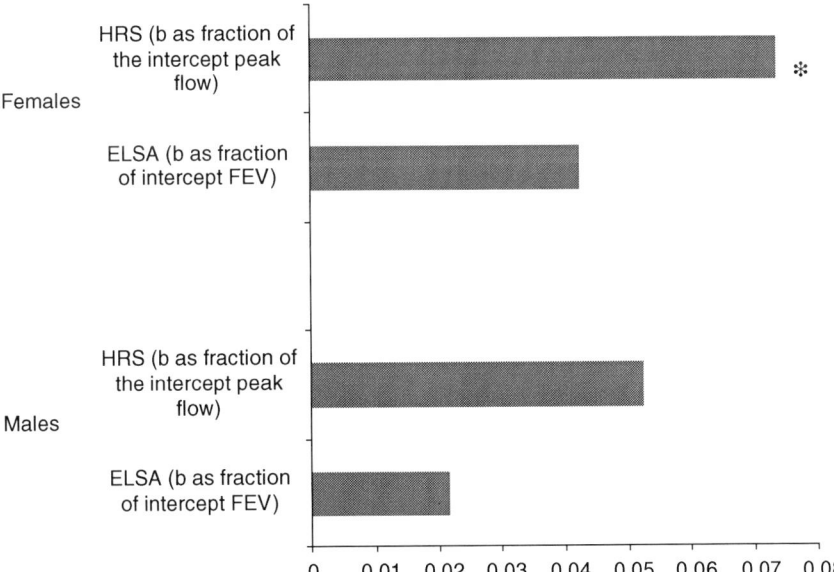

FIGURE 8-4C Association between partnership status and lung function for men and women.
NOTES: Statistical significance is indicated by an asterisk, FEV = forced expiratory volume.
SOURCES: Authors' calculations from the Health and Retirement Study (2004) and the English Longitudinal Study of Ageing (2004) microdata.

men, low levels of negative interactions were associated with lower levels of obesity and diabetes and better lung function. Among U.S. women, negative interactions were associated with obesity, diabetes, heart disease, and lung function. English women with fewer negative interactions had significantly less hypertension and tended to have fewer chronic conditions, although these later associations were not statistically significant.

In each case, the 95 percent confidence intervals for the estimated coefficients of social network variables for the United States overlap with the confidence intervals in England. The current results do not therefore support the hypothesis that differences in the toxicity of current levels of social networks and integration explain current health differences between the two countries.

Other Psychosocial Factors and Health

We have been considering variables related to social contacts and interactions and their relationship with health outcomes. In the literature on inequalities in health, however, considerable attention has been given to a broader set of psychosocial factors that are argued to be relevant to health through neuroendocrine as well as behavioral pathways. The hypothesis is that stress, a lack of control over one's life, and even subjective social status itself lead to neuroendocrine dysregulation and/or high-risk behaviors, which are then risk factors for subsequent health (in particular heart disease) and mortality. Is it possible that differences in such factors across countries need to be factored into our comparative analysis?

In recent work, Banks et al. (n.d.) examined the impacts of a set of commonly used psychosocial factors to assess what role they might play in the much higher rates of morbidity in the United States compared with England. The study exploited ELSA and HRS data from 2004, which contain identical measures of both psychosocial risk factors and health for a sample of individuals ages 52+. The psychosocial factors included control at home and control at work (using items that were developed and are collected on an ongoing basis in the Whitehall study), subjective social status summarized in one's position on the ladder, and loneliness. In addition, the CASP-19 scale, a general quality-of-life instrument covering four broad dimensions (control, autonomy, self-realization, and pleasure) was included (Netuveli et al., 2005).

The analysis shows that differences in these psychosocial risk factors or their health consequences failed to explain higher prevalence of major health conditions in America relative to England. Measures of control and self-realization were strongly and consistently associated with health in both countries. But, much like the social network and contact indicators described previously, the mean levels of these factors and their distribution across age and sex groups differed only slightly between the two countries.

In addition, the direction and strength of their relationships with health were nearly identical in the United States and England. Simulations of disease prevalence, holding levels of psychosocial risk factors constant in the two countries, demonstrated that neither levels of psychosocial risk nor estimated differences in marginal effects of psychosocial risk factors on health were sufficiently different to explain any meaningful fraction of the differences in prevalence of disease between the two countries.

SOCIAL NETWORKS AND MORTALITY

In this section, we present our analysis of mortality in England and the United States using ELSA and HRS. Our models focus on effects of some basic social network and interaction variables in the two countries. The principal constructs of interest are measures of marital/partnership status, the amount and nature of support from family and friends, membership in clubs, and religious organizations. These are the same variables defined and discussed earlier and are derived from a self-completion leave-behind booklet administered to ELSA respondents in 2002 (N = 10,541) and to HRS respondents in 2004 (N = 3,084).

Tables 8-3 and 8-4 present our analysis of time to death of ELSA respondents between Wave 1 (interviews took place between April 2002 and March 2003) and February 2008. Notification of deaths comes from the national death register and does not depend on subsequent participation in the follow-ups of ELSA. Table 8-3 contains models for both genders combined, with separate estimates depending on whether or not deaths within the first 12 months of the interview were included or not. The purpose of this distinction is to control at least partially for any social network reactions to impending deaths of a loved one that reflect reverse causality. Table 8-4 (which excludes those who died 12 months following the interview) contains separate models for men and women. For all models, we present a model that aggregates all social interaction variables into a single index and a model in which each unique dimension of the social interaction index is entered separately.

For completeness we briefly discuss nonsocial variables, all dated at baseline. Not surprisingly, men are at higher risk of death than women. A set of age group controls is included in all models, with the reference group being individuals ages 65-69. Individuals under age 50 at baseline (the younger partners of ELSA sample members) were omitted from the estimation sample. Not surprisingly, all models show a sharply increasing mortality risk with age. In the gender-specific models, age gradients are somewhat steeper for women than for men.

These empirical models also replicate the well-established strong association of smoking with mortality. In English mortality models, we distinguish four types of smoking behavior: (1) never smoked (the reference group),

TABLE 8-3 English Mortality Hazard Models: Time (months) to Death from ELSA Wave 1 Interview Month (by treatment of deaths within 12 months of interview)

	Early Deaths Excluded		Early Deaths Included	
	Hazard ratio p-value	Hazard ratio p-value	Hazard ratio p-value	Hazard ratio p-value
Male	1.460**	1.562**	1.517**	1.618**
	0.000	0.000	0.000	0.000
Ages 50-59	0.332**	0.340**	0.334**	0.340**
	0.000	0.000	0.000	0.000
Ages 60-64	0.650**	0.659**	0.625**	0.633**
	0.005	0.007	0.001	0.001
Ages 70-74	1.784**	1.741**	1.742**	1.704**
	0.000	0.000	0.000	0.000
Ages 75-79	2.919**	2.786**	2.893**	2.775**
	0.000	0.000	0.000	0.000
Ages 80-84	4.508**	4.181**	4.503**	4.208**
	0.000	0.000	0.000	0.000
Ages 85+	9.434**	8.514**	8.825**	8.054**
	0.000	0.000	0.000	0.000
Ex-smoker current	1.793**	1.711**	1.796**	1.714**
	0.000	0.000	0.000	0.000
Ex-smoker regular	1.294**	1.297**	1.288**	1.289**
	0.002	0.001	0.001	0.001
Ex-smoker occasional	1.029	1.027	1.013	1.013
	0.836	0.846	0.922	0.917
Medium-waist risk	1.353**	1.356**	1.260*	1.266*
	0.004	0.004	0.013	0.012
High-waist risk	1.544**	1.522**	1.381**	1.365**
	0.000	0.000	0.000	0.000
Wealth 1	1.421**	1.366**	1.621**	1.553**
	0.001	0.005	0.000	0.000
Wealth 2	1.580**	1.520**	1.659**	1.592**
	0.000	0.000	0.000	0.000
Wealth 3	1.417**	1.382**	1.433**	1.395**
	0.002	0.004	0.001	0.002
Wealth 4	0.990	0.986	1.014	1.008
	0.931	0.905	0.902	0.944
Positive support	0.988*	0.983**	0.985**	0.980**
	0.045	0.006	0.006	0.000
Negative interactions	1.008	1.009	1.008	1.008
	0.274	0.255	0.268	0.256
Index	0.956*		0.955**	
	0.014		0.004	
Frequency of meeting:				
Children		1.017		1.004
		0.655		0.914
Friends		1.022		1.021
		0.590		0.574

TABLE 8-3 Continued

	Early Deaths Excluded		Early Deaths Included	
	Hazard ratio p-value	Hazard ratio p-value	Hazard ratio p-value	Hazard ratio p-value
Other family		0.983		0.991
		0.679		0.804
Membership:				
Club other than below		0.918*		0.912*
		0.028		0.010
Sports club		0.696**		0.713**
		0.006		0.005
Religious organization		1.023		0.997
		0.798		0.968
Partner		0.765**		0.773**
		0.000		0.000
N	10,541	10,541	10,745	10,745
Number of deaths				

NOTES: Medium-waist risk: 94-102 cm (men), 80-88 cm (women). High-waist risk: > 102 cm (men), > 88 cm (women). Wealth quintiles are single/couple-specific quintiles of gross housing wealth. *p < 0.05, **p < 0.01.
SOURCE: Authors' calculations from English Longitudinal Study of Ageing microdata.

(2) currently smoke, (3) a current nonsmoker who regularly smoked in the past, and (4) a current nonsmoker who only occasionally smoked in the past. The relative risks of these patterns of smoking behaviors were as expected—compared with those who never smoked, the highest relative mortality risks were for current smokers (59 percent higher risk for men and almost double for women), followed by ex-smokers who smoked regularly in the past (25-30 percent higher risk). There apparently is no statistically significant extra risk from having been an occasional smoker in the past. These estimated effects were similar by gender.

We found elevated mortality risks for those with greater waist circumference, especially for women—men with high waist risk had a 45 percent higher mortality hazard, and for women a close to 70 percent one. Finally, these models include controls for five wealth quintiles, with the top (richest) quintile serving as the reference group.[1] For men, the relative risks increased with wealth quintiles, but at a highly nonlinear rate—that is, there is little

---

[1] Rather than worry about how wealth levels should be adjusted for household size or how to allocate household wealth across members of the married couple, we instead place individuals into quintiles of the wealth distribution according to their marital status. Thus, a single pensioner with a wealth of $200,000 might be in the third quintile of the wealth distribution for his or her type, whereas a couple with the same amount of wealth might only be in the second quintile.

TABLE 8-4 English Mortality Hazard Models: Time (months) to Death from ELSA Wave 1 Interview Month (deaths within 12 months of interview excluded)

	Men1 Hazard ratio p-value	Men2 Hazard ratio p-value	Women1 Hazard ratio p-value	Women2 Hazard ratio p-value
Ages 50-59	0.298**	0.303**	0.393**	0.404**
	0.000	0.000	0.000	0.000
Ages 60-64	0.599**	0.608*	0.733	0.745
	0.008	0.010	0.217	0.243
Ages 70-74	1.670**	1.652**	1.985**	1.886**
	0.001	0.001	0.001	0.002
Ages 75-79	2.426**	2.362**	3.743**	3.485**
	0.000	0.000	0.000	0.000
Ages 80-84	4.097**	3.977**	5.260**	4.672**
	0.000	0.000	0.000	0.000
Ages 85+	7.803**	7.099**	12.448**	10.925**
	0.000	0.000	0.000	0.000
Smoker current	1.683**	1.589**	1.936**	1.856**
	0.000	0.001	0.000	0.000
Ex-smoker regular	1.295*	1.279	1.252*	1.257*
	0.042	0.054	0.039	0.036
Ex-smoker occasional	0.870	0.861	1.191	1.197
	0.518	0.487	0.325	0.313
Medium-waist risk	1.257	1.277	1.491*	1.480*
	0.092	0.072	0.018	0.020
High-waist risk	1.451**	1.442**	1.690**	1.669**
	0.004	0.005	0.001	0.001
Wealth 1	1.572**	1.533**	1.282	1.226
	0.003	0.006	0.116	0.207
Wealth 2	1.741**	1.681**	1.378*	1.328
	0.000	0.001	0.043	0.080
Wealth 3	1.429*	1.406*	1.411*	1.378*
	0.021	0.030	0.032	0.049
Wealth 4	0.985	0.998	0.988	0.975
	0.927	0.989	0.945	0.881
Positive support	0.987	0.981*	0.992	0.988
	0.099	0.025	0.365	0.193
Negative interactions	1.008	1.008	1.008	1.008
	0.438	0.434	0.508	0.480
Index	0.977		0.936*	
	0.317		0.011	
Frequency of meeting:				
Children		1.062		0.966
		0.248		0.535
Friends		1.072		0.952
		0.201		0.408
Other family		0.965		1.008
		0.518		0.900

TABLE 8-4 Continued

	Men1	Men2	Women1	Women2
	Hazard ratio p-value	Hazard ratio p-value	Hazard ratio p-value	Hazard ratio p-value
Membership:				
Club other than below		0.933		0.901
		0.169		0.086
Sports club		0.724		0.657*
		0.057		0.046
Religious organization		1.053		1.015
		0.692		0.904
Partner		0.775*		0.741**
		0.012		0.010
N	4760	4760	5781	5781
Number of deaths				

NOTES: Medium-waist risk: 94-102 cm (men), 80-88 cm (women). High-waist risk: > 102 cm (men), > 88 cm (women). Wealth quintiles are single/couple-specific quintiles of gross housing wealth. *p < 0.05, **p < 0.01.
SOURCE: Authors' calculations from English Longitudinal Study of Ageing microdata.

evidence of any association above the third quintile. This association of mortality with baseline wealth was smaller among women.

Our main focus concerns the estimated mortality impacts of variables that measure aspects of the extent of social interactions reported by respondents. Our key variables can be conceptually divided into four groups: the extent of positive support and/or negative interactions, the presence of a spouse, the frequency of meeting with family and friends, and membership in clubs or organizations. In an alternative specification, the last three variables are also aggregated into a single measure of social interactions that we label the "index," which is equivalent to the index of social networks used in previous sections.

Consider first estimates that include measures of positive and negative social support and the index. For our English sample, negative interactions were never statistically significant in either the combined gender or the gender-specific models. The amount of positive interaction was statistically significant in several of the models, pointing to a potentially relevant role of the quality of interactions in relation to mortality risk. The coefficient per unit change in positive support is quite small, although the range of this variable, which is 0-27, needs to be borne in mind when interpreting the magnitude of the coefficient. Examination of the distribution of this variable in the two samples (which is similar in both countries) shows that the majority of individuals were located toward the upper ends of the scale—a movement from the 25th percentile to the 75th percentile, for example, would be an increase of around 7 points, from 15 to 22—suggesting a relatively small overall effect.

For our English sample, we found that the single aggregate social network index had a statistically significant protective effect on mortality. However, the estimated impacts of subcomponents are highly different and reject aggregation into a single index. Estimated impacts on subsequent mortality vary considerably across social network subcomponents. For men and women, presence of a spouse/partner was found to be highly protective of reduced future mortality. This replicates a widely found result in the literature. With this exception, we did not find any significant associations between any of the other social network measures and subsequent mortality. In this analysis, other than the spouse, we found no evidence that the frequency of meeting with children, friends, or other relatives has any impact on subsequent mortality.

Combining all different types of clubs (religious organizations, sports clubs, and all other types of clubs) into a single aggregate variable on club membership, we found a significant protective effect of clubs on subsequent mortality. However, the reason is apparent from disaggregation of club membership into its different forms. The only type of club that had a statistically significant negative impact on mortality is membership in sports clubs. A straightforward and plausible explanation for that association is not a social network effect, but that only healthier people are able or willing to join and remain members of sports clubs where exercise may be required. Membership of religious organizations or clubs (other than sports clubs or religious organizations) was not statistically significantly associated with mortality. This analysis demonstrates that it is essential to disaggregate club membership social network variables before drawing any conclusions about their potential health impacts.

Tables 8-5 and 8-6 contain parallel analysis for our U.S. HRS sample. We attempt to make our U.S. mortality analysis as close as possible to the English one, but some data differences remain. The key social network variables in HRS are in a 2004 psychosocial leave-behind module, so our analysis of U.S. mortality begins in 2004 and covers all deaths to the end of 2007, the most recent year of mortality follow-up. After excluding the first 12 months of follow-up, this provides approximately 2 or 3 years of mortality data for each respondent. Since our U.S. analysis is by necessity restricted to a random subsample of the full HRS sample that received the psychosocial leave-behind questionnaire, sample sizes are smaller than for the English ELSA, and the raw number of deaths in the analysis sample is also lower due to the shorter mortality follow-up period. Our empirical findings are somewhat less precise as a result.

While most variables are the same in English and U.S. samples, there are some differences. Variables that are identical include age groups, wealth

TABLE 8-5 U.S. Mortality Hazard Models: Time (months) to Death from HRS 2004 Wave Interview Month (by treatment of deaths within 12 months of interview)

	Early Deaths Excluded		Early Deaths Included	
	Hazard ratio p-value	Hazard ratio p-value	Hazard ratio p-value	Hazard ratio p-value
Male	1.225	1.219	1.387	1.378
	0.276	0.288	0.037	0.042
Ages 50-59	0.315**	0.322**	0.330**	0.334**
	0.004	0.005	0.002	0.002
Ages 60-64	0.632	0.638	0.820	0.821
	0.223	0.232	0.522	0.524
Ages 70-74	2.029**	2.056**	2.343**	2.375**
	0.018	0.016	0.001	0.001
Ages 75-79	2.879**	2.889**	3.334**	3.351**
	0.002	0.002	0.000	0.000
Ages 80-84	4.483**	4.550**	4.245**	4.290**
	0.000	0.000	0.000	0.000
Ages 85+	8.485**	8.802**	7.521**	7.692**
	0.000	0.000	0.000	0.000
Smoker current	1.402	1.415	1.216	1.221
	0.186	0.175	0.374	0.365
Ever smoked	1.615**	1.614**	1.566**	1.566**
	0.015	0.016	0.008	0.008
Vigorous exercise	0.582**	0.574**	0.455**	0.451**
	0.029	0.025	0.001	0.000
Vigorous exercise 1 to 3	0.471	0.480	0.567	0.573
	0.144	0.154	0.148	0.155
Wealth 1	3.161**	3.269**	2.786**	2.875**
	0.000	0.000	0.000	0.000
Wealth 2	2.179**	2.249**	2.047**	2.105**
	0.014	0.011	0.007	0.005
Wealth 3	2.030**	2.100**	1.756**	1.808**
	0.028	0.022	0.039	0.030
Wealth 4	1.522	1.545	1.404	1.412
	0.209	0.194	0.227	0.220
Positive support	1.031	1.032	1.020	1.020
	0.044	0.043	0.120	0.120
Negative interactions	1.025	1.024	1.014	1.012
	0.156	0.189	0.356	0.398
Index	0.959		0.984	
	0.318		0.662	
Frequency of meeting:				
Children		1.060		1.033
		0.500		0.668
Family		0.840		0.901
		0.081		0.217

continued

TABLE 8-5 Continued

	Early Deaths Excluded		Early Deaths Included	
	Hazard ratio p-value	Hazard ratio p-value	Hazard ratio p-value	Hazard ratio p-value
Friends		0.983		1.033
		0.853		0.675
Number of meetings	0.996	0.996	0.996	0.995
	0.149	0.133	0.085	0.070
Religion regularly	0.649**	0.658**	0.620**	0.621**
	0.034	0.041	0.006	0.007
Religion periodically	0.927	0.929	0.965	0.965
	0.738	0.744	0.852	0.849
Partner	1.012	0.966	0.892	0.880
	0.952	0.863	0.506	0.452
N	3007	3007	3062	3062
Number of deaths				

*p < 0.05, **p < 0.01.
SOURCE: Authors' calculations from English Longitudinal Study of Ageing microdata.

quintiles, positive support and negative interactions, having a partner, and frequency of meeting with children, family, or friends. The main difference in social network domain concerns the membership variables. In ELSA, membership means whether you are a member of each of various types of organizations. Although there is a single question asking, for all organization types, in total, how many meetings are attended in a year, this variable was not used, primarily because of the inability to split out religious attendance from attendance at other organizations. In HRS, the closest comparable question is "Not including attendance at religious services, how often do you attend meetings or programs of groups, clubs, or organizations that you belong to?" We converted the possible answers into numbers of days per year.[2]

Since religious services are excluded in this question phrasing but are included in ELSA organizational membership questions, we added two variables that measure whether or not one attends religious services regularly or attends periodically. The omitted group is those who did not attend at all. For participation in clubs or organizations, our English analysis indicated that it was crucial to separate out participation in sports clubs or organizations. Since we had no direct HRS measure of sports club participation, we

---

[2] Answers = more than once a week, once a week, 2 or 3 times a month, about once a month, less than once a month, never.

TABLE 8-6 U.S. Mortality Hazard Models: Time (months) to Death from HRS 2004 Wave Interview Month (deaths within 12 months of interview excluded)

	Men1	Men2	Women1	Women2
	Hazard ratio p-value	Hazard ratio p-value	Hazard ratio p-value	Hazard ratio p-value
Ages 50-59	0.380	0.386	0.216**	0.217**
	0.066	0.072	0.020	0.021
Ages 60-64	0.713	0.718	0.541	0.538
	0.515	0.525	0.264	0.261
Ages 70-74	1.999	1.982	2.147	2.164
	0.104	0.110	0.073	0.070
Ages 75-79	1.602	1.604	4.469**	4.447**
	0.370	0.369	0.001	0.001
Ages 80-84	2.967**	2.913**	6.289**	6.465**
	0.026	0.030	0.000	0.000
Ages 85+	8.184**	8.219**	10.365**	10.997**
	0.000	0.000	0.000	0.000
Smoker current	1.580	1.589	1.297	1.323
	0.193	0.186	0.500	0.469
Smoker ever	1.747	1.747	1.547	1.548
	0.123	0.123	0.076	0.075
Vigorous exercise	0.546	0.542	0.583	0.561
	0.062	0.060	0.162	0.134
Vigorous exercise 1 to 3	0.393	0.396	0.642	0.638
	0.201	0.205	0.541	0.536
Wealth 1	7.323**	7.274**	1.871	1.970
	0.001	0.001	0.105	0.082
Wealth 2	3.428**	3.408**	1.745	1.842
	0.033	0.035	0.152	0.118
Wealth 3	5.006**	4.979**	0.989	1.055
	0.004	0.004	0.980	0.900
Wealth 4	2.978	3.001	1.057	1.072
	0.064	0.062	0.895	0.870
Positive support	1.019	1.021	1.045**	1.044
	0.393	0.361	0.049	0.055
Negative interactions	1.039	1.037	1.011	1.007
	0.134	0.148	0.677	0.775
Index	0.972		0.954	
	0.669		0.398	
Frequency of meeting:				
Children		1.033		1.078
		0.812		0.517
Family		0.930		0.790
		0.646		0.076
Friends		0.936		1.024
		0.642		0.849
Number of meetings	0.995	0.995	0.996	0.995

continued

TABLE 8-6 Continued

	Men1	Men2	Women1	Women2
	Hazard ratio p-value	Hazard ratio p-value	Hazard ratio p-value	Hazard ratio p-value
	0.252	0.263	0.262	0.212
Religion regularly	1.106	1.124	0.456**	0.455**
	0.740	0.703	0.004	0.004
Religion periodically	0.843	0.856	0.976	0.958
	0.643	0.675	0.934	0.883
Partner	0.797	0.762	1.208	1.158
	0.444	0.351	0.484	0.582
N	1262	1262	1745	1745
Number of deaths				

*$p < 0.05$, **$p < 0.01$.
SOURCE: Authors' calculations from English Longitudinal Study of Ageing microdata.

added two variables measuring the extent of vigorous exercise.[3] Finally, with regard to the other controls, we were unable to measure waist circumference in the U.S. sample, since in-person interviews to collect biomarker data did not start in HRS until 2006. Our categorization of smoking is also slightly different from the English specification presented earlier. More specifically, we included a dummy variable to capture whether an individual has ever smoked (regardless of their current smoking status), and then an additional variable to capture whether they are currently smoking. In addition, there is no measure of past smoking frequency, so there is no distinction between the two types of "ever-smoker" (i.e., regular and occasional).

The U.S. mortality analysis is presented in Table 8-5 and Table 8-6 using the same structure as the English mortality results. Consider briefly the nonsocial interaction and social support variables. Similar to our English results, mortality increased sharply with age, and there was a significant wealth gradient in mortality. In aggregate, smokers did have significantly elevated mortality rates, although the additional mortality risk for current smokers over and above past smokers was not statistically significant in this sample (presumably reflecting either inadequate statistical power or the relatively short follow-up period). With regard to physical activity, vigorous or intermediate exercise was associated with lower mortality risk.

Turning to social support variables for the U.S. sample, the evidence indicates that negative interactions had no statistically significant effect on subsequent mortality. Surprisingly, people who reported more positive

---

[3] Vigorous exercise is defined as participating in sports or activities that are vigorous, such as running or jogging, swimming, cycling, aerobics or gym workout, tennis, or digging with a spade or shovel once a week or more than once a week. The second vigorous exercise variable uses the same categories but for 1-3 times a month.

support were at elevated mortality risk during the follow-up. In gender-stratified models, this association was found for women but not for men. Similar to our English results, we found no statistically significant results for frequency of meeting with children, friends, or other relatives. Finally, the number of meetings of organizations or friends also appears to have no effect on subsequent mortality in America.

Attending religious services regularly but not periodically was associated with much lower subsequent mortality risk among women but not men. The concentration of a health promotion association of strong religious attendance among women is a common finding in U.S. samples (see, for example, Hummer et al., 2004; Deaton, 2009; Idler, 2009). There is as yet little consensus about what mechanisms may underlie that association, although some of the more obvious candidates, such as smoking, have been controlled in the analysis. Finally, having a partner was protective for mortality, but only for men. This contrasts with ELSA, in which we found a protective effect of partnership for both men and women.

In sum, we found relatively small or inconsistent effects of social interaction and network-type measures on subsequent mortality in either country with the length of follow-up period in cohorts to date. In some cases, we found associations that are inconsistent with well-established prior results (e.g., increased mortality among recipients of positive support). However, coupled with the lack of substantial differences in the distribution of social ties across the two countries, these results suggest that differences in social interactions across countries are quite unlikely to be a cause of longevity or life-expectancy differences between the United States and England.

VARIATIONS IN OTHER EUROPEAN COUNTRIES

Differences in life expectancy between England and the United States are less marked than between the United States and other industrialized countries. For example, in 2006, male life expectancy was 75 in the United States and 77 in the United Kingdom, while among women it was 80 for the United States and 81 for the United Kingdom (World Health Organization, 2009). Diverging trends between the United States and other countries are considerably more marked for populations in Sweden (79 for men and 83 for women), Switzerland (79 for men and 84 for women), Japan (79 for men and 86 for women), and Italy (78 for men and 84 for women) (World Health Organization, 2009). Similarly, as our analysis shows, the differences between England and the United States in the extent of social networks and kinds of interactions are small and in some cases quite subtle.

To explore the hypothesis that variations in social networks and interactions might explain cross-country variations in life expectancy in industrialized countries, we examined variations in social ties and life expectancy in 28 countries, including Japan, the United States, and several European countries. In this exploratory analysis, we used data from the Gallup World Survey to examine variations in distributions of social connections and social participations across countries. Although the Gallup survey includes data for a much larger array of developing and developed countries, we focused on 28 member states of the Organisation for Economic Co-operation and Development and the European Union as a first step. We chose these countries because our purpose here is to understand diverging trends in life expectancy primarily among industrialized nations.

We used data from the Gallup World Survey to examine variations in distributions of social connections and social participations across countries. We discuss both first-order correlations and a simple descriptive model of aggregate levels of social connections and social participation and World Health Organization (WHO) data on life expectancy at birth. These analyses are not meant to be conclusive and aim only to broaden the research agenda by illustrating the potential to use cross-country variations in social networks to understand their role in explaining health variations among populations. We regard this analysis as descriptive, with the aim of opening the discussion about these associations and not at establishing any inferences of causality.

Measures

Social integration measures were obtained from the Gallup Survey (2006 and 2007) based on the following survey questions: (1) Have you attended a place of worship or religious service within the last 7 days? (2) What is your current marital status? (Marital status was measured as a dichotomous variable: married or living in a domestic partnership or not.) (3) Approximately how many hours did you spend, socially, with friends or family yesterday? (4) Have you done any of the following in the past month? . . . How about volunteered your time to an organization?

Life-expectancy measures for both men and women at birth and at ages 15, 50, and 65 were obtained for 2006 from the WHO Statistical Information System (see http://apps.who.int/whosis/data/Search.jsp?countries=[Location]. Members [accessed June 2010]). Results did not vary when Gallup measures for social integration (questions listed above) were assessed against life expectancy at these different ages, so, in the final analyses, only life expectancy at birth was used.

Distribution of Social Integration Across Countries

Tables 8-7 and 8-8 list mean levels of social integration and life expectancy for each of the 28 countries in the Gallup data. To highlight com-

TABLE 8-7 Distribution of Social Network Measures in 28 Countries Participating in the Gallup Survey, Women

	Married or Living with Partner	Attended Religious Services Past Week	Social Time with Friends/ Family Yesterday (hours)	Volunteered Time to an Organization in Past Month	Life Expectancy
Austria (2006)	0.63	0.37	7.31	0.25	82.7
Belgium (2007)	0.62	0.28	7.55	0.29	82.2
Canada (2005)	0.63	0.33	—	0.42	82.9
Cyprus (2006)	0.64	0.60	5.54	0.17	81.9
Czech Republic (2007)	0.55	0.15	4.50	0.19	79.9
Denmark (2007)	0.64	0.21	7.26	0.25	81.0
Estonia (2006)	0.47	0.12	5.10	0.17	78.5
Finland (2006)	0.67	0.15	5.84	0.27	82.8
France (2006)	0.55	0.19	6.50	0.28	84.2
Germany (2007)	0.49	0.42	8.21	0.23	82.3
Greece (2007)	0.56	0.38	3.52	0.07	82.5
Ireland (2006)	0.59	0.63	5.27	0.41	81.9
Italy (2007)	0.62	0.59	8.66	0.21	84.0
Japan (2007)	0.67	0.23	10.75	0.24	85.9
Latvia (2006)	0.46	0.19	5.11	0.18	76.3
Lithuania (2006)	0.46	0.29	4.10	0.15	77.1
Netherlands (2007)	0.59	0.26	8.33	0.38	82.0
Norway (2006)	0.64	0.15	7.69	0.36	82.7
Poland (2007)	0.61	0.71	7.56	0.09	79.5
Portugal (2006)	0.61	0.50	5.41	0.11	82.3
Romania (2007)	0.62	0.43	7.51	0.05	76.1
Slovakia (2006)	0.51	0.53	5.28	0.13	78.3
Slovenia (2006)	0.58	0.37	5.34	0.28	81.7
Spain (2007)	0.59	0.33	7.83	0.16	84.1
Sweden (2007)	0.67	0.14	8.44	0.12	83.0
Switzerland (2006)	0.56	0.33	6.80	0.29	84.2
United Kingdom (2007)	0.45	0.29	7.53	0.25	81.3
United States (2007)	0.51	0.46	—	0.43	80.4

SOURCE: Authors' calculations from Gallup World Survey (2006-2007).

parisons with our previous analysis, means for the United Kingdom and the United States appear in the last two rows. These tables show considerable variation among the industrialized countries in these social outcome measures. For example, the highest percentage of married/partnered women and men was found in Finland, Japan, and Sweden, where about 65 percent or more of people were married. The lowest percentages are in the United Kingdom and several countries in Eastern Europe or the former Soviet Union, where about 50 percent were married/partnered.

TABLE 8-8 Distribution of Social Network Measures in 28 Countries Participating in the Gallup Survey, Men

	Married or Living with Partner	Attended Religious Services Past Week	Social Time with Friends/ Family Yesterday (hours)	Volunteered Time to an Organization in Past Month	Life Expectancy
Austria (2006)	0.61	0.28	7.13	0.35	77.2
Belgium (2007)	0.67	0.22	7.97	0.30	76.6
Canada (2005)	0.60	0.29	—	0.33	78.3
Cyprus (2006)	0.69	0.36	5.29	0.15	78.8
Czech Republic (2007)	0.54	0.07	4.59	0.18	73.5
Denmark (2007)	0.59	0.14	7.08	0.23	76.2
Estonia (2006)	0.53	0.06	5.46	0.16	67.4
Finland (2006)	0.65	0.12	5.23	0.32	75.8
France (2006)	0.61	0.14	6.86	0.29	77.2
Germany (2007)	0.52	0.37	8.41	0.23	77.0
Greece (2007)	0.58	0.24	3.59	0.07	77.4
Ireland (2006)	0.46	0.51	4.96	0.40	77.3
Italy (2007)	0.60	0.51	8.41	0.22	78.4
Japan (2007)	0.66	0.21	7.55	0.26	79.2
Latvia (2006)	0.58	0.09	5.43	0.19	65.3
Lithuania (2006)	0.61	0.15	4.87	0.11	65.3
Netherlands (2007)	0.57	0.21	6.60	0.36	77.7
Norway (2006)	0.63	0.19	7.76	0.42	78.1
Poland (2007)	0.55	0.62	7.23	0.12	70.9
Portugal (2006)	0.65	0.31	5.71	0.13	75.5
Romania (2007)	0.61	0.30	7.28	0.06	69.2
Slovakia (2006)	0.58	0.34	5.00	0.13	70.4
Slovenia (2006)	0.64	0.27	5.11	0.36	74.4
Spain (2007)	0.57	0.23	7.46	0.13	77.5
Sweden (2007)	0.64	0.10	8.14	0.13	78.7
Switzerland (2006)	0.57	0.27	5.58	0.39	79.1
United Kingdom (2007)	0.54	0.20	7.16	0.21	77.0
United States (2007)	0.58	0.46	—	0.43	75.5

SOURCE: Authors' calculations from Gallup World Survey (2006-2007).

There is even wider variation in attendance at religious ceremonies. In Ireland, Italy, and Poland, between 50 and 60 percent of people attended a religious ceremony in the past week. In the United States, 46 percent of men and women reported similar attendance, but only 29 percent of the English did so. At the other extreme, attendance was 15 percent or below for France, Sweden, and several Eastern European or former Soviet countries. Turning to social time with family and friends, there was much variation across countries. Japan, Switzerland, and the Netherlands reported among the highest levels of social time, while Greece and the Czech Republic reported relatively low levels. This question was not asked in U.S. and Canadian samples. Time volunteered to an organization in the past month also varied widely among countries, with the United States ranking highest for both men and women (43 percent), followed by Ireland, the Netherlands, and Norway. In several countries, less than 15 percent of the population reported volunteering, among them Greece and Romania.

Associations with Life Expectancy

To illustrate a simple first-order relationship between life expectancy and measures of social integration, Figures 8-5, 8-6, 8-7, and 8-8 show plots of life expectancy at birth for men and women against country-level means or percentages for four types of social connections or social participation: religious attendance, partnership status, social time with friends and relatives, and volunteered time. Table 8-9 presents a simple multivariate model predicting country-level life expectancy that includes all social network variables.

Countries with higher percentages of ties with regard to marriage had higher life expectancy (Figures 8-5A and 8-5B). However, in our model that controls for all measures of social ties and participation, this association was statistically significant for women ($p = .05$) but not for men ($p = .35$). Countries with high levels of social time also had higher life expectancy (Figures 8-7A and 8-7B), but these associations were not significant in multivariate models (the effect is positive but the p-values are around 0.2). A higher percentage who volunteered their time was associated with higher life expectancy (Figures 8-8A and 8-8B), and this association was significant for men ($p = .02$) and of borderline significance for women ($p = .06$). Finally, there is no correlation between life expectancy and religious attendance (Figures 8-6A and 8-6B) or in the results shown in Table 8-9.[4]

This analysis indicates large variability across these countries both in life expectancy and aggregate levels and distribution of social integration and social ties and participation. While our results indicate that some measures of social integration might be correlated with life expectancy, aggregated Gallup data for these industrialized countries by themselves were not able to distinguish sufficiently among alternative measures of social integration, even without placing into these models other relevant health behaviors on which countries differ. Even if we take these results at face value, their

---

[4]When gross domestic product was controlled for in analyses conducted by Deaton that included a much larger number of countries in the Gallup poll, significant correlations were reported for many analyses, especially for women.

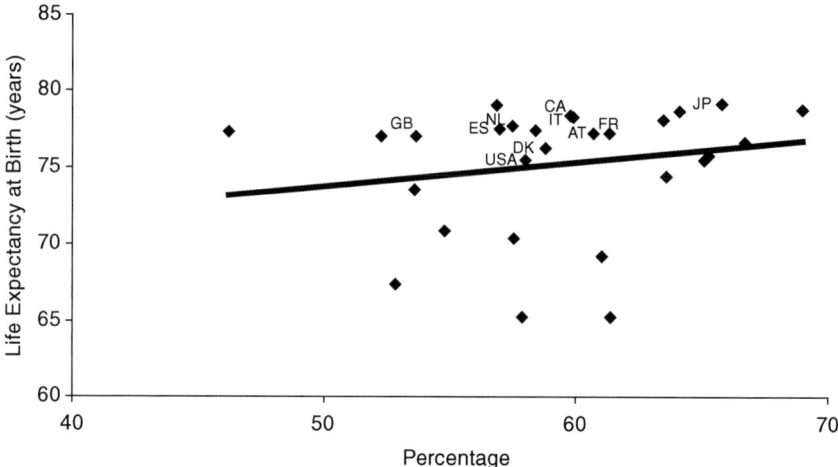

FIGURE 8-5A Life expectancy and marriage/living with partner for men in 28 countries.
NOTE: AT = Austria, CA = Canada, DK = Denmark, ES = Estonia, FR = France, GB = Great Britain, IT = Italy, JP = Japan, NL = the Netherlands, USA = United States.
SOURCE: Authors' calculations from the Gallup World Survey (2006-2007).

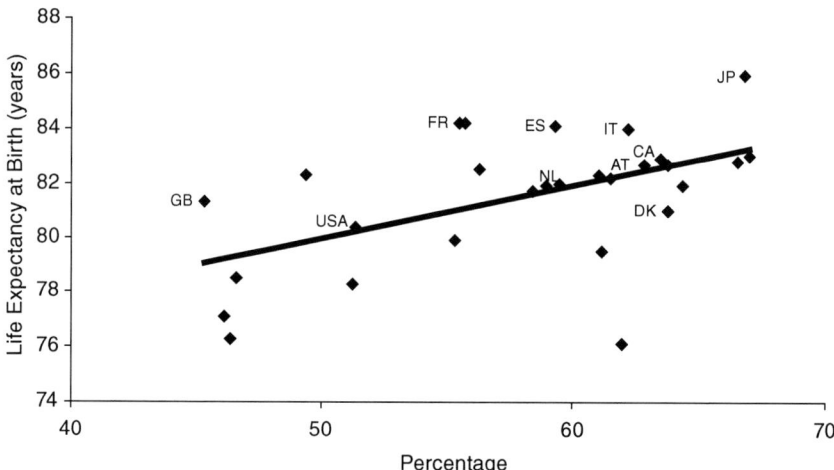

FIGURE 8-5B Life expectancy and marriage/living with partner for women in 28 countries.
NOTE: AT = Austria, CA = Canada, DK = Denmark, ES = Estonia, FR = France, GB = Great Britain, IT = Italy, JP = Japan, NL = the Netherlands, USA = United States.
SOURCE: Authors' calculations from the Gallup World Survey (2006-2007).

VARIATIONS IN SOCIAL INTEGRATION AND SOCIAL INTERACTIONS   249

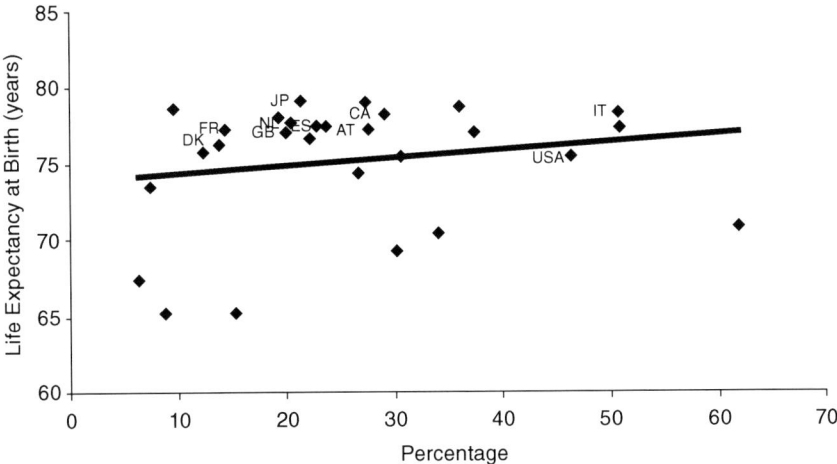

FIGURE 8-6A Life expectancy and religious attendance in past week for men in 28 countries.
NOTE: AT = Austria, CA = Canada, DK = Denmark, ES = Estonia, FR = France, GB = Great Britain, IT = Italy, JP = Japan, NL = the Netherlands, USA = United States.
SOURCE: Authors' calculations from the Gallup World Survey (2006-2007).

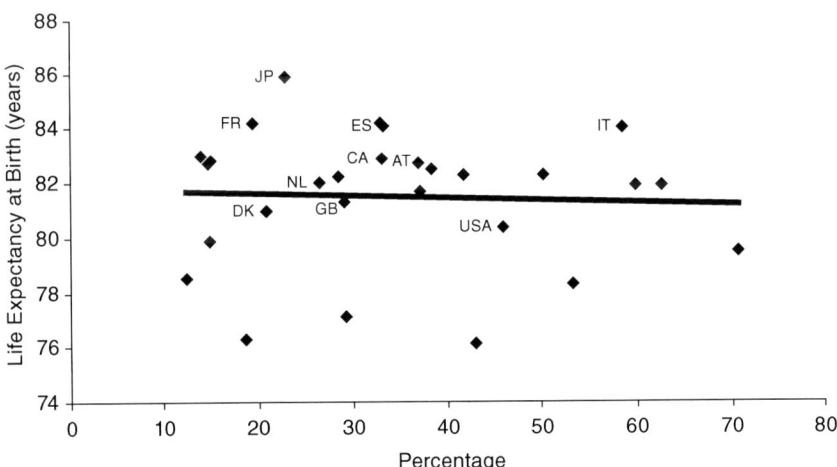

FIGURE 8-6B Life expectancy and religious attendance in past week for women in 28 countries.
NOTE: AT = Austria, CA = Canada, DK = Denmark, ES = Estonia, FR = France, GB = Great Britain, IT = Italy, JP = Japan, NL = the Netherlands, USA = United States.
SOURCE: Authors' calculations from the Gallup World Survey (2006-2007).

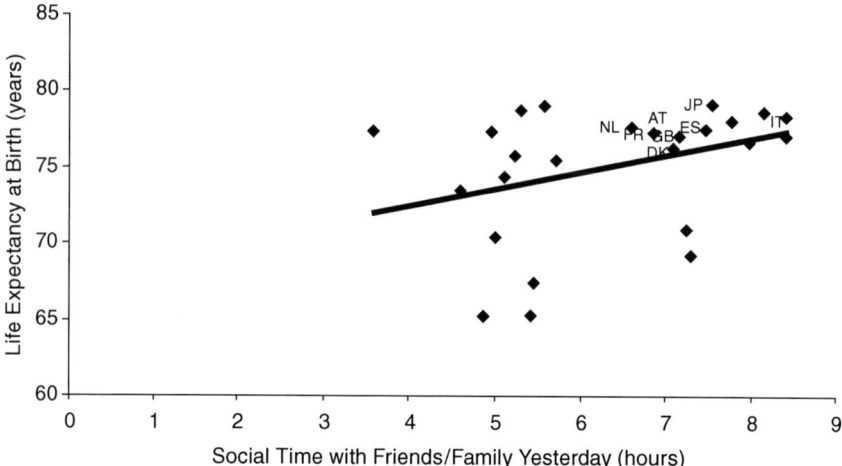

FIGURE 8-7A Life expectancy and social time for men in 28 countries.
NOTE: AT = Austria, CA = Canada, DK = Denmark, ES = Estonia, FR = France, GB = Great Britain, IT = Italy, JP = Japan, NL = the Netherlands, USA = United States.
SOURCE: Authors' calculations from the Gallup World Survey (2006-2007).

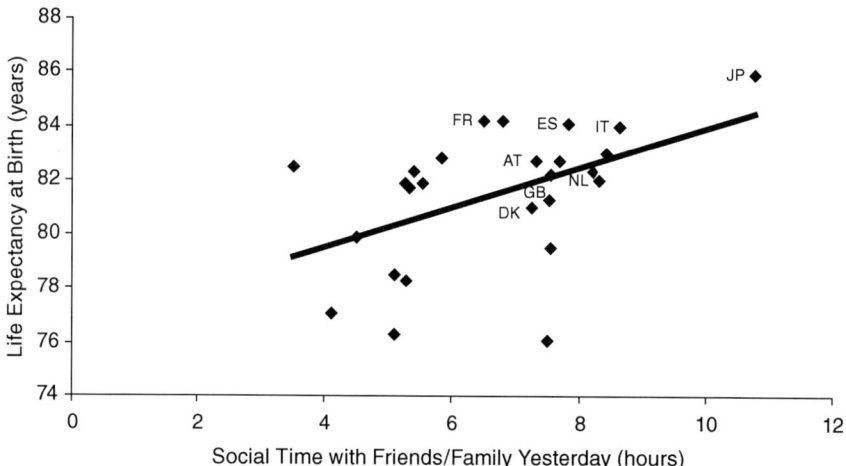

FIGURE 8-7B Life expectancy and social time for women in 28 countries.
NOTE: AT = Austria, CA = Canada, DK = Denmark, ES = Estonia, FR = France, GB = Great Britain, IT = Italy, JP = Japan, NL = the Netherlands, USA = United States.
SOURCE: Authors' calculations from the Gallup World Survey (2006-2007).

VARIATIONS IN SOCIAL INTEGRATION AND SOCIAL INTERACTIONS   251

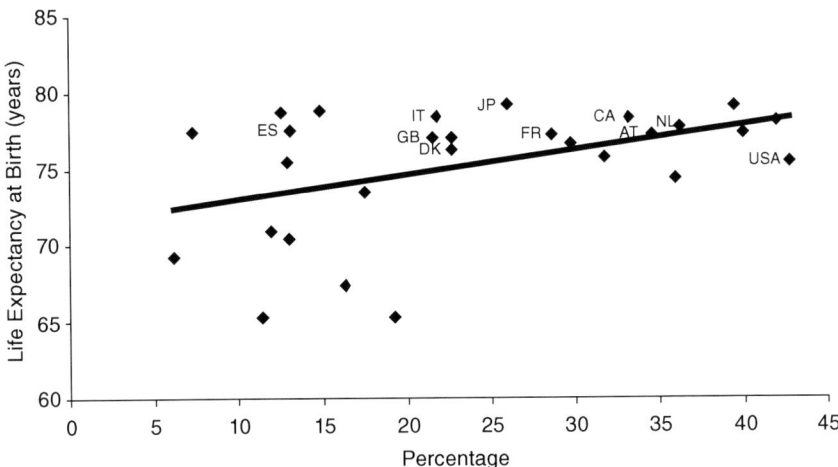

FIGURE 8-8A Life expectancy and volunteered time to organization in past month for men in 28 countries.
NOTE: AT = Austria, CA = Canada, DK = Denmark, ES = Estonia, FR = France, GB = Great Britain, IT = Italy, JP = Japan, NL = the Netherlands, USA = United States.
SOURCE: Authors' calculations from the Gallup World Survey (2006-2007).

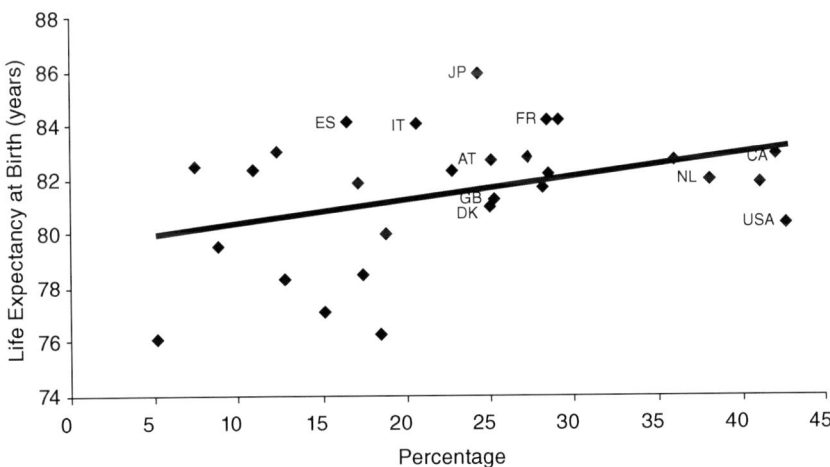

FIGURE 8-8B Life expectancy and volunteered time to organization in past month for women in 28 countries.
NOTE: AT = Austria, CA = Canada, DK = Denmark, ES = Estonia, FR = France, GB = Great Britain, IT = Italy, JP = Japan, NL = the Netherlands, USA = United States.
SOURCE: Authors' calculations from the Gallup World Survey (2006-2007).

TABLE 8-9 Linear Regression Model of Country Life Expectancy on Social Participation and Ties: Gallup and World Health Organization Data

		Coefficient	S.E.	p-value
Men	(Intercept)	54.82		
	Religious services	5.39	5.61	0.348
	Married or living with partner	17.18	14.81	0.259
	Social time with friends/family	0.76	0.57	0.198
	Volunteered time	16.80	7.01	0.026
Women	(Intercept)	68.92		
	Religious services	0.10	2.49	0.969
	Married or living with partner	13.98	6.83	0.053
	Social time with friends/family	0.37	0.28	0.195
	Volunteered time	9.06	4.59	0.062

NOTES: Coefficients indicate the change in life expectancy for a change from 0 to 1 in the probability of the social contact variable.
SOURCE: Authors' calculations from Gallup World Survey (2006-2007).

implications for explaining the U.S. health disadvantage are far from clear. While America might rank relatively low on some measures of social integration, such as marriage and social ties, it ranks relatively high on other measures, such as religious attendance and especially volunteering. Finally, the extent to which these associations are causal, produced by reverse causation, or are the result of underlying variations in third factors, such as gross domestic product, needs to be adequately examined in future research. Our purpose is to illustrate the window of opportunity to examine these issues by capitalizing on variations across countries in social integration and life expectancy.

IMPLICATIONS

In this chapter we attempt to assess whether aspects of social relationships and social participation might account for country differences in morbidity and life expectancy. The findings from our cross-sectional analyses and 3- to 5-year follow-ups suggest that current differences in these social conditions between the United States and England do not explain current differences in mortality or morbidity. First, observed differences in social networks and support between these two countries are small. Second, we found weak and inconsistent effects of the social network and support variables on the health outcomes we considered, with few associations reaching conventional levels of statistical significance.

Our analyses highlight the difficulty in undertaking comparative analyses in these domains. Even with tightly harmonized studies, such as HRS and ELSA, some differences in measurement remain, and mortality follow-up periods for studies with relevant social network constructs remain relatively short—5 years for ELSA and 3 years for HRS. Only time will tell whether these factors affect our results, as future data waves become available. The potential contribution of future data and analysis derived from long-term follow-ups of these and other, even more tightly harmonized cohorts is clear.

We found remarkable similarities in the cross-sectional distributions of social contacts and participation between the United States and England. We focused on these two countries because comparable data on social contacts and health were available for these populations, and recent research has demonstrated that health differences in morbidity are large. However, given the similarity in the two distributions, this focus also limited our ability to detect the potential role that these factors might have in a context of wider variation in social contacts and support. Our descriptive analysis based on the Gallup survey illustrates this limitation by pointing out the much larger variability in social contacts in other industrialized nations. Our analysis of England and the United States might not reveal the full potential contribution of social networks and social support to health differences across a broader set of countries. In exploring whether social networks might account for cross-country differences, priority should therefore be given to harmonizing data across countries that allow us to test this hypothesis in a broader international context.

A second issue refers to what the appropriate measures of social networks and participation might be. We have focused here on self-reports of frequency of contacts and levels of positive and negative support in England and America. Beyond these measures, there may be other key aspects, including how close relationships truly are and whether individuals feel they can rely on a social network. These less tangible aspects of social networks might have health effects not captured by the measures in our surveys. For example, some studies suggest that it might be the perception of social connectedness rather than the actual level of social support that influences health outcomes (Ashida and Heaney, 2008). Others have argued that one special friend or relative is the key concept, implying that the nature of the relations with others may not be relevant. Compared with many areas of determinants of health, the development of conceptual measures of social networks and support is relatively recent. It is fair to say that the field has not yet reached a consensus on the most appropriate set of conceptual measures, especially harmonized measures in an international comparative context.

Besides social networks and integration, other aspects of social behavior not incorporated into our study could be important in explaining health differences among countries. In addition, social contacts may influence health via several distinct mechanisms, including social regulation and behavioral norms; direct contagion of disease; transfer of material resources or information; positive emotional experiences, such as feeling loved, valued, or "belonging" to a group; or negative emotional experiences, such as shame or loneliness (Berkman and Glass, 2000). The importance of each pathway may depend on the specific health outcome—for example, smoking behavior may be very responsive to norms and social regulation, whereas they may be less relevant for breast cancer survival rates. Our study focuses primarily on whether networks and support have an overall association with health outcomes, but future studies should examine whether other social mechanisms might contribute to health differences across countries.

A fourth issue refers to differences in reporting styles among countries. While we found no differences in levels of social support and networks between English and U.S. respondents, many measures rely on subjective scales that have been shown in other contexts to exhibit considerable international variation (Kapteyn, Smith, and VanSoest, 2007). Individuals in each country might report their level of contact using different reporting thresholds, which may in turn influence their answers to these subjective questions. Additional investigations, perhaps including the use of vignettes, are needed in order to evaluate heterogeneity in reporting styles and, if such heterogeneity exists, to identify true differences in the distribution of social networks and support among countries.

A final set of issues relates to the fact that our analysis has been predominantly cross-sectional in nature, out of necessity given the availability of comparable data. As such, we can neither investigate nor control for intertemporal or, for that matter, intergenerational issues. This has a number of consequences. First, we can say nothing about how current differences across countries (to the extent they exist) in social integration and interactions might affect future life expectancy, nor how past trends in social integration are related to past trends in life expectancy. Second and closely related, to the extent that there are differences among countries in the level and trajectories of past social interactions and this history matters for current health and mortality outcomes, these differences are uncontrolled for in our study. Once again, when one extends the set of countries being analyzed beyond the United States and England, this may be an even more important issue than when considering these two countries alone. For example, to the extent that historical trajectories in Europe and the former Soviet Union countries differ for marriage, age of childbearing, and single parenthood, there may well be knock-on effects onto past trajectories of social support and integration, which could plausibly affect life-course health and mortality outcomes, and hence life expectancy, in these countries. Given the data available, investigation of such a hypothesis is beyond the scope or capacity of our analysis. Similarly, it is also impossible to investigate the hypothesis that one possible role of social integration and support is alleviating or mitigating the consequences of adverse shocks when they happen, given the lack of internationally comparable historical data. The intuitive plausibility of such intertemporal hypotheses suggests that data collection activities should be prioritized in order to facilitate analyses of these issues in the future.

Taken together, the analyses of this chapter and the caveats in the discussion above suggest that future research should focus on identifying multiple measures that can capture the most relevant aspects of the lifecourse trajectories of social networks, integration, and support that might be important to health, as well as developing strategies to make these measures comparable across countries. Until that happens, claims about the power of social network constructs to explain international health differences are still premature. Such an approach might also yield a new line of research that will allow the testing of the role of social networks and support in explaining diverging trends in life expectancy in a wider set of industrialized nations.

REFERENCES

Ashida, S., and Heaney, C.A. (2008). Differential associations of social support and social connectedness with structural features of social networks and the health status of older adults. *Journal of Aging Health, 20*(7), 872-893.

Banks, J., Marmot, M., McMunn, A., and Smith, J.P. (n.d.). *The English Are Healthier Than Americans: Do Social Risk-Factors Contribute?* Manuscript in preparation.

Banks, J., Marmot, M., Oldfield, Z., and Smith, J.P. (2006). Disease and disadvantage in the United States and in England. *Journal of the American Medical Association, 295*(17), 2037-2045.

Berkman, L.F., and Glass, T. (2000). Social integration, social networks, social support, and health. In L.F. Berkman and I. Kawachi (Eds.), *Social Epidemiology* (pp. 137-173). New York: Oxford University Press.

Berkman, L.F., and Syme, S.L. (1979). Social networks, host resistance, and mortality: A nine-year follow-up study of Alameda County residents. *American Journal of Epidemiology, 109*(2), 186-204.

Berkman, L.F., Melchior, M., Chastang, J.F., Niedhammer, I., Leclerc, A., and Goldberg, M. (2004). Social integration and mortality: A prospective study of French employees of Electricity of France-Gas of France: The GAZEL Cohort. *American Journal of Epidemiology, 159*(2), 167-174.

Blazer, D.G. (1982). Social support and mortality in an elderly community population. *American Journal of Epidemiology, 115*(5), 684-694.

Deaton, A. (2009). *Aging, Religion, and Health*. NBER Working Paper w15271. Cambridge, MA: National Bureau of Economic Research.

Fuhrer, R., and Stansfeld, S.A. (2002). How gender affects patterns of social relations and their impact on health: A comparison of one or multiple sources of support from "close persons." *Social Science & Medicine, 54*(5), 811-825.

Fuhrer, R., Stansfeld, S.A., Chemali, J., and Shipley, M.J. (1999). Gender, social relations and mental health: Prospective findings from an occupational cohort (Whitehall II study). *Social Science & Medicine, 48*(1), 77-87.

House, J.S., Robbins, C., and Metzner, H.L. (1982). The association of social relationships and activities with mortality: Prospective evidence from the Tecumseh Community Health Study. *American Journal of Epidemiology, 116*(1), 123-140.

Hummer, R.A., Ellison, C.G., Rogers, R.G., Moulton, B.E., and Romero, R.R. (2004). Religious involvement and adult mortality in the United States: Review and perspective. *Southern Medical Journal, 97*(12), 1223-1230.

Idler, E., Contrada, R.J., Boulifard, D.A., Labouvie, E.W., Chen, Y., and Krause, T.J. (2009). Looking in the black box of "attendance at services": Exploring an old dimension for religion and health research. *International Journal for the Psychology of Religion, 9*, 1-20.

Juster, F.T., and Suzman, R. (1995). An overview of the Health and Retirement Study. *Journal of Human Resources, 30*, S7-S56.

Kaplan, G.A., Salonen, J.T., Cohen, R.D., Brand, R.J., Syme, S.L., and Puska, P. (1988). Social connections and mortality from all causes and from cardiovascular disease: Prospective evidence from eastern Finland. *American Journal of Epidemiology, 128*(2), 370-380.

Kapteyn, A., Smith, J.P., and VanSoest, A. (2007). Vignettes and self-reported work disability in the US and the Netherlands. *American Economic Review, 97*(1), 461-473.

Khang, Y.H., and Kim, H.R. (2005). Explaining socioeconomic inequality in mortality among South Koreans: An examination of multiple pathways in a nationally representative longitudinal study. *International Journal of Epidemiology, 34*(3), 630-637.

Marmot, M., Banks, J., Blundell, R., Lessof, C., and Nazroo, J. (Eds.). (2002). *Health, Wealth, and Lifestyles of the Older Population in England: The 2002 English Longitudinal Study of Ageing.* London, England: Institute for Fiscal Studies.

Netuveli, G., Wiggins, R.D., Hildon, Z., Montgomery, S.M., and Blane, D. (2005). Functional limitation in long standing illness and quality of life: Evidence from a national survey. *British Medical Journal, 331*(7529), 1382-1383.

Orth-Gomer, K., and Johnson, J.V. (1987). Social network interaction and mortality: A six-year follow-up study of a random sample of the Swedish population. *Journal of Chronic Diseases, 40*(10), 949-957.

Orth-Gomer, K., Unden, A.L., and Edwards, M.E. (1988). Social isolation and mortality in ischemic heart disease: A 10-year follow-up study of 150 middle-aged men. *Acta Medica Scandinavica, 224*(3), 205-215.

Orth-Gomer, K., Rosengren, A., and Wilhelmsen, L. (1993). Lack of social support and incidence of coronary heart disease in middle-aged Swedish men. *Psychosomatic Medicine, 55*(1), 37-43.

Orth-Gomer, K., Horsten, M., Wamala, S.P., Mittleman, M.A., Kirkeeide, R., Svane, B., Ryden, L., and Shenck-Gustafsson, K. (1998). Social relations and extent and severity of coronary artery disease: The Stockholm Female Coronary Risk Study. *European Heart Journal, 19*(11), 1648-1656.

Penninx, B.W., Guralnik, J.M., Ferrucci, L., Simonsick, E.M., Deeg, D.J., and Wallace, R.B. (1998). Depressive symptoms and physical decline in community-dwelling older persons. *Journal of the American Medical Association, 279*(21), 1720-1726.

Sugisawa, H., Liang, J., and Liu, X. (1994). Social networks, social support, and mortality among older people in Japan. *Journal of Gerontology, 49*(1), S3-S13.

Welin, L., Tibblin, G., Svardsudd, K., Tibblin, B., Ander-Peciva, S., Larsson, B., and Wilhelmsen, L. (1985). Prospective study of social influences on mortality: The study of men born in 1913 and 1923. *Lancet, 1*(8434), 915-918.

World Health Organization. (2009). *WHO Statistical Information System.* Available: http://apps.who.int/whosis/data/ [accessed August 2009].

Part III

The U.S. Health System

9

Low Life Expectancy in the United States: Is the Health Care System at Fault?

Samuel H. Preston and Jessica Ho

The United States falls well behind the world's leaders in life expectancy at birth. Some of the discrepancy is attributable to relatively high infant mortality and some to high mortality from violence among young adults. But the bulk of the discrepancy is attributable to mortality above age 50, an age to which 94 percent of newborns in the United States will survive according to the 2006 U.S. life table. Life expectancy at age 50 in the United States ranked 29th highest in the world in 2006 according to the World Health Organization (2009). It falls 3.3 years behind the leader, Japan, and more than 1.5 years behind Australia, Canada, France, Iceland, Italy, Spain, and Switzerland. About 4 million Americans reach age 50 each year, so an average loss of 1.5 years of life years per person means that some 6 million years of potential life are being lost annually. At the conventional value of $100,000 per additional year of life (Cutler, 2004), the relative loss of life in the United States above age 50 is valued at roughly $600 billion annually. Using Japan as a standard, the loss is $1.3 trillion.

The U.S. medical system is often blamed for this poor life-expectancy ranking. But measures of population health such as life expectancy do not depend solely on what transpires within the health care system—the array of hospitals, doctors, and other health care professionals, the techniques they employ, and the institutions that govern access to and utilization of them. Such measures also depend on a variety of personal behaviors that affect an individual's health, such as diet, exercise, smoking, and compliance with medical protocols. The health care system could be performing exceptionally well in identifying and administering treatment for various diseases, but a country could still have poor measured health if personal health care practices were unusually deleterious. This could be the case in the United States, which had the highest level of cigarette consumption per capita in the developed world over a 40-year period ending in the mid-1980s (Forey et al., 2002). Smoking in early life has left an imprint on mortality patterns that remains visible as cohorts age (Haldorsen and Grimsrud, 1999; Preston and Wang, 2006). One recent study estimated that, if deaths attributable to smoking were eliminated, the ranking of U.S. men and women in life expectancy at age 50 among 21 countries of the Organisation for Economic Co-operation and Development (OECD) would improve sharply (Preston, Glei, and Wilmoth, Chapter 4, in this volume). Recent trends in obesity are also more adverse in the United States than in other developed countries (Cutler, Glaeser, and Shapiro, 2003; Organisation for Economic Co-operation and Development, 2008).

This chapter begins with a review of previous international studies of the comparative performance of health care systems in disease identification and treatment. The review is focused on the major diseases of adulthood, cancer and cardiovascular disease, in the belief that disease-level analyses are more likely to reveal the forces at work than more highly aggregated studies (Garber, 2003). In 2005, cancer and major cardiovascular diseases were responsible for 61.0 percent of deaths in the United States at ages 45+ (National Center for Health Statistics, 2008). Because our concern is with mortality per se, the criterion we employ is effectiveness at preventing death, rather than cost-effectiveness or efficiency of resource deployment. These latter criteria have been used in several other recent comparative studies describing features of the U.S. health care system that appear inefficient by international standards (Garber and Skinner, 2008; McKinsey Global Institute, 2008). A comprehensive evaluation of the U.S. health care system would need to consider patient physical and emotional welfare, a much broader concept than survival, which is the sole focus of this chapter.

Health care systems can prevent death from a particular disease either by preventing it from developing or by effectively treating it once it has developed. A key element in effective treatment is accurate diagnosis. However, almost no internationally comparable data exist on the actual incidence of various diseases, which is the appropriate measure of the success of prevention. While cancer appears to be an exception because "incidence" data are published for various cancer registry sites (e.g., at the website of the International Agency for Research on Cancer), the data refer not to the origin of a disease but to its detection, a process that combines actual patterns of incidence with the mechanics of identification. And even if pure measures of it were available, actual disease incidence reflects not only features of a health care system but also many other factors of behavioral, social, and genetic origin.

Disease prevalence—the proportion of the population that has been diagnosed with a disease—is even more difficult to interpret. The United

States has a higher prevalence than Europe of the major adult diseases, including cancer, heart disease, and diabetes (Avendano et al., 2009; Thorpe, Howard and Galactionova, 2007a). But higher prevalence could reflect higher incidence, better detection, or longer survival resulting from more successful treatment. Because of these limitations of data and interpretation, our review focuses primarily on disease identification and treatment, elements that are customarily considered to be the provenance of health care systems.

A valuable but not unimpeachable indicator of the effectiveness of treatment is the comparative survival rate of individuals once a disease has been detected. Relatively high survival rates imply either that the disease has been detected unusually early or that treatment is unusually successful. Early detection is valuable to the extent that it permits better therapy. However, if early detection did not alter the clinical course of a disease but only increased the expected length of time from detection to death (so-called lead-time bias), then it would not be associated with reductions in mortality at the population level despite raising 5-year survival rates (e.g., Gatta et al., 2000).

Because they are not subject to this potential bias, we pay special attention to mortality rates. In particular, in the second half of the chapter we investigate comparative mortality trends for prostate cancer and breast cancer. We document that:

- effective methods of screening for these diseases have been developed relatively recently;
- these diagnostic methods have been deployed earlier and more widely in the United States than in most comparison countries;
- effective methods are being used to treat these diseases; and
- the United States has had a significantly faster decline in mortality from these diseases than comparison countries.

INTERNATIONAL STUDIES OF CANCER

The United States does well in international comparisons of the frequency of cancer screening. The OECD (2006, 2007) provides 2000-2005 data on the percentage of women ages 20-69 in 15 countries who had been screened for cervical cancer during the preceding 3 years. The United States has the highest percentage of women who have been screened in both tabulations.[1] We present evidence below that the United States also

---

[1] Ages vary somewhat, but the variation is thought to be a "minor threat" to the validity of comparisons (Organisation for Economic Co-operation and Development, 2006, p. 69). The 15 countries include 6 for whom the recall period is greater than 3 years, the period used in the United States.

has exceptionally high screening rates for prostate cancer and breast cancer. Quinn (2003) reports U.S. colorectal screening rates that are "quite high" in comparison to Europe but does not provide comparative data. Gatta et al. (2000, p. 899) also suggest that access to and use of sigmoidoscopy, colonoscopy, and fecal occult blood tests are more common in the United States than in Europe. This difference is supported by the finding that colorectal cancer patients in the United States have less advanced disease at diagnosis than patients in Europe (Ciccolallo et al., 2005).

A higher rate of screening for cancer would produce a higher prevalence of ever-diagnosed cancer in the population, ceteris paribus. The elevated prevalence would occur simply because a higher fraction of the population would know about their disease. An additional boost to prevalence would be provided if early detection resulted in reduced mortality. Thus, in view of the higher frequency of screening in the United States, we would expect its reported prevalence of diagnosed cancer to be higher than in Europe.

That expectation is confirmed by data from the Health and Retirement Survey and its English and European counterparts. Thorpe et al. (2007a) found that 12.2 percent of Americans over age 50 reported having been diagnosed by physicians with cancer, compared with only 5.4 percent in a composite of 10 European countries. Avendano et al. (2009) reported similar figures for the age range 50-74, with England intermediate between the United States and Europe but closer to Europe. Some fraction of these very large differences in prevalence could, of course, be attributable to real differences in disease incidence or to reporting differences, which are discussed briefly below.

Thanks to a large number of cancer registries that record new cancer diagnoses and follow individuals forward from the point of diagnosis, 5-year survival rates for people initially diagnosed with cancer are widely available to provide evidence about the success of detection and treatment. Because of their relative comparability and pertinence to a major disease process, these data are among the best indicators of comparative health care system performance. In this summary, we use 5-year relative survival rates, which compare the survival of those diagnosed with cancer to that of an average person of the same age and sex as the person diagnosed.

International comparisons of cancer survival rates show a distinct advantage for the United States. Using cancer registry data, researchers from the Eurocare Working Group compare 5-year survival rates for cancers of 12 sites that were diagnosed between 1985 and 1989 (Gatta et al., 2000). The aggregate of 41 European registries, which were drawn from 17 countries, had lower survival rates than the United States from all cancer sites except the stomach, where differences were small and attributed to differences between the distributions of sites within the stomach. The U.S. data were drawn from the National Cancer Institute's Surveillance, Epidemiology and

End Results (SEER) database, a population-based cancer registry covering approximately 14 percent of the U.S. population. For the major sites of lung, breast, prostate, colon, and rectum cancers, U.S. survival rates were the highest of any of the 18 countries investigated. Cancers first diagnosed on the death certificate (5 percent in Europe and 1 percent in the United States) were excluded from analysis; if they had been included, the U.S. survival advantage would have increased. The authors discount the possibility that the U.S. advantage was attributable to statistical or registration artifacts.

An updated analysis reached similar conclusions. Based on period survival data for 2000-2002 from 47 European cancer registries, 5-year survival rates were found to be higher in the United States than in a European composite for cancer at all major sites (Verdecchia et al., 2007). Table 9-1 presents the comparative data for all sites for which the U.S. 95 percent confidence interval was < 0.025. For men (all sites combined), 47.3 percent of Europeans survived 5 years, compared with 66.3 percent of Americans. For women, the contrast was 55.8 versus 62.9 percent. The male survival difference was much greater than the female primarily because of the very large difference in survival rates from prostate cancer.

Scattered data for cancer of various sites indicate that tumors are typically detected at an earlier stage in the United States (Ciccolallo et al., 2005; Gatta et al., 2000; Sant et al., 2004). Thus, the United States appears to screen more vigorously for cancer than Europe, and people in the United States who are diagnosed with cancer have higher 5-year survival probabilities. Of course, all of these phenomena could be the exclusive product of lead-time bias if early detection afforded no benefit for the clinical course

TABLE 9-1 5-Year Relative Survival Rates for Cancer of Different Sites, U.S. and European Cancer Registries[a]

Site	5-Year Survival Rate (%)	
	United States	Europe
Prostate	99.3	77.5
Skin melanoma	92.3	86.1
Breast	90.1	79.0
Corpus uteri	82.3	78.0
Colorectum	65.5	56.2
Non-Hodgkin lymphoma	62.0	54.6
Stomach	25.0	24.9
Lung	15.7	10.9
All malignancies (men)	66.3	47.3
All malignancies (women)	62.9	55.8

[a]Based on period survival data for 2000-2002.
SOURCE: Adapted from Verdecchia et al. (2007).

of the disease. Below, we present evidence that innovations in diagnosis and treatment of prostate and breast cancer were associated with faster declines in mortality in the United States than in OECD countries. Such a pattern would not be observed if lead-time bias were the only factor at work, that is, if early detection conferred no advantage.

INTERNATIONAL STUDIES OF CARDIOVASCULAR DISEASE

In contrast to cancer, nations do not have registries for heart disease and stroke. So information about the comparative performance of medical systems with respect to cardiovascular disease is not as systematic and orderly as it is for cancer. One useful source of comparative data is the Health and Retirement Survey (HRS) and its European counterpart, the Survey of Health, Ageing and Retirement in Europe (SHARE). Thorpe et al. (2007a) compared the United States with a composite of 10 European countries on the frequency with which people with a particular diagnosis reported using medication. Of people ages 50+ diagnosed with heart disease, 60.7 percent of Americans and 54.5 percent of Europeans reported being on medication. The proportions using medication after a stroke are comparable at 45.1 and 44.6 percent, respectively. Of those reporting high cholesterol levels, 88.1 percent of Americans report being medicated versus 62.4 percent of Europeans.[2] Crimmins, Garcia, and Kim (Chapter 3, in this volume) show that a much higher fraction of Americans are using lipid-lowering drugs at a particular age than in Italy, Japan, or the Netherlands, even though the proportions with elevated cholesterol in these countries are similar to or higher than that in the United States.

Among those reporting high blood pressure in HRS and SHARE, the proportions reporting taking medication for the condition are similar in the United States (88.0 percent) and Europe (88.9 percent) (Thorpe et al., 2007a). However, when actual measures of blood pressure are used rather than self-reports, the U.S. position improves. Wolf-Maier et al. (2004) employed regional or national samples in the United States, Canada, and five European countries. Hypertension was defined as the population of persons who have systolic blood pressure of 160+ or diastolic blood pressure of 95+ or who are using antihypertensive medication. Of persons ages 35-64 with hypertension, 77.9 percent were being treated in the United States, compared with a range of 41.0 to 62.4 percent in the other six countries. Among those with hypertension, 65.5 percent were being *successfully* treated in the United States (i.e., their levels were reduced below the hypertension-defining threshold), compared with 24.8 to 49.1 percent in the other countries.

---

[2]The U.S. figure for cholesterol is drawn from the Medicare Expenditure Panel Survey because HRS did not gather this information.

Survival data for cardiovascular disease start not from the point of diagnosis but from an acute event of heart attack or stroke. An OECD study, following up on a study by the Technological Change in Health Care Research Network, computed 1-year case fatality rates for people hospitalized for acute myocardial infarction in Australia, Canada, Denmark, Finland, Sweden, Great Britain, and the United States. The samples were sometimes regionally rather than nationally representative. Among the seven countries in 1996, the United States had the third-lowest case fatality rate for men ages 40-64 and the second-lowest rate for men ages 85-89. For women at these ages, the United States ranked fourth and first (Moise, 2003). Part of the explanation for why the U.S. performs better may be related to its unusually aggressive treatment regime. Of the seven countries, the United States had the highest proportion of male and female patients in both age intervals undergoing revascularization operations (percutaneous transluminal coronary angioplasty or coronary artery bypass graft) (Moise, 2003; see also Technological Change in Health Care (TECH) Research Network, 2001).[3]

One study has explicitly linked more aggressive surgical treatment in the United States to better outcomes. It compared Canadians and Americans who had just experienced an acute myocardial infarction and who enrolled in a drug trial (Kaul et al., 2004). Data are not nationally representative but rather reflect the patient base of hospitals participating in the trial. Americans had a small but statistically significant advantage in 5-year survival. Controlling many baseline characteristics, the hazard rate was 17 percent higher in Canada. When revascularization was added to the model, it was associated with a 28 percent reduction in the hazard rate and its addition reduced the international difference to an insignificant 7 percent. The authors conclude that "our findings are strongly suggestive of a survival advantage for the U.S. cohort based on more aggressive revascularization" (Kaul et al., 2004, p. 1758).

The OECD (2003) has conducted a large international study of ischemic stroke, which accounts for roughly 88 percent of stroke cases except in Japan, where it represents about 70 percent. They calculate in-hospital 7-day and 30-day survival rates for patients newly admitted with ischemic stroke. For both men and women ages 65-74, the U.S. ranking on 7-day survival rates was third out of nine; at ages 75+, it was second out of nine for both sexes. For 30-day hospital survival rates at ages 65-74, the United States was second for women and tied for second with two others among men. At ages 75+, the U.S. 30-day survival rate was first for men and second for women. Counting all deaths, not simply deaths in the hospital, and limiting comparison to six regions, including two in Canada, the U.S. survival

---

[3]Data on treatments at ages 85-89 were not available for Spain or the United Kingdom.

rate ranked first for men ages 65-74 and 75+ and second for women in these ages. However, the U.S. 1-year survival rate among this set of populations was considerably poorer, ranking fifth out of six for men ages 65-74 and fourth out of six for men ages 75+. For women at these two ages, the rankings were fourth and third. Consistently in these rankings, the U.S. position was better at ages 75+ than at ages 65-74.

Carotid endarterectomy (surgical removal of plaque from inside the carotid artery) is used to prevent stroke or the recurrence of stroke. Such surgery is much more common in the United States than in any of 11 comparison OECD countries (Organisation for Economic Co-operation and Development, 2003). We are unaware of any studies linking this surgery to international patterns of stroke mortality, but a randomized clinical trial reported a large survival advantage for persons undergoing the procedure (Halliday et al., 2004).

In summary, persons with high blood pressure or high serum cholesterol are more likely to be treated for these conditions in the United States than in other countries. Survival rates following a heart attack are somewhat above average in the United States, whereas survival rates following a stroke are comparable to those of comparison countries. The evidentiary basis for international comparisons of the treatment of cardiovascular diseases is much weaker than in the case of cancer.

CONTRARY EVIDENCE? "MORTALITY AMENABLE TO MEDICAL CARE"

The Commonwealth Fund (2008) has recently issued a "scorecard" on U.S. health care system performance that consists of 37 indicators. A prominent indicator is "mortality amenable to medical care," on which the United States currently ranks last among 19 countries. This index was developed and applied in Nolte and McKee (2008), in which amenable deaths are described as "deaths from certain causes that should not occur in the presence of timely and effective health care" (p. 59). Only deaths below age 75 are included; these constitute 43.2 percent of deaths in the United States in 2005 (National Center for Health Statistics, 2008). For some causes of death, an earlier age cutoff is used.

The distribution of major causes of death included among the "amenable causes" is provided for the United States, the United Kingdom, and France (Nolte and McKee, 2008). A majority of amenable deaths in all three countries is attributed to ischemic heart disease and other circulatory diseases, even though only half of ischemic heart disease deaths are included because some are believed not to be amenable to health care. That rule of thumb is clearly a poor substitute for an effort to attribute international variation in mortality from ischemic heart disease to its various components, including health care systems and behavioral and social factors.[4] The authors note that a similar rule of thumb could have been introduced for cerebrovascular diseases, which constitute at least a quarter of the "amenable" deaths in the United States and the United Kingdom. But it would have been no more satisfactory for that cause of death.

In view of the studies that show that the United States does relatively well in treating cardiovascular disease, it seems inaccurate to attribute its high death rates from these causes to a poorly performing medical system. And these diseases contribute a majority of their set of amenable deaths, rendering the totality of amenable causes problematic. On one hand, a related objection could be raised to the inclusion of diabetes deaths in the set. On the other hand, prostate cancer is excluded from the list of amenable causes despite the fact that the 5-year survival rate from prostate cancer in the United States is above 99 percent and the disease can be readily identified (see below).

According to Nolte and McKee (2008), males in the United States had a faster fall in mortality from nonamenable causes of death (an 8 percent decline) than from amenable ones (4 percent) between the latest two readings, 1997-1998 and 2002-2003. This anomaly suggests either flaws in the index or the unimportance of medical care relative to other factors that are operating.

Causes of death whose inclusion in Nolte and McKee's list of amenable causes at older ages is more defensible are influenza and pneumonia. Mortality from both causes is heavily influenced by smoking (Centers for Disease Control and Prevention, 2002), so the international distribution of mortality is a product of factors beyond the health care system. However, influenza is partially immunizable, and death from pneumonia can often be avoided through administration of vaccines or antibiotics or improvements in hospital sanitation.

The United States ranks ninth out of 23 OECD countries in the proportion of the population above age 65 offered an annual influenza vaccination (Organisation for Economic Co-operation and Development, 2007). Figure 9-1 demonstrates that the 2000-2004 age-standardized death rate from influenza at ages 50+ in the United States is among the lowest of the 16 countries investigated. The United States fares less well in mortality from pneumonia, having sixth highest rates among the 16 countries investigated (see Figure 9-2). However, the ranking is somewhat deceiving because its death rate is closer to all but one of the better ranked countries than to the five countries with higher rates. The U.S. death rate from pneumonia at

---

[4]The strategy adopted by Nolte and McKee is no different from saying that genetic factors play some role in cardiovascular mortality and, as a consequence, attributing half of international variation in cardiovascular mortality to genetic factors.

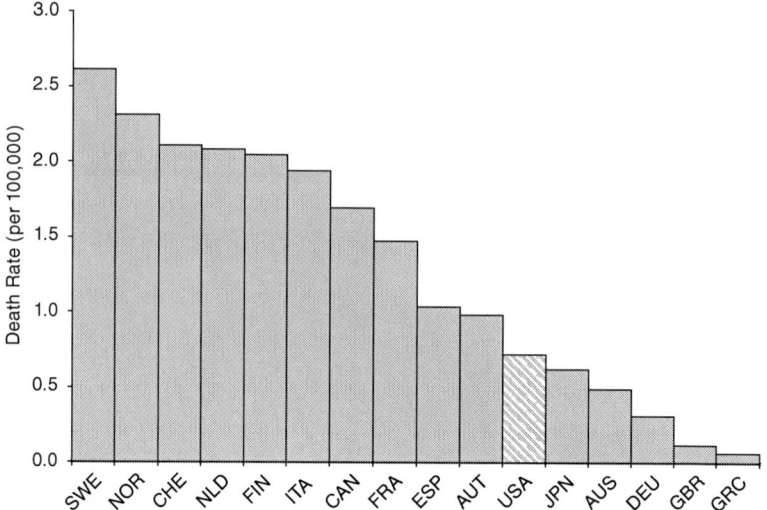

FIGURE 9-1 Age-standardized death rates at ages 50+ from influenza, 2000-2004.
NOTE: AUS = Australia, AUT = Austria, CAN = Canada, CHE = Switzerland, DEU = Germany, ESP = Spain, FIN = Finland, FRA = France, GBR = Great Britain, GRC = Greece, ITA = Italy, JPN = Japan, NLD = the Netherlands, NOR = Norway, SWE = Sweden, USA = United States.

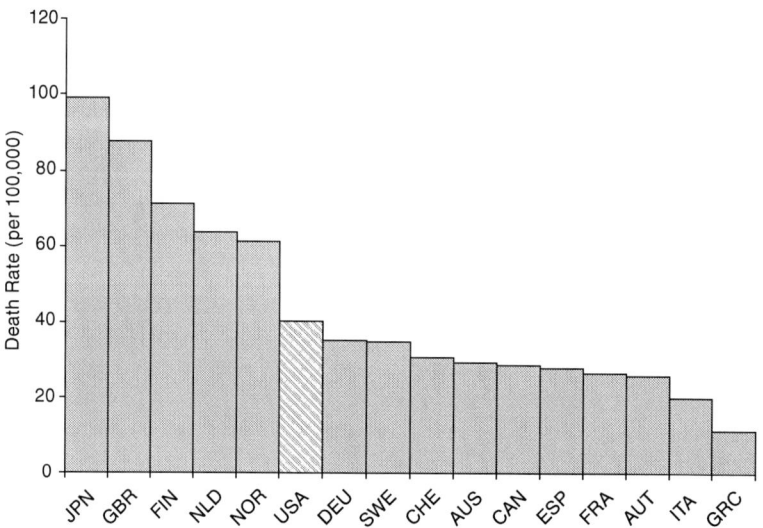

FIGURE 9-2 Age-standardized death rates at ages 50+ from pneumonia, 2000-2004.
NOTE: AUS = Australia, AUT = Austria, CAN = Canada, CHE = Switzerland, DEU = Germany, ESP = Spain, FIN = Finland, FRA = France, GBR = Great Britain, GRC = Greece, ITA = Italy, JPN = Japan, NLD = the Netherlands, NOR = Norway, SWE = Sweden, USA = United States.

ages 50+ is actually below the weighted or unweighted mean for the other 15 countries.

DISEASE PREVENTION

Medical procedures and survival rates are indicators of what happens to individuals whose health problems come to the attention of the health care system. But a health care system can also help prevent serious health problems from occurring in the first place. Of course, early identification of a disease is also preventive medicine in the sense that it may prevent death. But access to preventive medicine would appear to be an especially problematic area in the United States because 47 million people lack any form of health insurance (DeNavas-Walt, Proctor, and Smith, 2007).[5] Such people are less likely to see a doctor and thus to receive routine testing that might detect the early stages of a disease and prevent its clinical manifestations (Institute of Medicine, 2001). They are also less likely to receive advice about health maintenance and disease prevention (Institute of Medicine, 2001). While this chapter focuses on ages above 50, the mortality levels in this age range reflect the conditions to which individuals have been exposed throughout their lives. Preventive medicine may have a large role to play at younger ages as well as older ones.

An additional factor that may inhibit disease prevention in the United States is the shortage of primary care physicians. The United States scores in the bottom group of 6 out of 18 OECD countries on a scale of the adequacy of primary care (Macinko, Starfield, and Shi, 2003). The scale is built from items relating to policy, finances, and personnel. In turn, the adequacy of primary care may be related to disease prevention (Macinko, Starfield, and Shi, 2003).

The best indication of the success of prevention is disease incidence—but international data on disease incidence are nil. As noted earlier, disease prevalence is higher in the United States than in a European composite for cancer, heart disease, stroke, chronic lung disease, and diabetes (Thorpe et al., 2007a). Such a difference could result from higher incidence, better detection, or longer survival after detection in the United States. It could also result from reporting differences, for example, a greater inclination to report disease in the United States. But a careful study by Banks et al. (2006) using biomarkers suggests that morbidity differences between England and the United States at ages 55-64 are real and not a result of differences in reportage. A related study found that, faced with the same set of health-

---

[5]It has been claimed that this number includes 10 million people who are in fact covered by Medicaid insurance but who fail to report it (Ohsfeldt and Schneider, 2006).

related vignettes, Americans were less likely to report themselves as disabled than the Dutch (Kapteyn, Smith, and van Soest, 2007).

Even if incidence data were available, analysts would have to disentangle the role of personal behavioral and social histories from that of health system performance. And these are not always readily distinguishable. Are the historically high rates of smoking in the United States attributable to the failure of the U.S. public health system to stem the smoking tide? The fact that Canada had for many years the second highest consumption of cigarettes per adult (Forey et al., 2002) makes it appear that geographic factors, perhaps related to conditions for growing or importing tobacco, had more to do with consumption patterns than did health care systems. And public health authorities were not passive in the United States. The U.S. surgeon general's 1964 report on the health hazards of cigarette smoking was the first major indictment of the habit by a government authority (U.S. Department of Health, Education, and Welfare, 1964), and it was quickly followed up with a massive antismoking media campaign (Cutler and Glaeser, 2006). The United States had the largest reduction in manufactured cigarettes consumed per adult of any country between 1970 and 2000 (Forey et al., 2002). Some of that decline was likely attributable to public health efforts (Cutler and Glaeser, 2006).

However it is achieved, the high prevalence of disease in the United States adds considerably to health expenditure. Thorpe et al. (2007b) combine comparative prevalence data on 10 conditions in HRS (in the United States) and SHARE (in Europe) with U.S. Agency for Healthcare Research and Quality data on expenditure per medical condition for the population ages 50+. Their 95 percent confidence intervals on the per capita cost of higher disease prevalence in the United States are $1,195 to $1,750 per year, or 12.7 to 18.7 percent of total personal health care spending among those ages 50+. Inefficiencies in the U.S. health care system are not solely responsible for high per capita health expenditures; the high prevalence of major diseases is also substantially implicated (see also Michaud et al., 2009).

CASE STUDY I: PROSTATE CANCER

Accounting for 31,000 deaths in 2000, prostate cancer was, after lung cancer, the second leading cause of cancer deaths among U.S. men that year (National Center for Health Statistics, 2002). Unlike most chronic diseases, it is not associated with cigarette smoking (Lumey et al., 1997). A link with exercise has been suggested in several studies, but a review article found that "conclusions were quite variable . . . odds ratios [of developing prostate cancer] for men engaged in high levels of activity ranged from 0.2 to over 2.0" (Torti and Matheson, 2004). Dietary risk factors are suspected but not well established. The risk of prostate cancer is somewhat higher for men with a high body mass index, but the risk is less than for other cancers (Crawford, 2003). Genetic factors, some of them associated with race, appear to be important in the risk of developing prostate cancer (Li et al., 2007). Its relatively flat landscape of behavioral risk factors, together with its medical preventability, make mortality from prostate cancer a purer indicator of health care system performance than mortality from many other chronic diseases of adulthood.

Prostate Cancer Screening

The Digital Rectal Examination (DRE) and Prostate Specific Antigen (PSA) test are the primary screening tools for prostate cancer. As a screening test, DRE is of limited value because it cannot investigate the entire prostate gland (Ilic et al., 2006). It is more difficult to detect cancer with DRE than with the PSA test (Harris and Lohr, 2002). The PSA test has the added benefits of being easy to perform, relatively inexpensive, and reproducible (Constantinou and Feneley, 2006).

The PSA blood test for the presence of prostate cancer was approved by the Food and Drug Administration in 1986 (Shampo, 2002). The test enables the detection of high and/or rapidly increasing levels of an antigen that often signal the presence of prostate cancer. High levels of the antigen can also be produced by other conditions; confirmation of cancer is made by transrectal ultrasound-guided biopsy (TRUS).

The PSA test is somewhat controversial. One reason is that, like many other medical screens, the PSA test can produce a false positive—a report of potential cancer when it is not present. According to a summary of studies of the sensitivity and specificity of PSA testing, an average of 75 percent of those with PSA readings above 4.0 ug/l have prostate cancer and 71 percent of men with prostate cancer have a PSA reading above 4.0 ug/l (Bunting, 2002). However, the main reservation about the use of the PSA test is that treatment for prostate cancer can produce impotence and/or incontinence. Because of these side effects, several organizations have recommended against PSA testing for men over 75 (U.S. Preventive Services Task Force, 2008). However, the American Cancer Society and the American Urological Association recommend that the PSA test should be offered annually to men over age 50 with at least a 10-year life expectancy.

By reputation the United States has been the world leader in PSA testing, especially in the early years after the test was developed (Bouchardy et al., 2008; De Koning et al., 2002; Hsing, Tsao, and Devesa, 2000; Vercelli et al., 2000). Table 9-2 compiles data on the frequency of PSA testing in various countries or regions. The age ranges used and the survey dates are not identical from country to country, preventing exact comparisons. The United States has the highest recorded percentage ever tested at older

TABLE 9-2 Indicators of Frequency of PSA Testing Among Men

A. Percentage of Men Ever Receiving a PSA Test

Country	Percentage of Men Ever Receiving a PSA Test	Year	Age Group
Australia	49	2003	40+
Austria	54.6	2006-2007	40+
Canada	47.5[a]	2000-2001	50+
France	36	2005	40-74
Italy	31.4	2003	50+
Netherlands (Rotterdam)	12.7[a]	1994	55-74
Switzerland (Vaud and Neuchâtel Cantons)	10	Early 1990s	65+
United States	75 (BRFSS)	2001	50+
	62.7 (NHIS)[b]	2005	50-79

B. Percentage of Men Recently Receiving a PSA Test

Country	Percentage of Men Receiving a PSA Test in the Past x Years	x	Year	Age Group
Australia	27	2	1995/1996	50+
Austria	31.1	1	2006-2007	40+
Belgium (Limburg Province)	23	1	1996-1998	40+
Canada	26	1	2000-2001	40+
Italy	15.9	1	2002	50+
Netherlands (Rotterdam)	20.2	3	1997-2000	55-74
Norway (3 counties)	7	1	1999	50-65
Spain (Getafe City)	20.9	2	1997-1999	55+
Sweden	25.3[c]	1	2002	50+
United Kingdom	7	1	1999-2001	45-84
United States	57 (BRFSS)	1	2001	50+
	48.4 (NHIS)[b]	2	2005	50-79

NOTE: BRFSS = Behavioral Risk Factor Surveillance System; NHIS = National Health Interview Survey.

[a]Of the two sources of U.S. data presented in Table 9-2, the data from the Centers for Disease Control and Prevention's Behavioral Risk Factor Surveillance System are less reliable because they are based on a telephone survey with a low response rate.

[b]This figure does not include men with a history of prostate cancer.

[c]According to Sennfalt, Carlsson, and Varenhorst (2006), 430,000 PSA tests were performed in Sweden in 2002. We assume that all were performed on men ages 50+. The UN Population Division's estimates for Sweden's male population (ages 50+) for 2000 and 2005 were retrieved from the UN Statistics Division's Common Database and interpolated to give a figure for 2002 of 1,699,442.

SOURCES: Adapted from Beaulac, Fry, and Onysko (2006); Beemsterboer et al. (2000); D'Ambrosio et al. (2004); Eisinger et al. (2008); Gibbons and Waters (2003); Holden et al. (2006); Klimont, Ktir, and Leitner (2007); Levi et al. (1998); Lousbergh et al. (2002); Melia et al. (2003); Otto et al. (2003); Páez et al. (2002); Ross, Berkowitz, and Ekweume (2008); Sennfalt, Carlsson, and Varenhorst (2006); Sirovich, Schwartz, and Woloshin (2003); Smith and Armstrong (1998); Zappa et al. (2003).

ages (prevalence) as well as the highest percentage tested in a recent period (incidence).[6] An analysis of survey data from HRS and SHARE at ages 50-64, 65-74, and 75+ shows that, among 16 OECD countries in 2004, the United States ranked either first or second in the proportion of the population having had a PSA test in the past year (Howard, Richardson, and Thorpe, 2009).

Evidence about the efficacy of PSA testing from randomized controlled trials has been mixed. The Prostate, Lung, Colorectal, and Ovarian (PLCO) Cancer Screening Trial began in 1993 and involved 76,693 U.S. men ages 55-74. After 7 to 10 years of follow-up, the death rate from prostate cancer did not differ significantly between the study and the control groups. As noted by the authors, one possible explanation of the negative result is that PSA testing is already so frequent in the United States (see Table 9-2) that high levels of screening were already present among the control group. Furthermore, many cancers had already been identified in both the study and the control groups (Andriole et al., 2009). Results of the study are most reasonably interpreted as addressing the question of whether mortality advantages would pertain to *extending* PSA testing in a population in which half of men are already being tested every two years.

The second trial, the European Randomized Study of Screening for Prostate Cancer, was more than twice as large and was conducted in a region where prostate cancer screening is much less common. The trial began in the early 1990s in seven European countries and included a total of 162,243 men between the ages of 55 and 69. The study found that offering PSA screening to the treatment group reduced the death rate from prostate cancer by 20 percent (rate ratio of 0.73, 95% CI, 0.56 to 0.90). The absolute reduction was 0.71 prostate cancer deaths per 1,000 men. The median and average follow-up times were 9 and 8.8 years, respectively; death rates in the two study groups began diverging after 7 to 8 years and continued to diverge subsequently (Schröder et al., 2009).

The Goteborg, Sweden, component of the European trial followed 20,000 randomly selected men ages 50-66 for 10 years. Half were invited for biennial PSA testing, with 10,000 men serving as passive controls for whom diagnosis of metastatic prostate cancer was monitored by using the Swedish Cancer Registry. The risk of being diagnosed with metastatic (i.e., advanced) prostate cancer was reduced by 48.9 percent in the PSA treatment group relative to controls ($p < .01$) (Aus et al., 2007).

According to the SEER database, after the PSA test was introduced in the late 1980s, the recorded incidence of prostate cancer in the United States rose from 119 per 100,000 in 1986 to a peak of 237 per 100,000

---

[6]Of the two sources of U.S. data presented in Table 9-2, the data from the Center for Disease Control and Prevention's Behavioral Risk Factor Surveillance System are less reliable because they are based on a telephone survey with a low response rate.

in 1992 (National Cancer Institute, 2008).[7] The proportion of tumors that are metastatic was 25 percent of newly diagnosed tumors in 1980 and only 4 percent in 2002 (Etzioni et al., 2008). Consistent with more extensive screening, the United States identifies prostate cancer at an earlier stage, on average, than Sweden (Stattin et al., 2005), Japan (Ogawa et al., 2008), or the United Kingdom (Collin et al., 2008). Stage at diagnosis is particularly important in prognosis—if detected at an early stage, prostate cancer can be treated by radical prostatectomy or radiotherapy.

Prostate Cancer Treatment

Once prostate cancer is detected, a variety of treatments can be employed, including radical prostatectomy, radiation by beam (external beam radiotherapy) or implanted seeds (brachytherapy), or hormone therapy. "Watchful waiting" is also an option. Since 1991, radical prostatectomy has been the most common treatment for localized prostate cancer in the United States. It serves as the initial treatment for over a third of newly diagnosed patients (Harris and Lohr, 2002). Observational studies have described apparent survival advantages from radical prostatectomy and radiation therapy (e.g., Trock et al., 2008; Wong et al., 2006) but not always from hormone therapy alone (Lu-Yao et al., 2008). The questions of possible selection bias that are always present in observational studies add uncertainty to these results.

Uncertainty has been reduced by several recent reports of randomized clinical trials. A key study of Scandinavian men examined survival after diagnosis of prostate cancer. Men were randomly assigned to radical prostatectomy or to watchful waiting (Bill-Axelson et al., 2005). Some of those assigned to prostatectomy did not have the operation, and some of those assigned to watchful waiting pursued radiation or hormonal therapy. Nevertheless, after a median follow-up period of 8.2 years, the group assigned to prostatectomy had cumulative proportions of death from prostate cancer that were lower by 44 percent, rates of disease progression that were lower by 67 percent, and rates of distant metastasis that were lower by 40 percent. All comparisons were statistically significant (Bill-Axelson et al., 2005). After a median follow-up period of 10.8 years, the group assigned to prostatectomy had relative reductions of 35 percent in risk of prostate cancer death and 35 percent in risk of distant metastases (Bill-Axelson et al., 2008). In summary, radical prostatectomy was found to reduce prostate cancer mortality and risk of metastases, although no further increase in benefit was observed 10+ years after surgery.

---

[7]The data are for males and refer to the age-adjusted rates for all ages.

A randomized trial of variation in radiation dosage reported a highly significant beneficial effect on survival of heavier doses (Pollack et al., 2002). This study did not compare those radiated to those unradiated. Another randomized trial of adjuvant radiotherapy enrolled 425 men with pathologically advanced prostate cancer who had undergone radical prostatectomy between 1988 and 1997. Adjuvant radiotherapy significantly reduced the risk of PSA relapse and disease recurrence, although improvements in survival were not statistically significant (Thompson et al., 2006).

Several randomized clinical trials evaluate the use of hormone therapy as an adjunct to surgery or radiation in high-risk patients; the value of hormone therapy used alone or as primary therapy has been assessed only by observational studies. A population-based cohort study found that primary androgen deprivation therapy does not improve survival in elderly men compared with conservative management (no surgery, radiation, or hormone therapy) (Lu-Yao et al., 2008). However, three Phase III randomized trials have shown that a combination of radiotherapy and androgen suppression improve survival relative to radiotherapy alone (Bolla et al., 2002; Hanks et al., 2003; Pilepich et al., 2005).

Antonarakis and colleagues (2007) conducted a systematic review of studies published between 1986 and 2006 on hormone therapy for nonmetastatic prostate cancer. They extracted survival probabilities for men with localized or locally advanced prostate cancer receiving immediate hormone therapy as adjunct to radiation therapy, adjunct to radical prostatectomy, or stand-alone therapy. They found that survival in patients treated with hormone therapy for nonmetastatic prostate cancer may be longer than has been previously estimated. Men receiving hormone therapy alone had estimated 5-year disease-free survival (DFS) of 57 percent (median = 6.0 years) and overall survival (OS) of 70 percent (median = 7.0 years). Of the 10 studies used to estimate the DFS and OS for hormone therapy alone, 7 were Phase III randomized controlled trials and 3 were observational. The median follow-up was between 3.9 and 10.4 years. Comparative figures from two meta-analyses of primary hormone therapy in men with metastatic prostate cancer are a 5-year OS of 25 percent, a 10-year OS of 6 percent, and a median OS of 1.7-3.3 years (Antonarakis et al., 2007).

Thus far, few studies have compared all the standard treatment regimens in terms of overall survival and disease-specific survival. Zhou and colleagues (2009) used linked Ohio Cancer Incidence Surveillance System, Medicare, and death certificate files to examine overall and disease-specific survival for 10,179 men ages 65+ who were diagnosed with prostate cancer between 1999 and 2001 and received radical prostatectomy, brachytherapy, external beam radiotherapy, androgen deprivation therapy, or no treatment within 6 months after the initial diagnosis. At 7 years of follow-up and controlling for age, race, comorbidities, stage, and Gleason score, patients with localized disease who received radical prostatectomy or brachytherapy had a significantly lower risk of dying from prostate cancer compared with patients who received no treatment (HR = 0.25, p < 0.0001 for radical prostatectomy, and HR = 0.45, p < 0.02 for brachytherapy). In this study, radical prostatectomy and brachytherapy significantly improved overall and disease-specific survival compared with no treatment, suggesting that earlier curative treatment is better than no treatment (Zhou et al., 2009).

Population-based information about the frequency of various treatments of prostate cancer is much skimpier than information about the use of the PSA test. Among U.S. men ages 65-80 in SEER who were diagnosed with low-grade tumors between 1991 and 1999, 25.5 percent received no treatment within 6 months of diagnosis, 9.6 percent received hormone therapy, and the remaining 64.8 percent received either radiation or prostatectomy (Wong et al., 2006).

Scandinavian countries rarely use radical therapies—radical prostatectomy or radiation—and rely primarily on watchful waiting or hormone therapy for palliation (Fleshner, Rakovitch, and Klotz, 2000; Sandblom et al., 2000). For example, the fraction of patients treated with curative intent in Norway was only 3 percent in 1985-1989 and rose to 6 percent in 1990-1994. In 1990-1994, radical prostatectomy was used to treat only 3.0 and 3.3 percent of all patients diagnosed with prostate cancer in Norway and Sweden, respectively (Kvåle et al., 2007). Low levels of surgery and radiation therapy are also reported in Japan (Ogawa et al., 2008).

Differences in treatment approach also exist between the United States and the United Kingdom, with U.S. approaches generally being more aggressive, particularly in the use of surgery (Collin et al., 2008). A survey of U.S. and Canadian urologists indicated that American urologists tended to have a more aggressive approach to case identification and surgical intervention. They were also more likely to perform radical prostatectomy on patients over the age of 70 (Fleshner, Rakovitch, and Klotz, 2000).

Prostate Cancer Survival

The combination of earlier detection and aggressive treatment in the United States has produced greatly improved survival chances for men diagnosed with prostate cancer. The 5-year relative survival rates in the United States increased from 71 to 83 percent between 1984-1986 and 1987-1989, whereas European rates improved from 55 to 59 percent during the same period (Post et al., 1998). According to the National Cancer Institute (2008), the U.S. 5-year relative survival rate had increased to 99.2 percent for those diagnosed in 2000.

Gatta et al. (2000) compared international survival rates for cancers diagnosed between 1985 and 1989. All of the European countries considered had lower prostate cancer survival rates than the United States. European patients had a 4.1 times greater risk of dying in the first year after diagnosis, suggesting that earlier diagnosis plays an important role in these survival differences (Gatta et al., 2000). The updated study whose results are presented in Table 9-1 found that 5-year survival rates for prostate cancer in 2000-2002 were 99.3 percent in the United States compared with 77.5 percent in Europe.

Prostate Cancer Mortality

Population-level data on mortality have one distinct advantage over data on survival rates among those newly diagnosed: they are not subject to lead-time bias. If one country is diagnosing cancer sooner than another but early diagnosis does not alter the clinical course of the disease and delay or prevent death, then that country will enjoy no advantage in mortality as a result of its earlier diagnoses. When early diagnosis improves prognosis, population-level mortality is responsive to the timeliness of diagnosis. It is also responsive to the efficacy of treatments employed, regardless of stage at diagnosis. Mortality data have a similar advantage relative to recorded incidence and prevalence data, both of which are subject to lead-time bias.

In order to investigate whether the relatively aggressive use of PSA testing and therapy in the United States has produced an unusually rapid decline in mortality from prostate cancer, we have used World Health Organization (WHO) data on deaths by cause and population by 5-year age groups. We have chosen a group of 15 economically developed OECD countries for purposes of comparison: Australia, Austria, Canada, Finland, France, Germany, Greece, Italy, Japan, the Netherlands, Norway, Spain, Sweden, Switzerland, and the United Kingdom.

Figure 9-3 compares levels of age-standardized death rates per 100,000 (all ages combined) in the United States to the unweighted mean death rate in these 15 comparison countries.[8] With the exception of 1985, the United States had higher death rates each year from 1980 to 1995. Beginning in 1996, the United States had lower rates and the U.S. advantage grew every year thereafter. By 2003, the United States had death rates that were 20.4 percent lower than the mean of the comparison countries. Mortality rates among men ages 60-79 were lower in 1997 than in any year since 1950 (Tarone, Chu, and Brawley, 2000). Baade, Coory, and Aitken (2004) note that changes in risk factors and in the accuracy of procedures for recording cause-of-death information are unlikely to be responsible for the observed trends.

---

[8]These rates are taken from the International Agency for Research on Cancer (http://www.dcp.iarc.fr/ [accessed June 2010]), which extracts the World Health Organization mortality data and standardizes the rates to the world population in 1960 (Segi world standard).

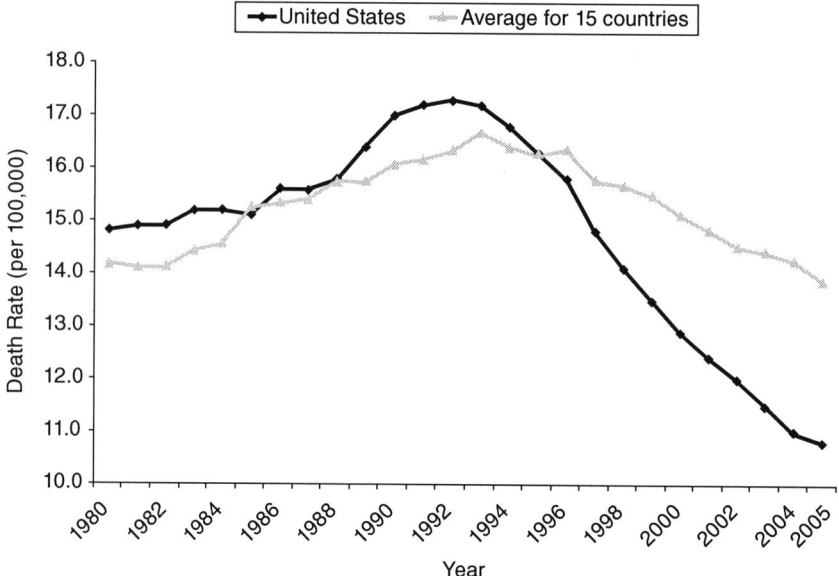

FIGURE 9-3 Age-standardized death rates from prostate cancer, 1980-2005.

Declines in prostate cancer mortality have been attributed to both PSA screening and improvements in treatment (Baade, Coory, and Aitken, 2004; Bouchardy et al., 2008; Collin et al., 2008; Kvåle et al., 2007; Potosky, Feuer, and Levin, 2001). An individual-level population model that used counterfactuals to simulate U.S. mortality and incidence of advanced-stage prostate cancer concluded that two-thirds of the decline in mortality between 1990 and 1999, and 80 percent of the decline in distant-stage incidence, was attributable to expanded PSA testing (Etzioni et al., 2008).

To test whether the faster mortality decline in the United States was statistically significant, we use a negative binomial regression in a fixed-effects model applied to data for these 15 countries for the period 1982-2005. The dependent variable is the log of the number of deaths from prostate cancer in a particular age, country and year cell, with population size in a particular cell used as the exposure. Independent variables are a set of age group identifiers, a set of period identifiers, a dummy variable for the United States, and a set of U.S./period interactions. Six 4-year-wide time periods are used, beginning with 1982-1985 and ending with 2002-2005. The period before PSA testing was begun, 1982-1985, was chosen as the reference period. Significance tests recognize the clustering of observations by country. Results are presented in Table 9-3.

The coefficient of the interactive variable for U.S. observations during

TABLE 9-3 Coefficients of Negative Binomial Regression Predicting the Log of the Number of Deaths from Prostate and Breast Cancer

		Coefficient (standard error)	
Variable		Prostate Cancer	Breast Cancer
Constant		−10.37***	−7.657***
		(0.079)	(0.067)
Age	50-54	0.000	0.000
		(−)	(−)
	55-59	1.166***	0.247***
		(0.026)	(0.013)
	60-64	2.159***	0.413***
		(0.026)	(0.019)
	65-69	3.013***	0.550***
		(0.032)	(0.024)
	70-74	3.744***	0.721***
		(0.034)	(0.029)
	75-79	4.384***	0.925***
		(0.038)	(0.032)
	80-84	4.942***	1.157***
		(0.041)	(0.038)
	85+	5.455***	1.520***
		(0.047)	(0.046)
Period	1982-1985	0.000	0.000
		(−)	(−)
	1986-1989	0.0586***	0.0350***
		(0.010)	(0.011)
	1990-1993	0.103***	0.0276
		(0.016)	(0.015)
	1994-1997	0.0837***	−0.00241
		(0.023)	(0.028)
	1998-2001	0.0242	−0.0741*
		(0.029)	(0.037)
	2002-2005	−0.0529	−0.114**
		(0.036)	(0.042)
Observation from United States		0.125	0.108
		(0.080)	(0.082)
Observation from United States in	1982-1985	0.000	0.000
		(−)	(−)
	1986-1989	−0.0229*	−0.0216*
		(0.010)	(0.011)
	1990-1993	−0.00278	−0.0225
		(0.015)	(0.015)
	1994-1997	−0.0850***	−0.0585*
		(0.023)	(0.028)
	1998-2001	−0.215***	−0.0892*
		(0.029)	(0.036)
	2002-2005	−0.274***	−0.126**
		(0.036)	(0.040)

*$p < 0.05$, **$p < 0.01$, ***$p < 0.001$.

the period 2002-2005 is –0.274, which is significant at p < .001. Compared with expectations based on country and year, the United States had roughly 27 percent lower mortality in 2002-2005 than it did in 1982-1985. (The U.S./2002-2005 variable is always significant at p < 0.001 regardless of reference period used.) Likewise, the coefficient of the U.S./period interactive variable for the 1998-2001 period is –0.215 and is also significant at p < .001. So the United States had significantly faster declines in mortality from prostate cancer than did comparison countries between 1982-1985 and both 1998-2001 and 2002-2005.

Mortality trends from prostate cancer may be affected by "attribution bias": people who have had prostate cancer detected may be more likely to have their death ascribed to it, even though some other morbid process was actually responsible (Feuer, Merrill, and Hankey, 1999). Such bias, combined with more aggressive screening, would produce a rise rather than a fall in prostate cancer mortality. This bias may account for the rise in prostate cancer mortality in the late 1980s and early 1990s (see Figure 9-3), but it obviously would minimize rather than accentuate the actual decline that is observed between 1982-1985 and 2002-2005.

African Americans have prostate cancer death rates that are among the highest in the world (Crawford, 2003). Perhaps the most prominent explanation of the racial disparity is that dark skin inhibits the absorption of Vitamin D, which is highly protective against prostate cancer (Li et al., 2007). A more tenuous connection to the health care system among African Americans is probably also a factor. Nevertheless, a sharp decline in prostate cancer mortality in the United States is evident among both whites and African Americans. Both whites and African Americans had rates that peaked in the early 1990s. Between 1992-1993 and 2004-2005, the death rate declined by 32.2 percent for African Americans and by 36.3 percent for whites (Li et al., 2007). The absolute decline in rates was much larger for African Americans: their 5-year survival rate increased from 68.4 percent for those diagnosed in 1986, the year PSA testing was approved, to 97.0 percent for those diagnosed in 2000. Among whites, the improvement was from 79.0 to 99.8 percent (National Cancer Institute, 2008).

CASE STUDY II: BREAST CANCER

Breast cancer is the most common cause of cancer death among women in a majority of high-income countries (Vainio and Bianchini, 2002). In contrast to prostate cancer, there are important behavioral risk factors for breast cancer. These include childlessness or low parity, late age at first birth, obesity, and use of hormone replacement therapy (Das, Feuer, and Mariotto, 2005; Levi et al., 2005). Thus, trends in mortality are more difficult to interpret as exclusively reflecting medical factors. But, like prostate cancer, breast cancer is highly amenable to medical intervention through screening and therapy.

Breast Cancer Screening

Mammography, breast self-examination, clinical breast examination (CBE), and magnetic resonance imaging (MRI) are used to screen for breast cancer. No randomized trials of CBE alone have been completed, and case-control and ecological studies have provided only limited evidence for its efficacy in reducing mortality from breast cancer (Vainio and Bianchini, 2002). Breast self-examination is an appealing screening method because it is noninvasive, but it has weak ability to detect breast cancer (Elmore et al., 2005). Two randomized trials of breast self-examination have been conducted, and neither found evidence of mortality reduction. The International Agency for Research on Cancer (IARC) has concluded that there is inadequate evidence for the efficacy of CBE and breast self-examination in reducing breast cancer mortality (Vainio and Bianchini, 2002). The U.S. Preventive Services Task Force also found evidence from trials involving CBE and breast self-examination to be inconclusive (Humphrey et al., 2002). The third technique, MRI, is mainly employed in high-risk patients and after conventional diagnostic procedures have already been conducted (Veronesi et al., 2005). Because of its high cost (approximately 10 times that of mammography) and its relatively low specificity, MRI is not a feasible tool for routine screening in the general population (Elmore et al., 2005).

Thus, mammography is currently the most important diagnostic tool for breast cancer. It is the only screening test that has been shown to reduce mortality from breast cancer in randomized trials and population studies (Veronesi et al., 2005; Wells, 1998). The IARC concluded that there is sufficient evidence from randomized trials that offering of mammography to a treatment group reduces breast cancer mortality in women ages 50-69, by an average of 25 percent. After adjusting for the effect of nonacceptance of the screening invitation, this figure rises to 35 percent (Vainio and Bianchini, 2002). The U.S. Preventive Services Task Force reviewed eight randomized controlled trials of offering mammograms to treatment groups and concluded that, for studies that were designated as of fair quality or better, the relative mortality risk for women ages 40-74 was 0.84 (95% CI, 0.77 to 0.91) (Humphrey et al., 2002; see also Gøtzsche and Nielsen, 2009). While some concerns have been raised concerning flaws in the trials' design and execution, in-depth independent reviews have concluded that they do not negate the trials' results (Quinn, 2003).

The National Cancer Institute and the American Cancer Society issued the first formal guidelines for mammography in 1977, advocating screening for all women over the age of 50 (Wells, 1998). Currently, all major U.S.

medical organizations recommend screening mammography for women over the age of 40 (Ahern and Shen, 2009; Elmore et al., 2005). The United States is the only country that strongly endorses screening mammography for women under age 50 (Jatoi and Miller, 2003); recent evidence has supported the efficacy of screening in the age group 40-49 (Humphrey et al., 2002).

Use of mammographic screening in the United States increased very rapidly; the percentage of women ages 50-64 who reported having a mammogram in the past 2 years increased from 31.7 percent in 1987 to 73.7 percent in 1998 (Breen et al., 2001). Screening programs generally began later in Europe than in the United States (Møller et al., 2005). The start dates for organized screening programs in the countries under investigation range from 1986 to 1999 (Jatoi and Miller, 2003; Shapiro et al., 1998).

Table 9-4 presents international data on the frequency of screening for breast cancer in recent years. In the early to mid-1990s, the United States had the highest frequency of mammograms in the nine countries for which we are able to locate data. The OECD has collected more recent data showing that, while the frequency of mammograms has increased in the United States, it has grown faster in a number of other countries. The most recent tabulations, using data from HRS and SHARE, show that, among 11 OECD countries in 2004, the United States had the highest proportion of the population receiving a mammogram within the past 2 years at ages 50-64, 65-74, and 75+ (Howard, Richardson, and Thorpe, 2009).

Consistent with the relatively high frequency of mammograms in the United States, Sant et al. (2004) found that breast cancer is diagnosed at what is, on average, a later stage in Europe than in the United States.

Breast Cancer Treatment

In OECD countries, the large majority of cases of breast cancer are treated surgically. Surgery is often supplemented with some combination of radiotherapy, hormone therapy, and chemotherapy (i.e., adjuvant therapy). Descriptions of the Halsted mastectomy, which served as the treatment of choice for breast cancer for almost a century, were first published in 1894 (Veronesi et al., 2002). It was later replaced by the modified radical mastectomy, which was popular in the 1980s (Cotlar, Dubose, and Rose, 2003). Neither the original Halsted radical mastectomy nor the modified radical mastectomy was introduced on the basis of evidence from randomized clinical trials; however, observational studies confirm an enormous survival advantage for surgery relative to no surgery (e.g., Sant et al., 2004).

In most high-income countries, breast-conserving surgery (BCS, also known as lumpectomy) is currently the most common primary treatment for breast cancer (Veronesi et al., 2005). Relative to total mastectomy, its

TABLE 9-4 Percentage of Women Receiving a Mammogram in Previous 2 Years: 1994 and 2003[a]

Country	Earlier Year			Later Year		
	% Screened	Year	Age Group	% Screened	Year	Age Group
Australia	51.4	1996-1997	50-69	55.6	2003-2004	50-69
Austria	23.1	1995	40-79			
	35.7		50-54			
Belgium	49.2	1997	50-69	54.0	2003	50-69
Canada	50.0	1994	50+	70.6	2003	50-69
Finland				87.7	2003	50-59
France				72.8	2003	50-69
Hungary				60.2	2003	45-65
Iceland				62.0	2003	40-69
Ireland				79.5	2003	50-64
Italy				29.0	2000	55-69
Japan				2.6	2003	50-69
Luxembourg				62.4	2003	50-69
Netherlands	53.2	1994	50-69	79.0	2003	50-75
New Zealand				62.3	2003	50-64
Norway				98.0	2003	50-69
Portugal				60.1	2003	50-69
Spain	28.0	1994	40-70			
Sweden				83.6	2004	50-74
Switzerland[b]	20.0	1992-1993	50-64	27.0	2002	50-69
United Kingdom[c]	63.9	1995	50-64	74.7	2003	50-64
United States	66.5	1994	50-64	76.0	2003	50-69

[a]For later years, when there are two observations for the same country, we use survey rather than program data in order to maximize comparability with the United States (this affected only Canada and the Netherlands).

[b]For 1992-1993, the data for Switzerland is for the canton of Vaud only, and the screening interval is 1 year.

[c]For the United Kingdom, the recall period is 3 years.

SOURCES: Adapted from Australian Institute of Health and Welfare (2008); Bulliard, De Landtsheer, and Levi (2003); Capet, Arbyn, and Abarca (2003); Centraal Bureau voor de Statistiek (2009); Department of Health (1999); Luengo et al. (1996); National Center for Health Statistics (2000); Organisation for Economic Co-operation and Development (2006, 2008); Snider et al. (1997); Vutuc, Haidinger, and Waldhoer (1998).

advantages are reduced disfigurement and morbidity rather than further reductions in mortality (Wood, 1994). After 20 years of follow-up in a randomized trial, Fisher et al. (2002) reported finding no differences in disease-free survival, distant-disease-free survival, or overall survival between women who underwent lumpectomy alone compared with those having a total mastectomy (see also Veronesi et al., 2002). In 1990, the

National Institutes of Health Consensus Development Conference recommended breast conservation therapy for the majority of women with Stage I or II breast carcinoma (Lazovich et al., 1999).

Since radiation treatment of breast cancer was first used in 1896, equipment and techniques have improved substantially, particularly since the 1960s (Ragaz et al., 1997). The Early Breast Cancer Trialists' Collaborative Group conducted a meta-analysis of 36 trials of radiotherapy. They found that the local recurrence rate with radiotherapy and surgery was three times lower than with surgery alone, and that radiotherapy was associated with a 6 percent reduction in the relative risk of death due to breast cancer (odds ratio, 0.94) (Early Breast Cancer Trialists' Collaborative Group, 1995). Ragaz et al. (1997) found that, after 15 years of follow-up, women assigned to chemotherapy plus radiotherapy had a 33 percent reduction in the recurrence rate and a 29 percent reduction in mortality from breast cancer compared with women treated with chemotherapy alone.

Adjuvant systemic multiagent chemotherapy and the drug tamoxifen have been estimated to reduce mortality (in terms of the relative reduction of the annual odds of death) by 27 percent and 47 percent, respectively (Early Breast Cancer Trialists' Collaborative Group, 1998a, 1998b). These figures are derived from the meta-analyses of all randomized trials of any aspect of treatment for early breast cancer that began before 1990. There were 47 trials of adjuvant polychemotherapy involving 18,000 women (Early Breast Cancer Trialists' Collaborative Group, 1998a). Greater benefits were reported in women under age 50, who experienced significant reductions in recurrence and mortality of 35 and 27 percent, respectively. For women between ages 50 and 69, these figures were 20 and 11 percent, respectively (Early Breast Cancer Trialists' Collaborative Group, 1998a).

Cole et al. first reported the clinical efficacy of tamoxifen for disseminated breast cancer in 1971. The Early Breast Cancer Trialists' Collaborative Group summarized the results of 55 randomized controlled trials involving more than 37,000 women. Compared with a placebo, adjuvant tamoxifen resulted in annual reductions of 26 percent in recurrence and 14 percent in death. Among women treated for 5 years, these figures rose to 50 and 28 percent, respectively (Early Breast Cancer Trialists' Collaborative Group, 1998b; Osborne, 1998). Tamoxifen produces significant benefits in women of all age groups (Early Breast Cancer Trialists' Collaborative Group, 1998b; Jaiyesimi et al., 1995). Following pharmacological and clinical evaluations, the U.S. Food and Drug Administration approved tamoxifen for the treatment of metastatic breast cancer in postmenopausal women in 1977. Tamoxifen was also approved as the initial endocrine therapy for disseminated breast cancer in premenopausal women.

Together, these studies constitute a substantial body of evidence supporting the effectiveness of treatment for breast cancer. A number of randomized trials have demonstrated that surgical options, radiation therapy, chemotherapy, and tamoxifen reduce recurrence rates and breast cancer mortality.

Information on international differences in breast cancer treatment is limited. A comparison of the Eurocare and SEER registry data found that 97 percent of women in SEER were treated surgically compared with 90 percent in the Eurocare registries. Rates of lymphadenectomy (surgical removal of one or more groups of lymph nodes) were slightly more extensive in the United States, and more axillary lymph nodes were examined in the United States (Sant et al., 2004). Hughes (2003) compared patterns of breast cancer care in Belgium, Canada (Manitoba and Ontario), France, Italy, Norway, Sweden, the United Kingdom (England), and the United States. During the latest period investigated, 1990-1993, at least 90 percent of women diagnosed with breast cancer received a mastectomy or breast-conserving surgery in all areas except Ontario, where the figure was 82 percent, and England (71 percent). The use of radiotherapy with BCS has also risen over time and varied considerably among countries. Among women receiving BCS in 1995-1997, Belgium, Canada, France, and the United Kingdom had the highest proportions of women receiving radiation therapy. The United States ranked below these countries and above Sweden and Italy (Hughes, 2003).

Adjuvant chemotherapy became standard treatment for breast cancer patients in the United States in the late 1970s (Ragaz et al., 1997). Tamoxifen began to be widely used in the late 1970s and early 1980s, after the Nolvadex Adjuvant Trial Organization trials demonstrated its effectiveness (Mariotto et al., 2002). It has since become the most widely prescribed antineoplastic agent for treatment of breast cancer in the United States and Great Britain (Jaiyesimi et al., 1995). Between 1975 and 2000, the percentage of breast cancer patients receiving chemotherapy in the United States increased from essentially 0 to 80 percent, while tamoxifen use increased from 0 to 50 percent (Berry et al., 2006). Starting in the mid-1980s, tamoxifen use in the United Kingdom also increased rapidly. By 1990, 50 percent of women with breast cancer over the age of 50 in the Thames region were receiving tamoxifen (Blanks et al., 2000). We have not found comparable international data on the use of chemotherapy and tamoxifen. Variations in stage and type of tumor, age of patient, type of surgery, and other factors make it impossible to reliably compare the few national or regional data that exist.

Breast Cancer Survival

Several studies have compared international survival rates from breast cancer. As noted above, the survival advantage of U.S. breast cancer patients compared with their European counterparts is well documented. The U.S. survival advantage is particularly sharp among older women (Hughes, 2003). International differences in survival are challenging to interpret, but three studies using cancer registry data for European and American women have attributed the survival differences from breast cancer to earlier diagnosis and more aggressive care in the United States. These factors have also been introduced to explain better breast cancer survival rates in the United States than in Canada (Ugnat et al., 2005).

Gatta et al. (2002) found that European breast cancer patients diagnosed in 1985-1989 had significantly lower 5-year relative survival rates than American patients (73 versus 82 percent). None of the 17 European countries had higher 5-year relative survival than the United States. In the first year after diagnosis, the risk of death from breast cancer was much higher in European than American patients. Survival rates fell with increasing age at diagnosis in both the United States and Europe, but the fall was more marked in Europe. Gatta et al. suggest that the survival rate differences may be attributable to earlier diagnosis in the United States.

The most thorough study compared American and European women diagnosed with breast cancer between 1990 and 1992 (Sant et al., 2004). The 5-year survival rate was higher in the United States than in Europe (89 versus 79 percent), and survival for each stage-at-diagnosis category was also higher in the United States. Early-stage tumors were more frequent in the United States (41 percent of cases) than in Europe (29 percent). Treatment was more aggressive in the United States, where 97.1 percent of women underwent surgery compared with 90.2 percent in Europe. In the United States, 50.7 percent of women had 15+ lymph nodes evaluated for metastasis, compared with 27.8 percent in Europe. The overall relative risk of death was 37 percent higher among European women (95 percent confidence interval, 25-50 percent). The excess risk was reduced to 20 percent by adjustment for surgical intervention, which was associated with a 90 percent reduction in mortality. Adjustment for stage at diagnosis reduced the relative risk to 12 percent, and further adjustment for the number of lymph nodes evaluated to determine cancer progression reduced the excess risk of death among the European women to an insignificant 7 percent. Introducing information on the use of radiotherapy did not alter the relative risk of European women. Thus, the higher survival rate in the United States appears to be a result both of earlier diagnosis and more aggressive treatment.

The most recent study compared cancer survival differences between Europe and the United States in 2000-2002 based on period rather than cohort survival data. As shown in Table 9-1, the 5-year survival rate for breast cancer was 79.0 percent in Europe, compared with 90.1 percent in the United States. Verdecchia et al. (2007) hypothesize that these differences were most likely due to differences in timeliness of diagnosis.

Trends in screening and in survival in the United States are consistent with the idea that earlier screening improves survival. The percentage of American women ages 50-64 who had received a mammogram in the previous two years increased from 32 percent in 1987 to 74 percent in 1998 and was accompanied by an increase in 5-year survival rates from 79 percent for those diagnosed in 1985 to 91 percent for those diagnosed in 2000 (National Cancer Institute, 2008).

Breast Cancer Mortality

In many developed countries, breast cancer mortality rates began declining around 1990 (Botha et al., 2003; Veronesi et al., 2005). It is unlikely that the declines in mortality were caused by changes in the major risk factors for the disease. In fact, the risk factor profile of women in high-income countries has, if anything, become less favorable over the past few decades as a result of rising obesity and delayed and reduced childbearing (Levi et al., 2005). Reductions after 2002 in the use of hormone replacement therapy could work in the opposite direction, but the risk is sufficiently small (Chlebowski et al., 2003; Writing Group for the Women's Health Initiative Investigators, 2002), and lags sufficiently long, that the decline should not be reflected in a data series that ends in 2005. Chu et al. (1996) rule out changes in coding or ascertainment as contributors to the mortality decline in the United States, noting that there had been no coding changes affecting breast cancer and that no systematic problems with ascertainment were identified after 1989.

Studies of trends in breast cancer mortality have attributed the declines mainly to earlier detection—in particular, rising rates of mammographic screening—and improved treatment (Chu et al., 1996; Levi et al., 2005; Veronesi et al., 2005). A careful, detailed simulation for the United States by Berry and colleagues (2006) concluded that "we can say with high probability that both screening and adjuvant therapy have contributed to the reductions in U.S. breast cancer mortality observed from 1975 (and especially from 1990) to 2000. Our best estimate is that about two-thirds of the reduction is due to therapy and one-third to screening" (p. 36). Using less precise methods, Blanks and colleagues (2000) reached a similar conclusion about the decline in breast cancer mortality in England and Wales from 1990 to 1998. Evidence that states with greater use of mammography had greater mortality declines between 1992 and 1999 supports the link between screening and mortality (Das et al., 2005).

We hypothesize that the United States has had a faster decline in breast cancer mortality than the comparison countries because it took better advantage of technological advances in screening and treatment. Mortality data alone do not permit us to distinguish between the effects of screening and treatment, but that distinction is not central to our argument.

Figure 9-4 shows the annual age-standardized death rate in the United States and the unweighted mean for our 15 OECD countries since 1980. Clearly, the United States has had a faster decline in breast cancer mortality than average among the comparison countries. Is the faster decline in the United States statistically significant? To answer this question, we repeat the approach used for prostate cancer, using WHO data files on deaths by cause and population by 5-year age groups. We employ negative binomial regression on data at ages 50+ (in 5-year-wide age groups until 85+). The dependent variable is the log of the number of deaths from breast cancer in a certain age group for a particular country and time period. Independent variables are a set of age group identifiers, a set of period identifiers, a dummy variable for the United States, and a set of U.S./period interactions. We designate six 4-year-wide time periods, beginning with 1982-1985 and ending with 2002-2005, and choose 1982-1985 as the reference period. Because of the rapid increase in the proportion of women receiving mammograms from less than a third in 1987 to 74 percent in 1998, a reference period in the early 1980s appears appropriate. Significance tests recognize the clustering of observations by country. Results are presented in Table 9-3.

Using 1982-1985 as the reference period, we find that the U.S./2002-2005 interaction term is significant at .01. With a coefficient of −.126, the coefficient implies that mortality in the United States has fallen 13 percent faster since 1982-1985 than in other countries. U.S. interactive coefficients

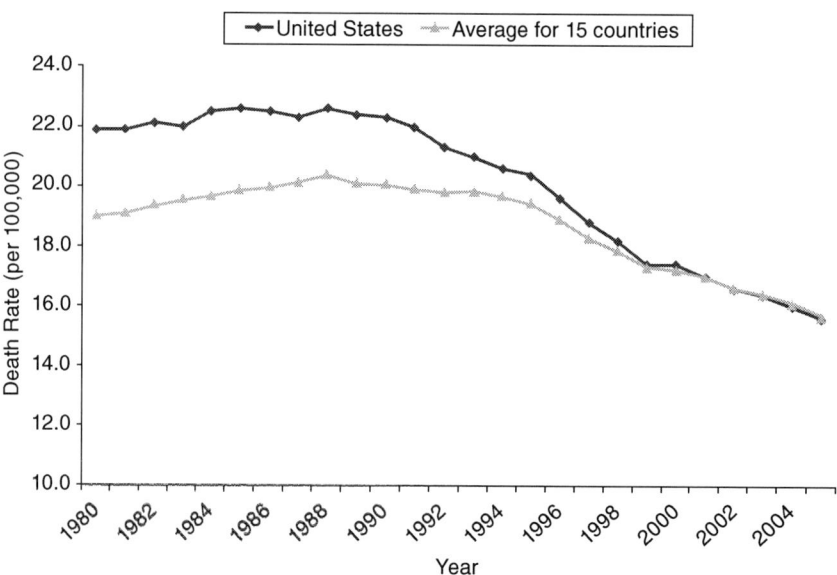

FIGURE 9-4 Age-standardized death rates from breast cancer, 1980-2005.

for 1994-1997 and 1998-2001 are also negative and significant at 5 percent. The interactive variable, U.S./2002-2005, is always significant at p < 0.01 regardless of which date is selected as the reference period (not shown). Thus, the United States has experienced a significantly faster decline in breast cancer mortality than comparison countries.

SUMMARY

We have demonstrated that mortality reductions from prostate cancer and breast cancer have been significantly more rapid in the United States than in a set of peer countries. We have argued that these unusually rapid declines are attributable to wider screening and more aggressive treatment of these diseases in the United States. It appears that the U.S. medical care system has worked effectively to reduce mortality from these important causes of death.

This conclusion is consistent with other evidence that we have reviewed on the performance of the U.S. health care system in enhancing survival: screening for other cancers also appears unusually extensive; 5-year survival rates from all of the major cancers are very favorable; survival rates following heart attack and stroke are also favorable (although 1-year survival rates following stroke are not above average); the proportion of people with elevated blood pressure or cholesterol levels who are receiving medication is well above European standards.

These performance indicators pertain primarily to what happens after a disease has developed. It is possible that the U.S. health care system performs poorly in preventing disease in the first place; however, there are no satisfactory international comparisons of disease incidence. Individuals report a higher prevalence of cancer and cardiovascular disease in the United States than in Europe, and biomarkers confirm the higher prevalence of many disease syndromes in the United States compared with England and Wales. Higher disease prevalence is prima facie evidence of higher disease incidence, although it could also be produced by better identification (e.g., through screening programs) or better survival. The history of exceptionally heavy smoking in the United States, and the more recent massive increase in obesity, suggest that a high disease incidence in the United States could not be laid entirely at the feet of the health care system, unless that system were held responsible for all health-related behaviors.

Evidence that the major diseases are effectively diagnosed and treated in the United States does not mean that there may not be great inefficiencies in the U.S. health care system. A list of prominent charges include fragmentation, duplication, inaccessibility of records, the practice of defensive medicine, misalignment of physician and patient incentives, limitations of access for a large fraction of the population, and excessively fast adoption of unproven technologies (Garber and Skinner, 2008; Cebul et al., 2008; Commonwealth Fund, 2008). Some of these inefficiencies have been identified by comparing performance across regions of the United States. Of course, the fact that certain regions do poorly relative to others does not imply that the United States does poorly relative to other countries. And many of the documented inefficiencies of the U.S. health care system add to its costs rather than harm patients.

Just as we are not addressing issues of efficiency on the production side, we are not treating patient welfare as the main outcome. Practices that produce greater longevity do not necessarily enhance well-being. This potential disparity is central to the controversy involving PSA testing, which uncovers many cancers that would never kill patients but whose treatment often produces adverse side effects.

The question that we have posed is much simpler: Does a poor performance by the U.S. health care system account for the low international ranking of longevity in the United States? Our answer is "No."

ACKNOWLEDGMENTS

This research was supported by the U.S. Social Security Administration (SSA) through grant no. 10-M-98363-1-01 to the National Bureau of Economic Research (NBER) as part of the SSA Retirement Research Consortium. The findings and conclusions expressed are solely those of the authors and do not represent the views of SSA, any agency of the federal government, or the NBER. We are grateful to Beth Soldo, Jason Schnittker, Eileen Crimmins, and anonymous reviewers for useful comments and suggestions.

REFERENCES

Ahern, C.H., and Shen, Y. (2009). Cost-effectiveness analysis of mammography and clinical breast examination strategies: A comparison with current guidelines. *Cancer Epidemiology, Biomarkers & Prevention, 18*(3), 718-725.

Andriole, G.L., Grubb, R.L., Buys, S.S., Chia, D., et al. (2009). Mortality results from a randomized prostate-cancer screening trial. *New England Journal of Medicine, 360*, 1310-1319.

Antonarakis, E.S., Blackford, A.L., Garrett-Mayer, E., and Eisenberger, M.A. (2007). Survival in men with nonmetastatic prostate cancer treated with hormone therapy: A quantitative systematic review. *Journal of Clinical Oncology, 25*(31), 4998-5008.

Aus, G., Bergdahl, S., Lodding, P., Lilja, H., et al. (2007). Prostate cancer screening decreases the absolute risk of being diagnosed with advanced prostate cancer—Results from a prospective, population-based randomized controlled trial. *European Urology, 51*, 659-664.

Australian Institute of Health and Welfare. (2008). *BreastScreen Australia Monitoring Report 2004-2005.* Cancer series no. 42, cat. no. CAN 37. Canberra: Author.

Avendano, M., Glymour, M., Banks, J., and Mackenbach, J.P. (2009). Health disadvantage in U.S. adults ages 50 to 74 years: A comparison of the health of rich and poor Americans with that of Europeans. *American Journal of Public Health, 99*(3), 540-548.

Baade, P.D., M.D. Coory, and J.F. Aitken. (2004). International trends in prostate-cancer mortality: The decrease is continuing and spreading. *Cancer Causes & Control, 15*(3), 237-241.

Banks, J., Marmot, M., Oldfield, Z., and Smith, J.P. (2006). Disease and disadvantage in the United States and in England. *Journal of the American Medical Association, 295*(17), 2037-2045.

Beaulac, J.A., Fry, R.N., and Onysko, J. (2006). Lifetime and recent prostate specific antigen (PSA) screening of men for prostate cancer in Canada. *Canadian Journal of Public Health, 97*(3), 171-6.

Beemsterboer, P.M.M., de Koning, H.J., Kranse, R., Trienekens, T.H., van der Maas, P.J., and Schröder, F.H. (2000). Prostate specific antigen testing and digital rectal examination before and during a randomized trial of screening for prostate cancer: European Randomized Study of Screening for Prostate Cancer, Rotterdam. *Journal of Urology, 164,* 1216-1220.

Berry, D.A., Cronin, K.A., Plevritis, S.K., Fryback, D.G., et al. (2005). Effect of screening and adjuvant therapy on mortality from breast cancer. *New England Journal of Medicine, 353,* 1784-1792.

Berry, D.A., Inoue, L., Shen, Y., Venier, J., et al. (2006). Modeling the impact of treatment and screening on U.S. breast cancer mortality: A Bayesian approach. *Journal of the National Cancer Institute Monograph, 36,* 30-36.

Bill-Axelson, A., Holmberg, L., Ruutu, M., Haggman, M., Andersson, S., Bratell, S., Spangberg, A., Busch, C., Nordling, S., Garmo, H., Palmgren, J., Adami, H., Norlen, B., and Johansson, J. (2005). Radical prostatectomy versus watchful waiting in early prostate cancer. *New England Journal of Medicine, 352*(19), 1977-84.

Bill-Axelson, A., Holmberg, L., Filén, F., Ruutu, M., et al. (2008). Radical prostatectomy versus watchful waiting in localized prostate cancer: The Scandinavian prostate cancer group-4 randomized trial. *Journal of the National Cancer Institute, 100,* 1144-1154.

Blanks, R.G., Moss, S.M., McGahan, C.E., Quinn, M.J., et al. (2000). Effect of NHS breast screening programme on mortality from breast cancer in England and Wales, 1990-1998: Comparison of observed with predicted mortality. *British Medical Journal, 321,* 665-669.

Bolla, M., Collette, L., Blank, L., Warde, P., et al. (2002). Long-term results with immediate androgen suppression and external irradiation in patients with locally advanced prostate cancer (an EORTC study): A Phase III randomised trial. *Lancet, 360*(9327), 103-8.

Botha, J.L., Bray, F., Sankila, R., and Parkin, D.M. (2003). Breast cancer incidence and mortality trends in 16 European countries. *European Journal of Cancer, 39,* 1718-1729.

Bouchardy, C., Fioretta, G., Rapiti, E., Verkooijen, H.M., et al. (2008). Recent trends in prostate cancer mortality show a continuous decrease in several countries. *International Journal of Cancer, 123,* 421-429.

Breen, N., Wagener, D.K., Brown, M.L., Davis, W.W., et al. (2001). Progress in cancer screening over a decade: Results of cancer screening from the 1987, 1992, and 1998 National Health Interview Surveys. *Journal of the National Cancer Institute, 93*(22), 1704-1713.

Bulliard, J.-L., De Landtsheer, J.-P., and Levi, F. (2003). Results from the Swiss mammography screening pilot programme. *European Journal of Cancer, 39,* 1761-1769.

Bunting, P. (2002). Screening for prostate cancer with prostate-specific antigen: Beware the biases. *Clinica Chimica Acta, 315,* 71-97.

Capet, F., Arbyn, M., and Abarca, M. (2003). *Mammografische opsporing van borstkanker in België: analyse van de gezondheidsenquêtes 1997 en 2001.* IPH / EPI—REPORTS Nr. 2003-008. Brussels.

Cebul, R.D., Rebitzer, J.B., Taylor, L.J., and Votruba, M.E. (2008). Organizational fragmentation and care quality in the U.S. healthcare system. *Journal of Economic Perspectives,* 22(4), 93-113.

Centers for Disease Control and Prevention. (2002). Annual smoking-attributable mortality, years of potential life lost, and economic costs: United States, 1995-1999. *Morbidity and Mortality Weekly Report,* 51(14), 300-303.

Centraal Bureau voor de Statistiek. (2009). *Statline.* Available: http://statline.cbs.nl/StatWeb/default.aspx [accessed May 2010].

Chlebowski, R.T., Hendrix, S.L., Langer, R.D., et al. (2003). Influence of estrogen plus progestin on breast cancer and mammography in healthy postmenopausal women: The Women's Health Initiative randomised trial. *Journal of the American Medical Association,* 289, 3243-3253.

Chu, K.C., Tarone, R.E., Kessler, L.G., Ries, L.A.G., et al. (1996). Recent trends in U.S. breast cancer incidence, survival, and mortality rates. *Journal of the National Cancer Institute,* 88, 1571-1579.

Ciccolallo, L., Capocaccia, R., Coleman, M.P., Berrino, F., et al. (2005). Survival differences between European and U.S. patients with colorectal cancer: Role of stage at diagnosis and surgery. *Gut,* 54(2), 268-273.

Cole, M.P., Jones, C.T.A., Todd, I.D.H. (1971). A new anti-oestrogenic agent in late breast cancer. An early clinical appraisal of ICI 46474. *British Journal of Cancer,* 25, 270-275.

Collin, S.M., Martin, R.M., Metcalfe, C., Gunnell, D., et al. (2008). Prostate-cancer mortality in the USA and UK in 1975-2004: An ecological study. *Lancet Oncology,* 9, 445-452.

Commonwealth Fund Commission on a High Performance Health System. (2008). *Why Not the Best? Results from the National Scorecard on U.S. Health System Performance, 2008.* New York: Commonwealth Fund.

Constantinou, J., and Feneley, M.R. (2006). PSA testing: An evolving relationship with prostate cancer screening. *Prostate Cancer and Prostatic Diseases,* 9, 6-13.

Cotlar, A.M., Dubose, J.J., and Rose, D.M. (2003). History of surgery for breast cancer: Radical to the sublime. *Current Surgery,* 60(3), 329-337.

Crawford, E.D. (2003). Epidemiology of prostate cancer. *Urology,* 62(6 suppl 1), 3-12.

Cutler, D. (2004). *Your Money or Your Life.* New York: Oxford University Press.

Cutler, D.M., and Glaeser, E.L. (2006). *Why Do Europeans Smoke More Than Americans?* NBER working paper 12124. Cambridge, MA: National Bureau of Economic Research.

Cutler, D.M., Glaeser, E.L., and Shapiro, J.M. (2003). Why have Americans become more obese? *Journal of Economic Perspectives,* 17(3), 93-118.

D'Ambrosio, G., Samani, F., Cancian, M., and De Mola, C. (2004). Practice of opportunistic prostate-specific antigen screening in Italy: Data from the health search database. *European Journal of Cancer Prevention,* 13(5), 383-386.

Das, B., Feuer, E.J., and Mariotto, A. (2005). Geographic association between mammography use and mortality reduction in the US. *Cancer Causes and Control,* 16, 691-699.

De Koning, H.J., Liem, M.K., Baan, C.A., Boer, R., et al. (2002). Prostate cancer mortality reduction by screening: Power and time frame with complete enrollment in the European Randomised Screening for Prostate Cancer (ERSPC) Trial. *International Journal of Cancer,* 98(2), 268-273.

DeNavas-Walt, C., Proctor, B.D., and Smith, J. (2007). *Income, Poverty, and Health Insurance Coverage in the United States: 2006.* U.S. Census Bureau, Current Population Reports, P60-233. Washington, DC: U.S. Government Printing Office.

Department of Health. (1999). *Breast Screening Programme, England 1997-1998*. Available: http://www.dh.gov.uk/en/Publicationsandstatistics/Statistics/StatisticalWorkAreas/Statisticalhealthcare/DH_4016216 [accessed May 2010].

Early Breast Cancer Trialists' Collaborative Group. (1995). Effects of radiotherapy and surgery in early breast cancer: An overview of the randomized trials. *New England Journal of Medicine, 333*(22), 1444-1455.

Early Breast Cancer Trialists' Collaborative Group. (1998a). Polychemotherapy for early breast cancer: An overview of the randomised trials. *Lancet, 352,* 930-942.

Early Breast Cancer Trialists' Collaborative Group. (1998b). Tamoxifen for early breast cancer: An overview of the randomised trials. *Lancet, 351,* 1451-1467.

Eisinger, F., Blay, J.-Y., Morère, J.-F., Rixe, O., Calazel-Benque, A., Cals, L., Coscas, Y., Dolbeault, S., Namer, M., Serin, D., Roussel, C., and Pivot, X. (2008). Cancer screening in France: Subjects' and physicians' attitudes. *Cancer Causes and Control, 19*(4), 431-434.

Elmore, J.G., Armstrong, K., Lehman, C.D., and Fletcher, S.W. (2005). Screening for breast cancer. *Journal of the American Medical Association, 293,* 1245-1256.

Etzioni, R., Gulati, R., Falcon, S., and Penson, D. (2008). Impact of PSA screening on the incidence of advanced stage prostate cancer in the United States: A surveillance modeling approach. *Medical Decision Making, 28,* 323-331.

Feuer, E.J., Merrill, R.M., and Hankey, B.F. (1999). Cancer surveillance series: Interpreting trends in prostate cancer—Part II: Cause of death misclassification and the recent rise and fall in prostate cancer mortality. *Journal of the National Cancer Institute, 91*(12), 1025-1032.

Fisher, B., Anderson, S., Bryant, J., Margolese, R., et al. (2002). Twenty-year follow up of a randomized trial comparing total mastectomy, lumpectomy, and lumpectomy plus irradiation for the treatment of invasive breast cancer. *New England Journal of Medicine, 347*(16), 1233-1241.

Fleshner, N., Rakovitch, E., and Klotz, L. (2000). Differences between urologists in the United States and Canada in the approach to prostate cancer. *Journal of Urology, 163,* 1461-1466.

Forey, B., Hamling, J., Lee, P., and Wald, N. (Eds.) (2002). *International Smoking Statistics: A Collection of Historical Data from 30 Economically Developed Countries.* London, England: Oxford University Press.

Garber, A. (2003). Comparing health systems from the disease-specific perspective. In Organisation for Economic Co-operation and Development, *A Disease-Based Comparison of Health Systems: What Is Best and at What Cost?* (pp. 95-106). Paris: Organisation for Economic Co-operation and Development.

Garber, A.M., and Skinner, J. (2008). Is American health care uniquely inefficient? *Journal of Economic Perspectives, 22*(4), 27-50.

Gatta, G., Capocaccia, R., Coleman, M.P., Gloeckler Ries, L.A., et al. (2000). Toward a comparison of survival in American and European cancer patients. *Cancer, 89*(4), 893-900.

Gibbons, L., and Waters, C. (2003). Prostate cancer—Testing, incidence, surgery and mortality. *Health Reports, 14*(3), 19-20.

Gøtzsche, P.C., and Nielsen, M. (2009). Screening for breast cancer with mammography (review). *Cochrane Database of Systematic Reviews,* Issue 2, 1-90.

Haldorsen, T., and Grimsrud, T.K. (1999). Cohort analysis of cigarette smoking and lung cancer incidence among Norwegian women. *International Journal of Epidemiology, 28*(6), 1032-1036.

Halliday, A., Mansfield, A., Marro, J., Peto, C., et al. (2004). Prevention of disabling and fatal strokes by successful carotid endarterectomy in patients without recent neurological symptoms: Randomised controlled trial. *Lancet, 363*(9420), 1491-1502.

Hanks, G.E., Pajak, T.F., Porter, A., Grignon, D., et al. (2003). Phase III trial of long-term adjuvant androgen deprivation after neoadjuvant hormonal cytoreduction and radiotherapy in locally advanced carcinoma of the prostate: The radiation therapy oncology group protocol 92-02. *Journal of Clinical Oncology, 21*(21), 3972-3978.

Harris, R., and Lohr, K.N. (2002). Screening for prostate cancer: An update of the evidence for the U.S. Preventive Services Task Force. *Annals of Internal Medicine, 137*(11), 917-929.

Holden, C.A., Jolley, D.J., McLachlan, R.I., Pitts, M., Cumming, R., Wittert, G., Handelsman, D.J., and de Kretser, D.M. (2006). Men in Australia Telephone Survey (MATeS): Predictors of men's help-seeking behaviour for reproductive health disorders. *Medical Journal of Australia, 185*(8), 418-422.

Howard, D., Richardson, L., and Thorpe, K. (2009). Cancer screening and age in the U.S. and Europe. *Health Affairs, 28*(6), 1838-1847.

Hsing, A.W., Tsao, L., and Devesa, S.S. (2000). International trends and patterns of prostate cancer incidence and mortality. *International Journal of Cancer, 85*(1), 60-67.

Hughes, M. (2003). Summary of results from breast cancer disease study. In Organisation for Economic Co-operation and Development, *A Disease-Based Comparison of Health Systems: What Is Best and at What Cost?* (pp. 77-94). Paris: Organisation for Economic Co-operation and Development.

Humphrey, L.L., Helfand, M., Chan, B.K.S., and Woolf, S.H. (2002). Breast cancer screening: A summary of the evidence for the U.S. Preventive Services Task Force. *Annals of Internal Medicine, 137*(5, 1), 347-360.

Ilic, D., O'Connor, D., Green, S., and Wilt, T. (2006). Screening for prostate cancer. *Cochrane Database of Systematic Reviews*, Issue 3.

Institute of Medicine. (2001). *Coverage Matters: Insurance and Health Care.* Washington, DC: National Academy Press.

International Agency for Research on Cancer. (2008). *World Health Organization Mortality Data.* Lyon, France: Author.

Jaiyesimi, I.A., Buzdar, A.U., Decker, D.A., and Hortobagyi, G.N. (1995). Use of tamoxifen for breast cancer: Twenty-eight years later. *Journal of Clinical Oncology, 13*, 513-529.

Jatoi, I., and Miller, A.B. (2003). Why is breast-cancer mortality declining? *Lancet Oncology, 4*, 251-254.

Kapteyn, A., Smith, J.P., and van Soest, A. (2007). Vignettes and self-reports of work disability in the United States and the Netherlands. *American Economic Review, 97*(1), 461-473.

Kaul, P., Armstrong, P., Chang, W., Naylor, C., Granger, C., Lee, K., Peterson, I., Califf, R., Topol, E., and Mark, D. (2004). Long-term mortality of patients with acute myocardial infarction in the United States and Canada. *Circulation, 110*, 1754-1760.

Klimont, J., Ktir, J., and Leitner, B. (2007). *Österreichische gesundheitsbefragung 2006/2007: hauptergebnisse und methodische Dokumentation.* Statistik Austria. Federal Ministry of Health, Family and Youth. Available: http://www.bmgfj.gv.at [accessed July 2008].

Kvåle, R., Auvinen, A., Adami, H.-O., Klint, Å., et al. (2007). Interpreting trends in prostate cancer incidence and mortality in the five Nordic countries. *Journal of the National Cancer Institute, 99*(24), 1881-1887.

Lazovich, D., Solomon, C.C., Thomas, D.B., Moe, R.E., et al. (1999). Breast conservation therapy in the United States following the 1990 National Institutes of Health Consensus Development Conference on the Treatment of Patient with Early Stage Invasive Breast Carcinoma. *Cancer, 86*(4), 628-637.

Levi, F., La Vecchia, C., Randimbison, L., Erler, G., Te, V.-C., and Franceschi, S. (1998). Incidence, mortality, and survival from prostate cancer in Vaud and Neuchatel, Switzerland, 1974-1994. *Annals of Oncology, 9*(1), 31-35.

Levi, F., Lucchini, F., Negri, E., and La Vecchia, C. (2000). Recent trends in prostate cancer mortality in the European Union. *Epidemiology, 11*(5), 612.

Levi, F., Bosetti, C., Lucchini, F., Negri, E., et al. (2005). Monitoring the decrease in breast cancer mortality in Europe. *European Journal of Cancer Prevention, 14*, 497-502.

Li, H., Stampfer, M., Hollis, J., Mucci, L., Gaziano, J., Hunter, D., Giovannucci, E., and Ma, J. (2007). A prospective study of plasma vitamin D metabolites, vitamin D receptor polymorphisms, and prostate cancer. *Public Library of Science, 4*(3), 562-571.

Lousbergh, D., Buntinx, F., Geys, G., Du Bois, M., Dhollander, D., and Molenberghs, G. (2002). Prostate-specific antigen screening coverage and prostate cancer incidence rates in the Belgian province of Limburg in 1996-1998. *European Journal of Cancer Prevention, 11*(6), 547-549.

Luengo, S., Lazrao, P., Madero, R., Alvirac, F., et al. (1996). Equity in the access to mammography in Spain. *Social Science and Medicine, 43*(8), 1263-1271.

Lumey, L.H., Pittman, B., Zang, E.A., and Wynder, E.L. (1997). Cigarette smoking and prostate cancer: No relation with six measures of lifetime smoking habits in a large case-control study among U.S. whites. *Prostate, 33*(3), 195-200.

Lu-Yao, G., Albersen, P., Moore, D., Shih, W., Lin, Y., DiPaola, R., and Yao, S. (2008). Survival following primary androgen deprivation therapy among men with localized prostate cancer. *Journal of the American Medical Association, 300*(2), 173-181.

Macinko, J., Starfield, B., and Shi, L. (2003). The contribution of primary care systems to health outcomes within Organisation for Economic Co-operation and Development (OECD) Countries, 1970-1998. *Health Services Research, 38*(3), 831-865.

Mariotto, A., Feuer, E.J., Harlan, L.C., Wun, L.M., et al. (2002). Trends in use of adjuvant multiagent chemotherapy and tamoxifen for breast cancer in the United States: 1975-1999. *Journal of the National Cancer Institute, 94*, 1626-1634.

McKinsey Global Institute. (2008). *Accounting for the Cost of U.S. Health Care: A New Look at Why Americans Spend More.* Available: http://www.mckinsey.com/mgi/publications/us_healthcare/ [accessed May 2010].

Melia, J., Coulson, P., Johns, L., and Moss, S. (2003). *Report to the Department of Health: Study to Assess the Rate of PSA Testing in Men with No Previous Diagnosis of Prostate Cancer.* Surrey, England: Cancer Screening Evaluation Unit.

Michaud, P.C., Goldman, D., Lakdawalla, D., Gailey, A., and Zheng, Y. (2009). *International Differences in Longevity and Health and Their Economic Consequences.* Santa Monica, CA: RAND.

Moise, P. (2003). The heart of the health care system: Summary of the ischaemic heart disease part of the OECD Ageing-Related Diseases Study. In Organisation for Economic Co-operation and Development, *A Disease-Based Comparison of Health Systems: What Is Best and at What Cost?* (pp. 27-52). Paris: Organisation for Economic Co-operation and Development.

Møller, B., Weedon-Fekjær, H., Hakulinen, T., Tryggvadóttir, L., et al. (2005). The influence of mammographic screening on national trends in breast cancer incidence. *European Journal of Cancer Prevention, 14*(2), 1117-1128.

National Cancer Institute. (2008). *Surveillance, Epidemiology and End Results.* Available: http://seer.cancer.gov/ [accessed May 2010].

National Center for Health Statistics. (2000). *Health, United States, 2000.* Hyattsville, MD: Author.

National Center for Health Statistics. (2002). Deaths: Final data for 2000. *National Vital Statistics Reports, 50*(15).

National Center for Health Statistics. (2008). Deaths: Final data for 2005. *National Vital Statistics Reports, 56*(10).

Nolte, E., and McKee, C.M. (2008). Measuring the health of nations: Updating an earlier analysis. *Health Affairs, 27*(1), 58-71.

Ogawa, K., Nakamura, K., Sasaki, T., Onishi, H., et al. (2008). Radical external beam radiotherapy for prostate cancer in Japan: Differences in the patterns of care among Japan, Germany, and the United States. *Radiation Medicine, 26*, 57-62.

Ohsfeldt, R.L., and Schneider, J.E. (2006). *The Business of Health: The Role of Competition, Markets, and Regulation.* Washington, DC: AEI Press.

Organisation for Economic Co-operation and Development. (2003). *Stroke Care in OECD Countries: A Comparison of Treatment, Costs, and Outcomes in 17 Countries.* Health Working Paper #5. Paris: Author.

Organisation for Economic Co-operation and Development. (2006). *Health Care Quality Indicators Project: Initial Indicators Report.* OECD health working paper #22. Paris: Author.

Organisation for Economic Co-operation and Development. (2007). *Health Care Quality Indicators Project 2006: Data Collection Update Report.* Working paper #29. Paris: Author.

Organisation for Economic Co-operation and Development. (2008). *OECD Health Data 2008: How Does the United States Compare?* Paris: Author.

Osborne, C.K. (1998). Tamoxifen in the treatment of breast cancer. *New England Journal of Medicine, 339*(22), 1609-1618.

Otto, S.J., Van der Crusijen, I.W., Liem, M.K., Korfage, I.J., Lous, J.J., Schröder, F.H., and De Koning, H.J. (2003). Effective PSA contamination in the Rotterdam section of the European Randomized Study of Screening for Prostate Cancer. *International Journal of Cancer, 105*(3), 394-399.

Páez, A., Luján, M., Llanes, L., Romero, I., de la Cal, M.A., Miravalles, E., and Berenguer, A. (2002). PSA-use in a Spanish industrial area. *European Urology, 41*, 162-166.

Pilepich, M.V., Winter, K., Lawton, C.A., Krisch, R.E., et al. (2005). Androgen suppression adjuvant to definitive radiotherapy in prostate carcinoma: Long-term results of Phase III. RTOG 85-31. *International Journal of Radiation Oncology*Biology*Physics, 61*(5), 1285-1290.

Pollack, A., Zagars, G., Starkschall, G., Antolak, J., Lee, J., Huang, E., von Eschenback, A., Kuban, D., and Rosen, I. (2002). Prostate cancer radiation dose response: Results of the M.D. Anderson Phase III randomized trial. *International Journal of Oncology, Biology, Physics, 53*(5), 1097-1105.

Post, P.N., Damhuis, R.A.M., van der Meyden, A.P.M., and the EUROCARE Working Group. (1998). Variation in survival of patients with prostate cancer in Europe since 1978. *European Journal of Cancer, 34*(14), 2226-2231.

Potosky, A.L., Feuer, E.J., and Levin, D.L. (2001). Impact of screening on incidence and mortality of prostate cancer in the United States. *Epidemiologic Reviews, 23*(1), 181-186.

Preston, S., and Wang, H. (2006). Changing sex differentials in mortality in the United States: The role of cohort smoking patterns. *Demography, 43*(4), 413-434.

Quinn, M.J. (2003). Cancer trends in the United States—A view from Europe. *Journal of the National Cancer Institute, 95*(17), 1258-1261.

Ragaz, J., Jackson, S.M., Le, N., Plenderleith, I.H., et al. (1997). Adjuvant radiotherapy and chemotherapy in node-positive premenopausal women with breast cancer. *New England Journal of Medicine, 337*(14), 956-962.

Ross, L.E., Berkowitz, Z., and Ekwueme, D.U. (2008). Use of the prostate-specific antigen test among U.S. men: Findings from the 2005 National Health Interview Survey. *Cancer Epidemiology Biomarkers & Prevention, 17*(3), 636-644.

Sandblom, G., Dufmats, M., Nordenskjöld, K., and Varenhorst, E. (2000). Prostate carcinoma trends in three counties in Sweden 1987-1996: Results from a population-based national cancer register, south-east region prostate cancer group. *Cancer, 88*(6), 1445-1453.

Sant, M., Allemani, C., Berrino, F., Coleman, M.P., et al. (2004). Breast carcinoma survival in Europe and the United States: A population-based study. *Cancer, 100*(4), 715-722.

Schootman, M., Jeffe, D., Reschke, A., and Aft, R. (2004). The full potential of breast cancer screening use to reduce mortality has not yet been realized in the United States. *Breast Cancer Research and Treatment, 85*(3), 219-222.

Schröder, F.H., Hugosson, J., Roobol, M.J., Tammela, T.L.J., et al. (2009). Screening and prostate-cancer mortality in a randomized European study. *New England Journal of Medicine, 360,* 1320-1328.

Sennfalt, K., Carlsson, P., and Varenhorst, E. (2006). Diffusion and economic consequences of health technologies in prostate cancer care in Sweden, 1991-2002. *European Urology, 49,* 1028-1034.

Shampo, M. (2002). Development of the PSA test. *Journal of Pelvic Surgery, 8*(2), 123-126.

Shapiro, S., Coleman, E.A., Breeders, M., Codd, M., et al. (1998). Breast cancer screening programmes in 22 countries: Current policies, administration and guidelines. *International Journal of Epidemiology, 27,* 735-742

Sirovich, B.E., Schwartz, L.M., and Woloshin, S. (2003). Screening men for prostate and colorectal cancer in the United States: Does practice reflect the evidence? *Journal of the American Medical Association, 289,* 1414-1420.

Smith, D.P., and Armstrong, B.K. (1998). Prostate-specific antigen testing in Australia and association with prostate cancer incidence in New South Wales. *Medical Journal of Australia, 169,* 17-20.

Snider, J., Beauvais, J., Levy, I., Villeneueve, P., and Pennock, J. (1997). Trends in mammography and Pap smear utilization in Canada. *Chronic Diseases in Canada, 17*(3), 1-15.

Stattin, P., Johansson, R., Lodnert, R., Ove, A., et al. (2005). Geographical variation in incidence of prostate cancer in Sweden. *Scandinavian Journal of Urology and Nephrology, 39*(5), 372-379.

Tarone, R.E., Chu, K.C., and Brawley, O.W. (2000). Implications of stage-specific survival rates in assessing recent declines in prostate cancer mortality rates. *Epidemiology, 11*(2), 167-170.

Technological Change in Health Care (TECH) Research Network. (2001). Technological change around the world: Evidence from heart attack care. *Health Affairs, 20*(3), 25-42.

Thompson, I.M., Tangen, C.M., Paradelo, J., Lucia, M.S., et al. (2006). Adjuvant radiotherapy for pathologically advanced prostate cancer: A randomized clinical trial. *Journal of the American Medical Association, 296*(19), 2329-2335.

Thorpe, K.E., Howard, D.H., and Galactionova, K. (2007a). Differences in disease prevalence as a source of the U.S.-European health care spending gap. *Health Affairs, 26*(6), 678-686.

Thorpe, K.E., Howard, D.H., and Galactionova, K. (2007b). Technical appendix. On-line data supplement to Thorpe et al. (2007a).

Torti, D.C., and Matheson, G.O. (2004). Exercise and prostate cancer. *Sports Medicine, 34*(6), 363-369.

Trock, B., Han, M., Freedland, S., Humphreys, E., DeWeese, T., Partin, A., and Walsh, P. (2008). Prostate cancer-specific survival following salvage radiotherapy vs. observation in men with biochemical recurrence after radical prostatectomy. *Journal of the American Medical Association, 299*(23), 2760-2769.

Ugnat, A.-M., Xie, L., Semenciw, R., Waters, C., et al. (2005). Survival patterns for the top four cancers in Canada: The effects of age, region and period. *European Journal of Cancer Prevention, 14,* 91-100.

U.S. Department of Health, Education, and Welfare. (1964). *Smoking and Health: Report of the Advisory Committee to the Surgeon General of the Public Health Service.* Public Health Service Publication No. 1103. Washington, DC: Office of the Surgeon General.

U.S. Preventive Services Task Force. (2008). Screening for prostate cancer: U.S. Preventive Services Task Force Recommendation Statement. *Annals of Internal Medicine, 149*(3), 185-191.

Vainio, H., and Bianchini, F. (2002). *Breast Cancer Screening. IARC Handbooks of Cancer Prevention, Vol. 7.* Lyon, France: International Agency for Research on Cancer Press and World Health Organization.

Vercelli, M., Quaglia, A., Marani, E., and Parodi, S. (2000). Prostate cancer incidence and mortality trends among elderly and adult Europeans. *Critical Reviews in Oncology/Hematology, 35,* 133-144.

Verdecchia, A., Francisci, S., Brenner, H., Gatta, G., et al. (2007). Recent cancer survival in Europe: A 2000-2002 period analysis of EUROCARE-4 data. *Lancet Oncology, 8,* 784-796.

Veronesi, U., Cascinelli, N., Mariani, L., Greco, M., et al. (2002). Twenty-year follow-up of a randomized study comparing breast-conserving surgery with radical mastectomy for early breast cancer. *New England Journal of Medicine, 347*(16), 1227-1232.

Veronesi, U., Boyle, P., Goldhirsch, A., Orecchia, R., et al. (2005). Breast cancer. *Lancet, 365,* 1727-1741.

Vutuc, C., Haidinger, G., and Waldhoer, T. (1998). Prevalence of self-reported screening mammography and impact on breast cancer mortality in Austria. *Wien Klin Wsch, 110,* 485-490.

Wells, J. (1998). Mammography and the politics of randomised controlled trials. *British Medical Journal, 317*(31), 1224-1230.

Wilt, T.J., MacDonald, R., Rutks, I., Shamliyan, T.A., et al. (2008). Systematic review: Comparative effectiveness and harms of treatments for clinically localized prostate cancer. *Annals of Internal Medicine, 148*(6), 435-448.

Wolf-Maier, K., Cooper, R., Kramer, H., Banegas, J., Giampaoli, S., Joffres, M., Poulter, N., Primastesta, P., Stegmayr, B., and Thamm, M. (2004). Hypertension treatment and control in five European countries, Canada, and the United States. *Hypertension, 43*(10), 10-17.

Wong, Y.-N., Mitra, N., Hudes, G., Localio, R., et al. (2006). Survival associated with treatment vs. observation of localized prostate cancer in elderly men. *Journal of the American Medical Association, 296,* 2683-2693.

Wood, W.C. (1994). Progress from clinical trials on breast cancer. *Cancer, 74*(S9), 2606-2609.

World Health Organization. (2009). *World Health Organization Statistical Information System.* Available: http://www.who.int/whosis/whostat/en/ [accessed May 2010].

Writing Group for the Women's Health Initiative Investigators. (2002). Risks and benefits of estrogen plus progestin in healthy postmenopausal women: Principal results from the Women's Health Initiative randomized controlled trial. *Journal of the American Medical Association, 288,* 321-333

Zappa, M., Visioli, C., Crocetti, E., Buonamici, C., Baccini, A., Taddei, S., and Ciatto, S. (2003). Practice of opportunistic PSA screening in the Florence District. *Cancer Prevention, 12,* 201-204.

Zhou, E.H., Ellis, R.J., Cherullo, E., Colussi, V., et al. (2009). Radiotherapy and survival in prostate cancer patients: A population-based study. *International Journal of Radiation Oncology*Biology*Physics, 73*(1), 15-23.

10

Can Hormone Therapy Account for American Women's Survival Disadvantage?

Noreen Goldman

Although the United States had one of the world's highest life expectancies during the first half of the 20th century, this survival advantage gradually eroded during the ensuing decades. Of particular concern in the context of this volume is the recent stagnation in mortality improvement among middle-aged and older U.S. women relative to both U.S. men and to women in other wealthy nations (Meslé and Vallin, 2006; Vaupel, 2003). These mortality patterns suggest an appealing but as yet unexplored explanation: the use of postmenopausal hormone therapy (HT) among women in the United States. There is considerable evidence that, at least prior to 2002, estrogen-type hormones had been widely prescribed to U.S. women after the cessation of menses not only for relief of unpleasant symptoms associated with menopause but also increasingly for presumed protection against cardiovascular disease and bone loss.[1] National estimates suggest a

---

[1] Hormone therapy (known commercially as Premarin) was approved by the U.S. Food and Drug Administration for the treatment of menopausal symptoms in 1942. In 1986, it was approved for the prevention of osteoporosis. Although the Food and Drug Administration never approved Premarin or alternative forms of HT for the prevention of other chronic diseases, physicians began to widely prescribe it for these purposes because observational studies in the 1980s and 1990s suggested numerous health benefits, including cardiovascular disease and dementia prevention (Wysowski and Governale, 2005). For example, clinical guidelines in 1992 for counseling postmenopausal women indicated that those with coronary disease or at an increased risk of it would be likely to benefit from HT use; they suggested that long-term therapy would yield the most benefit for reduced risk of coronary disease and osteoporotic fractures. The guidelines also noted that "all women, regardless of race, should consider preventive hormone therapy" (American College of Physicians, 1992; Wysowski, Golden, and Burke, 1995).

steady increase in HT use since the early 1980s, with a prevalence of about 38 to 40 percent among women ages 50 to 74 in 1995. Data on numbers of prescriptions for all forms of HT reveal a continued increase from 1995 to 2001, with the annual number of prescriptions peaking at 92 million in 2000 (Hersh, Stefanick, and Stafford, 2004).[2]

The plausibility of the hypothesis that HT use underlies the U.S. survival disadvantage rests heavily on the assumption that it is a risk factor for overall mortality. If this assumption is valid, the strength of evidence implicating HT use depends on a second assertion, namely that its use has been more prevalent in the United States than in other Western populations. In this chapter, I evaluate the evidence for these assumptions.

Observational studies have generally reported substantially lower rates of heart disease—on the order of 35 to 50 percent—for long-term users of postmenopausal HT compared with nonusers (Grodstein, Manson, and Stampfer, 2006; Grodstein et al., 2000; Manson and Bassuk, 2007; Prentice and Anderson, 2008). For example, in 1992, a meta-analysis based on 32 observational studies concluded that ever-users of estrogen had a relative risk of coronary heart disease of 0.65 compared with never-users, a finding generally in line with two previous meta-analysis estimates of 0.55 and 0.58 (Grady et al., 1992). However, during the past decade, randomized controlled trials (RCTs) have challenged findings from observational studies regarding the harm and benefits of long-term use of HT. Although both types of studies are in general agreement about its benefits for colorectal cancer and hip fracture and the increased risk associated with breast cancer, they have produced widely discrepant estimates for coronary heart disease or CHD (Grodstein, Clarkson, and Manson, 2003; Nelson et al., 2002).

Data from the Women's Health Initiative (WHI), a well-publicized randomized trial that administered the two dominant forms of hormone therapy to healthy U.S. women ages 50 to 79,[3] suggested an increased incidence of CHD and thromboembolic events, as well as all cardiovascular disease combined, based on an average of 5.2 years of use of the estrogen-progestin regimen (Nelson et al., 2002; Writing Group for the Women's Health Ini-

---

[2] The two most common forms of HT in the United States are (1) a mixture of conjugated equine estrogens, typically referred to as unopposed estrogens, and (2) a combination of estrogen and progestin (a synthetic substance with effects similar to progesterone). In light of evidence suggesting an increased risk of uterine cancer associated with unopposed estrogens, women with an intact uterus have been using estrogen-progestin combinations. The majority of prescriptions in the United States have been for orally administered hormone therapy; transdermal and vaginal preparations have been used much less frequently (Hersh et al., 2004).

[3] Initiated in 1992, the WHI enrolled about 27,500 postmenopausal women into two parallel clinical trials designed to evaluate the consequences of hormone therapy for disease prevention (particularly CHD and fractures). Women without a uterus were randomly assigned to receive unopposed estrogens or a placebo, and women with an intact uterus were randomly assigned to receive an estrogen-progestin combination or a placebo.

tiative Investigators, 2002). In the second arm of the WHI, an average of 6.8 years of use of unopposed estrogens was significantly associated with increased risk of stroke and total cardiovascular disease, but not coronary heart disease (Women's Health Initiative Steering Committee, 2004). Both trials were terminated earlier than scheduled[4] because, on balance, hormone therapy appeared to be causing more harmful outcomes than beneficial ones (Fletcher and Colditz, 2002). Widely disseminated estimates from the WHI, along with similar evidence from other RCTs,[5] have led to guidelines against the routine use of hormone therapy for prevention of cardiovascular disease and to a dramatic reduction in the prevalence of postmenopausal hormone therapy beginning in 2002 or 2003 in the United States and other countries (Barbaglia et al., 2009; Coombs and Boyages, 2005; Du et al., 2007; Gayet-Ageron et al., 2005; Guay et al., 2007; Hersh et al., 2004; Townsend and Nanchahal, 2005; Waaseth, Bakken, and Lund, 2009).

The link between hormone therapy and cardiovascular disease is a salient one for this study because cardiovascular disease is the leading cause of death among women in the United States and most Western countries. Nevertheless, the evidence from RCTs fails to support the hypothesis that HT is an important source of female mortality stagnation for two reasons. First, despite what appears to be a modest increase in overall disease events[6] for users of estrogen-progestin (but not unopposed estrogen) in the WHI, the estimated risks of HT use roughly counteract the estimated benefits in terms of deaths from all causes. The WHI estimates of the hazard ratios for overall mortality, for HT use compared with a placebo, are 0.98 (95 percent CI of 0.82-1.18) for estrogen-progestin at about 6 years of use and 1.04 (95 percent CI of 0.88-1.22) for unopposed estrogen at about 7 years of use. Similarly, a meta-analysis based on about 27,000 participants in 30 RCTs conducted between 1966 and 2002 yielded an odds ratio for total mortality associated with HT of 0.98 (95 percent CI of 0.87-1.12); the average duration of these trials was 4.5 years (Salpeter et al., 2004). Thus, estimates of relative all-cause mortality risk associated with HT use are consistently close to 1.

---

[4]The WHI estrogen-progestin trial was terminated in July 2002, and the WHI estrogen-only trial was terminated in February 2004.

[5]The Heart and Estrogen/Progestin Replacement Study, which examined women with established heart disease, identified an increased risk of coronary events among HT users in the first year but not in subsequent years of the trial. The WISDOM trial in the United Kingdom demonstrated an elevation in CHD risk associated with estrogen-progestin (but not unopposed estrogen) in the first year of use; estimates for longer durations were never obtained because the trial was cancelled after the release of the WHI results.

[6]The WHI computed a global health index that included the first event for each participant of CHD, stroke, pulmonary embolism, breast cancer, endometrial cancer, colorectal cancer, hip fracture, and death due to other causes.

Second, the argument for increased mortality risk associated with HT use is weakened by new evidence casting doubt on the earlier WHI claims. This work suggests that the widely publicized discrepancies between observational studies and randomized controlled trials may be due in large part to differences in the timing of HT initiation relative to the onset of menopause: women taking it in observational studies usually began therapy in early menopause, whereas participants in randomized trials were typically assigned to HT use at a later stage. In particular, whereas the average age of menopause in the United States is 51 years (Manson et al., 2007), the average age of the WHI sample at baseline was about 63 years, and most participants were more than a decade past the onset of menopause (Grodstein, Manson, and Stampfer, 2006).[7] Similarly, the average baseline age of participants in the Heart and Estrogen/Progestin Replacement Study (HERS) was 67 (and, by study design, all began the trial with a diagnosis of CHD). In contrast, 80 percent of hormone users in the Nurses' Health Study, the most frequently cited cohort study examining the health consequences of HT use, initiated use within a 2- to 3-year period after the start of menopause (Manson and Bassuk, 2007).

A hypothesis currently under evaluation that is consistent with data from clinical trials and experimental data from nonhuman primates is that exogenous estrogen has counteracting effects on coronary function that may vary with the stage of atherosclerosis. Researchers have speculated that, at early stages, estrogen may lower coronary risk by improving lipid and endothelial function, but that the prothrombotic and proinflammatory effects of estrogen may result in clotting or rupture of plaque in the presence of advanced lesions, which are more likely to exist at later ages or durations since menopause (Manson and Bassuk, 2007).

There are several recent sources of evidence to support this theory. First, a secondary analysis[8] based on pooled data from the two WHI trials yielded a significant trend in relative risk for CHD, with women at higher durations since menopause onset experiencing higher relative risks than those initiating use closer to menopause (Rossouw et al., 2007). Second, a reanalysis of the Nurses' Health Study by duration since menopause revealed a similar pattern: women initiating HT near menopause had a significantly lower risk of CHD than never-users, whereas the group of women initiating use at least 10 years after menopause was statistically indistinguishable from never-users (Grodstein, Manson, and Stampfer, 2006). Third, in a separate analysis of the Nurses' Health Study, in which the authors used these

---

[7]Cost and sample size considerations, as well as the fact that clinicians were frequently prescribing HT to older women for disease prevention, supported the choice of a broad age range for the WHI.

[8]Data from the WHI trials were pooled because of the small number of women who were assigned to HT treatment close to the onset of menopause.

observational data to mimic the WHI, differences between the two sets of data were greatly attenuated after stratification by time of HT initiation (Hernan et al., 2008). Fourth, results from a recent meta-analysis indicated that, in RCTs of relatively young postmenopausal women or women within a decade of menopause onset, HT users had significantly lower CHD risk than nonusers, but this advantage was not present in studies of older women (Salpeter et al., 2006). Similarly, an earlier meta-analysis that examined mortality as an outcome found that HT was associated with lower total mortality for trials with a mean age of women under 60, but not for other trials (Salpeter et al., 2004). Fifth, data from the WHI Coronary Artery Calcium Study initiated in 2004 examined the amount of atherosclerotic calcification in the coronary arteries of women in their fifties. The results indicated that the calcified-plaque burden—a marker of total atherosclerotic plaque burden—was lower in those randomly assigned to estrogen use than in those assigned to a placebo (Manson et al., 2007), suggesting that estrogen therapy may be protective against coronary disease among women who recently began menopause.

In sum, several high-quality studies undertaken since the termination of the WHI trials suggest that HT use does not result in increased CHD risk for women initiating it at younger ages or close to menopause onset[9] and that use by these women may confer protection against CHD for short to moderate durations of use. Not all studies, however, support this "timing hypothesis." A recent analysis of clinical trial and observational data from the WHI examined health outcomes for women who initiated HT use within 5 years of menopause. Although the researchers underscored the need for cautious interpretation of results because of data limitations,[10] they found that, contrary to expectation, rates of coronary disease and overall mortality were not significantly different between women initiating HT near menopause onset and later initiators (Prentice et al., 2009). This ongoing controversy underscores the need for further research regarding the effects of the timing of HT onset, as well as the extent of vascular disease and duration of HT use on health outcomes.

Hormone therapy may have had a negative impact on diseases other than coronary heart disease. For example, estimates from both observational studies and randomized controlled trials indicate that HT use is

---

[9]Possible harmful effects of hormone therapy on cardiovascular health for women initiating use at older ages or durations since menopause onset may reflect the presence of significant vascular disease.

[10]The broad postmenopausal age distribution of the WHI trials means that relatively few women were within 5 years of menopause at the time of randomization. Thus, this study included women who had used hormone therapy prior to enrollment in the randomized controlled trials as well as women in the WHI observational study.

associated with increased risk of breast cancer.[11] Moreover, several studies identified reductions in breast cancer incidence subsequent to the drop in HT use that followed the publicity of the WHI findings in 2002. One U.S. study revealed a 7 percent drop in age-adjusted incidence of breast cancer in 2003 compared with 2002, but a leveling off in 2004 and thereafter (Ravdin et al., 2007). Another U.S. study indicated an 8.8 percent decrease in breast cancer incidence between 2000 and 2005 (Coombs et al., 2009). A reduction of a similar magnitude between 2001 and 2003 was reported in Australia (Canfell et al., 2008). Corresponding temporal associations between a decline in HT use and a drop in breast cancer incidence occurred in Canada, France, Germany, New Zealand, Norway, and Switzerland, but not all countries showed this relationship (Kumle, 2008; Ringa and Fournier, 2008). There is evidence that at least part of these declines can be attributed to reductions in HT use rather than to changes in mammography screening or other causes (Chlebowski et al., 2009a, 2009b; Ravdin et al., 2007). One study estimated that the 52 percent reduction in HT use that occurred between 2000 and 2005 in the United States resulted in a decrease in breast cancer incidence ranging between 2 and 8 percent, depending on assumptions regarding the relative risk of breast cancer associated with HT use (Coombs et al., 2010).

Although few researchers dispute the overall link between HT use and higher rates of breast cancer, it is important to keep in mind that death rates from breast cancer are far lower than those from cardiovascular disease, and thus the impact of HT-related breast cancer on overall adult female mortality is likely to have been modest. For example, for the period between 1960 and 2000, death rates for women ages 50 and older from breast cancer were about one-twelfth as high, on average, as those from cardiovascular disease. Moreover, there are likely to have been at least partly offsetting reductions in mortality from other diseases (e.g., colon cancer) as a result of HT use.

All in all, there is little evidence to date linking HT use to an increased risk of all-cause mortality in postmenopausal women.[12] Nevertheless, for completeness of the argument, I consider whether the limited data available suggest a higher prevalence of HT use in the United States than in other wealthy countries.

The MONICA Project of the World Health Organization (WHO) pro-

---

[11]A recent study based on combined RCTs and observational data from the WHI found that breast cancer risks were particularly high for women who initiated HT soon after menopause and used it for many years (Prentice and Anderson, 2008).

[12]A WHI postintervention study compared disease events and mortality between the estrogen-progestin group and the placebo group 3 years after the WHI trial was terminated. The HT group had higher mortality, although the difference between groups was not statistically significant. There was, however, a notable excess of deaths from lung cancer, especially nonsmall-cell lung cancer (Chlebowski et al., 2009a, 2009b; Heiss et al., 2008).

vides a unique source of information on the prevalence of hormone therapy across 32 nonnational populations in 20 countries; the majority of surveys were fielded between 1990 and 1995 (Lundberg et al., 2004). In most of these samples, women ages 45 to 64 were asked about HT use in the past month; no information was collected regarding the regimen or form of administration. The resulting age-standardized prevalence estimates range from a low in Moscow, Russia (0 percent) to a high in Newcastle, Australia, and Halifax, Canada (42 percent). The corresponding estimate for the United States (38 percent, derived from four communities in California) was above the average but below those for Australia and Canada and roughly equal to those for the sampled locations in France, Germany, and Iceland.

Additional estimates derived from prescription or survey data from several countries suggest that the United States is not unique in having had a high prevalence of hormone therapy. For example, estimates for women ages 50-69 in France, based on eight cohort studies, indicate that over half of the women in this age group received hormone therapy in the period prior to the publication of the WHI findings (Gayet-Ageron et al., 2005). Schneider (2002) reported that, in the period 1998-2001, HT prevalence was about twice as high in France as in the United States and Germany. Data from the United Kingdom (Million Women Study Collaborators, 2002; Townsend and Nanchahal, 2005) reveal only slightly lower proportions of postmenopausal women taking hormone therapy in the period 1996-2002 in Britain (36 percent) than in the United States (38-40 percent). Estimates from a cohort study in North Norway indicate a similarly high prevalence (38 percent) among postmenopausal women in 2002 (Waaseth, Bakken, and Lund, 2009). Nevertheless, there is little doubt that HT prevalence in the United States vastly exceeded that in some countries with high life expectancy. For example, results from a community survey in Japan suggest HT prevalence in 1992 as low as 2.5 percent for women ages 45-64 (Nagata, Matsushita, and Shimizu, 1996), and data for the Netherlands indicate a prevalence of 5.6 percent in 2001 for women ages 40-74 (de Jong-van den Berg, Faber, and van den Berg, 2006).

Although statistical comparisons across countries might shed some light on the strength of the association between HT prevalence and death rates for postmenopausal women, the paucity of reliable and comparable estimates of HT use preclude such analyses. Most estimates, including those from the WHO MONICA Project, are based on relatively small geographic areas and short time periods.[13] Moreover, there is substantial variation across samples and countries in the quality of the HT estimates as well as

---

[13]The available data suggest large variations in HT prevalence by time period, typically increasing prior to termination of the WHI study and declining substantially thereafter, as well as by region in a given country (see, for example, Heier's study of HT use in Germany—Heier et al., 2009).

definitions of HT use. In addition, the method of administration (oral or transdermal), dose, and formulation (estrogen-progestin combination versus unopposed estrogens as well as type of progestin) of exogenous hormones vary across countries and may affect health outcomes (Fournier, Berrino, and Clavel-Chapeton, 2008; Manson et al., 2006). High-quality data on the characteristics of HT are even scarcer than estimates of its prevalence.

Of particular relevance to this discussion is cross-country variation in the use of the transdermal patch. Whereas the transdermal patch is prescribed relatively infrequently in the United States, transdermal administration is the most prevalent form of hormone therapy in France and may be widely used in other countries (Fournier et al., 2008; Kim et al., 2007; Scarabin, Oger, and Plu-Bureau, 2003).[14] Transdermal delivery of hormone therapy is thought to have the advantage of bypassing some of the detrimental effects of oral administration that are associated with gut and hepatic metabolism (Kopper, Gudeman, and Thompson, 2009; Stevenson, 2009). In particular, several studies suggest that oral estrogens may be more strongly associated with cardiovascular risk (e.g., elevated C-reactive protein levels or an increase in triglycerides) than nonorally administered estrogens (L'Hermite et al., 2008; Vrablik et al., 2008). In addition, there is evidence that oral but not transdermal administration is associated with an increased risk of venous thromboembolism in postmenopausal women (Scarabin, Oger, and Plu-Bureau, 2003). Thus, it is plausible that, for a given level of HT use, the negative health consequences have been greater in the United States than in some other countries, but the paucity of relevant data make it impossible to reach a firmer conclusion.

In summary, there is little evidence to support the notion that higher use of HT in the United States than in other wealthy countries is likely to have resulted in mortality stagnation among middle-aged and older women. This argument is based on three sets of findings from recent studies in the United States and other wealthy countries: (1) HT use does not appear to have a notable impact on all-cause mortality; (2) HT use does not appear to be a significant risk factor for coronary heart disease and may be protective in this regard when initiated near the onset of menopause; and (3) although high, HT prevalence in the United States prior to the recent decline is similar to

---

[14]Data from Berlin, Germany, and Quebec, Canada, suggest that, as in the United States, transdermal application of HT has been much less common that oral administration in these locations (Du et al., 2009; Guay et al., 2007). There are differences in formulations across countries as well. For example, in the period just prior to the termination of the WHI, unopposed estrogens were prescribed more frequently than estrogen-progestin combinations for postmenopausal women in the United States and Australia (Hersh et al., 2004; Main and Robinson, 2008). However, the Million Women Study found that HT users in the period 1996-2000 in the United Kingdom were more likely to use estrogen-progestin combinations than estrogen alone (Million Women Study Collaborators, 2002).

rates of use in several countries that have experienced steady improvements in female life expectancy. Although the major RCTs related to hormone therapy have been terminated, research on the health consequences of HT use has not abated. Analyses based on continued follow-up of participants in the randomized trials, smaller scale trials examining the biological pathways linking HT to cardiovascular disease, and observational studies are likely to provide updated and longer term estimates of the consequences of HT for health and survival in the United States and elsewhere.

REFERENCES

American College of Physicians. (1992). Guidelines for counseling postmenopausal women about preventive hormone therapy. *Annals of Internal Medicine, 117,* 1038-1041.

Barbaglia, G., Macia, F., Comas, M., Sala, M., del Mar Vernet, M., Casamitjana, M., and Castells, X. (2009). Trends in hormone therapy use before and after publication of the Women's Health Initiative trial: 10 years of follow-up. *Menopause: Journal of the North American Menopause Society, 16*(5), 1061-1064.

Canfell, K., Banks, E., Moa, A.M., and Beral, V. (2008). Decrease in breast cancer incidence following a rapid fall in use of hormone replacement therapy in Australia. *Medical Journal of Australia, 188*(11), 641-644.

Chlebowski, R.T., Kuller, L.H., Prentice, R.L., Stefanick, M.L., Manson, J.E., Gass, M., Aragaki, A.K., Ockene, J.K., Lane, D.S., Sarto, G.E., Rajkovic, A., Schenken, R., Hendrix, S.L., Ravdin, P.M., Rohan, T.E., Yasmeen, S., Anderson, G., and the WHI investigators. (2009a). Breast cancer after use of estrogen plus progestin in postmenopausal women. *New England Journal of Medicine, 360*(6), 573-587.

Chlebowski, R.T., Schwartz, A.G., Wakelee, H., Anderson, G.L., Stefanick, M.L., Manson, J.E., Rodabough, R.J., Chien, J.W., Wactawski-Wende, J., Gass, M., Kotchen, J.M., Johnson, K.C., O'Sullivan, M.J., Ockene, J.K., Chen, C., and Hubbell, F.A. (2009b). Oestrogen plus progestin and lung cancer in postmenopausal women (Women's Health Initiative trial): A post-hoc analysis of a randomised controlled trial. *Lancet, 374*(9697), 1243-1251.

Coombs, N.J., and Boyages, J. (2005). Changes in HT prescriptions in Australia since 1992. *Australian Family Physician, 34*(8), 697-698.

Coombs, N.J., Cronin, K.A., Taylor, R.J., Freedman, A.N., and Boyages, J. (2010). The impact of changes in hormone therapy on breast cancer incidence in the U.S. population. *Cancer Causes and Control, 21*(1), 83-90.

de Jong-van den Berg, L.T.W., Faber, A., and van den Berg, P.B. (2006). HRT use in 2001 and 2004 in the Netherlands—A world of difference. *Maturitas, 54*(2), 193-197.

Du, Y., Doren, M., Melchert, H., Scheidt-Nave, C., and Knopf, H. (2007). Differences in menopausal hormone therapy use among women in Germany between 1998 and 2003. *BMC Women's Health, 7*(1), 19.

Du, Y., Schneidt-Nave, C., Schaffrath Rosario, A., Ellert, U., Doren, M., and Knopf, H. (2009). Changes of menopausal hormone therapy use pattern since 2000: Results of the Berlin Spandau Longitudinal Health Study. *Climacteric, 12*(4), 329-340.

Fletcher, S.W., and Colditz, G.A. (2002). Failure of estrogen plus progestin therapy for prevention. *Journal of the American Medical Association, 288,* 366-368.

Fournier, A., Berrino, F., and Clavel-Chapeton, F. (2008). Unequal risks for breast cancer associated with different hormone replacement therapies: Results from the E3N cohort study. *Breast Cancer Research and Treatment, 107*(1), 103-111.

Gayet-Ageron, A., Amamra, N., Ringa, V., Tainturier, V., Berr, C., Clavel-Chapelon, F., Delcourt, C., Delmas, P.D., Ducimetier, P., and Schott, A.M. (2005). Estimated numbers of postmenopausal women treated by hormone therapy in France. *Maturitas, 52*(3-4), 296-305.

Grady, D., Rubin, S.M., Petitti, D.B., Fox, C.S., Black, D., Ettinger, B., Ernster, V.L., and Cummings, S.R. (1992). Hormone therapy to prevent disease and prolong life in postmenopausal women. *Annals of Internal Medicine, 117*, 1016-1037.

Grodstein, F., Manson, J.E., Colditz, G.A., Willett, W.C., Speizer, F.E., and Stampfer, M.J. (2000). A prospective, observational study of postmenopausal hormone therapy and primary prevention of cardiovascular disease. *Annals of Internal Medicine, 133*, 933-941.

Grodstein, F., Clarkson, T.B., and Manson, J.E. (2003). Understanding the divergent data on postmenopausal hormone therapy. *New England Journal of Medicine, 348*, 645-650.

Grodstein, F., Manson, J.E., and Stampfer, M.J. (2006). Hormone therapy and coronary heart disease: The role of time since menopause and age at hormone initiation. *Journal of Women's Health, 15*, 35-44.

Guay, M., Dragomir, A., Pilon, D., Moride, Y., and Perreault, S. (2007). Changes in pattern of use, clinical characteristics and persistence rate of hormone replacement therapy among postmenopausal women after the WHI publication. *Pharmacoepidemiology and Drug Safety, 16*, 17-27.

Heier, M., Moebus, S., Meisinger, C., Jöckel, K., Völzke, H., Döring, A., and Alte, D. (2009). Menopausal hormone therapy in Germany: Results of three national surveys from 1997 to 2003. *Maturitas, 62*(1), 9-15.

Heiss, G., Wallace, R., Anderson, G.L., Aragaki, A., Beresford, S.A.A., Brzyski, R., Chlebowski, R.T., Gass, M., LaCroix, A., Manson, J.E., Prentice, R.L., Rossouw, J., Stefanick, M.L., and the WHI investigators. (2008). Health risks and benefits 3 years after stopping randomized treatment with estrogen and progestin. *Journal of the American Medical Association, 299*(9), 1036-1045.

Hernan, M.A., Alonso, A., Logan, R., Grodstein, F., Michels, K.B., Willett, W.C., Manson, J.E., and Robins, J.M. (2008). Observational studies analyzed like randomized experiments: An application to postmenopausal hormone therapy and coronary heart disease. *Epidemiology, 19*, 766-779.

Hersh, A.L., Stefanick, M.L., and Stafford, R.S. (2004). National use of postmenopausal hormone therapy: Annual trends and response to recent evidence. *Journal of the American Medical Association, 291*(1), 47-53.

Kim, J.K., Alley, D., Hu, P., Karlamangia, A., Seeman, T., and Crimmins, E.M. (2007). Changes in postmenopausal hormone therapy use since 1988. *Women's Health Issues, 17*(6), 338-341.

Kopper, N.W., Gudeman, J., and Thompson, D.J. (2009). Transdermal hormone therapy in postmenopausal women: A review of metabolic effects and drug delivery technologies. *Journal of Drug Design, Development and Therapy, 2*, 193-202.

Kumle, M. (2008). Declining breast cancer incidence and decreased HRT use. *Lancet, 372*(9639), 608-610.

L'Hermite, M., Simoncini, T., Fuller, S., and Genazzani, A.R. (2008). Could transdermal estradiol + progesterone be a safer postmenopausal HRT? A review. *Maturitas, 60*(3-4), 185-201.

Lundberg, V., Tolonen, H., Stegmayr, B., Kuulasmaa, K., and Asplund, K. (2004). Use of oral contraceptives and hormone replacement therapy in the WHO MONICA Project. *Maturitas, 48*(1), 39-49.

Main, P., and Robinson, M. (2008). Changes in utilisation of hormone replacement therapy in Australia following publication of the findings of the Women's Health Initiative. *Pharmacoepidemiology and Drug Safety, 17*(9), 861-868.

Manson, J.E., and Bassuk, S.S. (2007). Menopausal hormone therapy and the risk of coronary heart disease. Does the relation vary by age or time since menopause? *Monitor*, 17-22.

Manson, J.E., Bassuk, S.S., Mitchell Harman, S., Brinton, E.A., Cedars, M.I., Lobo, R., Merriam, G.R., Miller, V.M., Naftolin, F., and Santoro, N. (2006). Postmenopausal hormone therapy: New questions and the case for new clinical trials. *Menopause: Journal of the North American Menopause Society*, 13, 139-147.

Manson, J.E., Allison, M.A., Rossouw, J.E., Carr, J.J., Langer, R.D., Hsia, J., Kuller, L.H., Cochrane, B.B., Hunt, J.R., Ludlam, S.E., Pettinger, M.B., Gass, M., Margolis, K.L., Nathan, L., Ockene, J.K., Prentice, R.L., Robbins, J., Stefanick, M.L., and the WHI and WHI-CACS investigators. (2007). Estrogen therapy and coronary-artery calcification. *New England Journal of Medicine*, 356, 2591-2602.

Meslé, F., and Vallin, J. (2006). Diverging trends in female old-age mortality: The United States and the Netherlands versus France and Japan. *Population and Development Review*, 32(1), 123-145.

Million Women Study Collaborators. (2002). Patterns of use of hormone replacement therapy in one million women in Britain, 1996-2000. *BJOG: International Journal of Obstetrics and Gynaecology*, 109, 1319-1330.

Nagata, C., Matsushita, Y., and Shimizu, H. (1996). Prevalence of hormone replacement therapy and user's characteristics: A community survey in Japan. *Maturitas*, 25(3), 201-207.

Nelson, H.D., Humphrey, L.L., Nygren, P., Teutsch, S.M., and Allan, J.D. (2002). Postmenopausal hormone replacement therapy: Scientific review. *Journal of the American Medical Association*, 288, 872-881.

Prentice, R.L., and Anderson, G.L. (2008). The Women's Health Initiative: Lessons learned. *Annual Review of Public Health*, 29, 131-150.

Prentice, R.L., Manson, J.E., Langer, R.D., Anderson, G.L., Pettinger, M., Jackson, R.D., Johnson, K.C., Kuller, L.J., Lane, D.S., Wactawski-Wende, J., Brzyski, R., Allison, M., Ockene, J., Sarto, G., and Rossouw, J.E. (2009). Benefits and risks of postmenopausal hormone therapy when it is initiated soon after menopause. *American Journal of Epidemiology*, 170(1), 12-23.

Ravdin, P.M., Cronin, K.A., Howlader, N., Berg, C.D., Chlebowski, R.T., Feuer, E.J., Edwards, B.K., and Berry, D.A. (2007). The decrease in breast-cancer incidence in 2003 in the United States. *New England Journal of Medicine*, 356(16), 1670-1674.

Ringa, V., and Fournier, A. (2008). Did the decrease in use of menopausal hormone therapy induce a decrease in the incidence of breast cancer in France (and elsewhere)? *Revue d'Épidémiologie et de Santé Publique*, 56, e8-e12.

Rossouw, J.E., Prentice, R.L., Manson, J.E., Wu, L., Barad, D., Barnabei, V.M., Ko, M., LaCroix, A.Z., Margolis, K.L., and Stefanick, M.L. (2007). Postmenopausal hormone therapy and risk of cardiovascular disease by age and years since menopause. *Journal of the American Medical Association*, 297, 1465-1477.

Salpeter, S.R., Walsh, J.M.E., Greyber, E., Ormiston, T.M., and Salpeter, E.E. (2004). Mortality associated with hormone replacement therapy in younger and older women. *Journal of General Internal Medicine*, 19, 791-804.

Salpeter, S.R., Walsh, J.M.E., Greyber, E., and Salpeter, E.E. (2006). Brief report: Coronary heart disease events associated with hormone therapy in younger and older women. *Journal of General Internal Medicine*, 21, 363-366.

Scarabin, P., Oger, E., and Plu-Bureau, G. (2003). Differential association of oral and transdermal oestrogen-replacement therapy with venous thromboembolism risk. *Lancet*, 362, 428-432.

Schneider, H.P.G. (2002). Report on the 10th World Congress on Menopause. June 2002, Berlin, Germany. *Climacteric*, 5, 219-228.

Stevenson, J.C. (2009). Type and route of estrogen administration. *Climacteric*, 12, 86-90.

Townsend, J., and Nanchahal, K. (2005). Hormone replacement therapy: Limited response in the UK to the new evidence. *British Journal of General Practice, 55*(516), 555.

Vaupel, J. (2003). The future of human longevity: How important are markets and innovation? Testimony before the Senate Special Committee on Aging. *Science of Aging Knowledge Environment,* (26), 18.

Vrablik, M., Fait, T., Kovar, J., Poledne, R., and Ceska, R. (2008). Oral but not transdermal estrogen replacement therapy changes the composition of plasma lipoproteins. *Metabolism: Clinical and Experimental, 57*(8), 1088-1092.

Waaseth, M., Bakken, K., and Lund, E. (2009). Patterns of hormone therapy use in the Norwegian Women and Cancer Study (NOWAC) 1996-2005. *Maturitas, 63*(3), 220-226.

Women's Health Initiative Steering Committee. (2004). Effects of conjugated equine estrogen in postmenopausal women with hysterectomy: The Women's Health Initiative randomized controlled trial. *Journal of the American Medical Association, 291*, 1701-1712.

Writing Group for the Women's Health Initiative Investigators. (2002). Risks and benefits of estrogen plus progestin in healthy postmenopausal women: Principal results from the Women's Health Initiative randomized controlled trial. *Journal of the American Medical Association, 288*(3), 321-333.

Wysowski, D.K., and Governale, L.A. (2005). Use of menopausal hormones in the United States, 1992 through June, 2003. *Pharmacoepidemiology and Drug Safety, 14*, 171-176.

Wysowski, D.K., Golden, L., and Burke, L. (1995). Use of menopausal estrogens and medroxyprogesterone in the United States, 1982-1992. *Obstetrics and Gynecology, 85*(1), 6-10.

Part IV

Inequality

11

Do Americans Have Higher Mortality Than Europeans at All Levels of the Education Distribution?: A Comparison of the United States and 14 European Countries

Mauricio Avendano, Renske Kok, Maria Glymour, Lisa Berkman, Ichiro Kawachi, Anton Kunst, and Johan Mackenbach with support from members of the Eurothine Consortium

INTRODUCTION

Among industrialized countries, the United States ranks near the bottom on life expectancy at birth. In 2006, the average American man and woman could expect to live 75 and 80 years, respectively, while the average Western European man and woman could expect to live 77 and 83 years, respectively (World Health Organization, 2009; World Health Organization Regional Office for Europe, 2010). Although the extent to which this is attributable to differences in the health care system is unknown, the United States spends two to three times more than other industrialized countries on medical care (Anderson and Hussey, 2001; Organisation for Economic Co-operation and Development, 2006). This suggests that at least part of the causes of the U.S. disadvantage might lie elsewhere.

A plausible hypothesis is that disparities in mortality in the United States are larger than in other high-income countries, particularly in Western Europe. This implies that U.S. excess mortality might be attributable to higher excess mortality in those with low levels of education, while mortality levels for those with secondary or higher education might be comparable in Europe and the United States. Population composition is more diverse in the United States in terms of geography, race, and ethnicity, which may translate into larger health disparities than in Europe. Health care and social policies also differ dramatically between Europe and the United States. Most noticeably, while access to health care is nearly universal in Western Europe, about 41 million Americans remain uninsured (Adams, Dey, and

Vickerie, 2007). In addition, compared with European countries, the United States has lower provision of social transfers (e.g., social retirement benefits, unemployment compensation, sick pay) and fewer redistributive policies, resulting in substantially larger income and wealth inequalities (Organisation for Economic Co-operation and Development, 2008; Wolf, 1996). Whether the less generous U.S. policies translate into larger mortality inequalities has not yet been established.

The overall excess mortality in the United States compared with Western Europe is well documented (Organisation for Economic Co-operation and Development, 2006; World Health Organization, 2009). However, whether Americans of all education levels have higher mortality than comparable Europeans is yet unknown. Earlier mortality studies have focused only on the strength of education effects, yielding mixed results (Dahl et al., 2006; Kunst and Mackenbach, 1994; Mackenbach et al., 1999). Two recent studies suggest that although older Americans of all education, wealth, and income levels report poorer health than equivalent Europeans, the U.S. health disadvantage is largest among the poor and less educated (Avendano et al., 2009; Banks et al., 2006). Although based on cross-sectional and self-reported data, these findings support the hypothesis that larger health disparities in the United States partly explain the overall U.S. health disadvantage. A competing hypothesis is that Americans of all education levels experience higher mortality than equivalent Europeans. If true, one would expect U.S. residents of all education levels to have higher mortality rates than comparable Europeans.

In this study, we examined cross-national differences in mortality by education level in the United States and 14 European countries in the 1990s and compared the magnitude of the disparities in mortality by education among these populations.

DATA AND METHODS

European Data

We obtained data on mortality according to age, sex, education level, and cause of death from mortality registries. In most countries, data were collected in a longitudinal design, by linking mortality data to 1990s census data in a follow-up period using personal identifiers. However, for some Eastern European and Baltic countries, only cross-sectional data were available around the 2000 census. The data comprise entire national populations, except for the United Kingdom, with data for England and Wales only. For countries with a follow-up period of 10 years or longer, the baseline was ages 30-74. For countries with follow-up shorter than 10 years, the baseline age comprised a broader age group to avoid bias due to variations in age at the end of follow-up. For populations with a follow-up period of 5 years or shorter (Belgium and Denmark), the baseline was ages 30-79, and for populations with cross-sectional data (Eastern European and Baltic countries), the baseline was ages 35-79. Table 11-1 shows details of the European data sets. Further details on these data can be found elsewhere (Eurothine Group, 2007; Mackenbach et al., 2008).

U.S. Data

We used the mortality follow-up of the five waves (1989-1993) of the National Health Interview Survey (NHIS). The NHIS is a continuous household survey based on a nationally representative sample of the U.S. civilian noninstitutionalized population, covering around 80,000 individuals each year (Massey et al., 1989). In 2004, the National Center for Health Statistics (NCHS) completed a mortality follow-up for the 1986-2000 NHIS cohorts through December 31, 2002, based on linkage with the National Death Index (NDI) (Massey et al., 1989). From this linked data file, we selected respondents who had been interviewed in 1989 through 1993 and used their mortality follow-up data through 2002. The final sample comprised 286,759 individuals.

Analyses by the NCHS have shown that survival rates as observed in the NHIS mortality follow-up data are similar to the survival rates in the general U.S. population. Mortality tends to be slightly lower in the NHIS sample mainly due to the exclusion of the institutionalized population (Ingram, Lochner, and Cox, 2008). Although in most cases differences are not statistically significant, we estimated that overall underestimation might be around 9 percent for white men, negligible for white women, 14 percent for black men, and 11 percent for black women (Ingram, Lochner, and Cox, 2008). In sensitivity analyses, we found that accounting for this underestimation using weights had only marginal effects on our results.

Analyses were conducted separately for whites and blacks, using appropriate sampling weights and adjusting standard errors for sample clustering (Massey et al., 1989).

Education Level

Information on education for Europe came from each national or regional census, while for the United States it came from the NHIS interview survey. In Europe, this classification corresponded approximately to the International Standard Classification of Education (ISCED) levels 0-2 (lower secondary or lower), 3 (upper secondary), and 4-6 (postsecondary). In the United States, corresponding levels were obtained based on years of schooling: ≤ 11 years (lower secondary or lower), upper secondary (12-15

TABLE 11-1 Overview of European and U.S. Data Sets on Socioeconomic Status and Mortality, 1990-2003

Country	Baseline	Follow-Up	Person-Years	Deaths	Type of Study
United States of America (NHIS)	1989-2003	2002	3,109,161	33,587	National, longitudinal, mortality study for a representative sample of the population
Finland	1990	2000	25,874,201	270,130	National, longitudinal, census-linked mortality study
Sweden	1991	2000	43,042,216	393,038	National, longitudinal, census-linked mortality study
Norway	1990	2000	19,956,768	213,022	National, longitudinal, census-linked mortality study
Denmark	1996	2000	14,619,326	183,281	National, longitudinal, census-linked mortality study
England and Wales	1991	1999	2,295,029	21,234	National, longitudinal, census-linked mortality study for a representative sample of 1 percent of the population of England and Wales
Belgium	1991	1995	24,860,995	283,325	National, longitudinal, census-linked mortality study
Switzerland[a]	1990	2000	27,910,587	255,270	National, longitudinal, census-linked mortality study
France[b]	1990	1999	2,478,782	20,215	National, longitudinal, census-linked mortality study for a representative sample of 1 percent of population
Slovenia	1991	2000	9,647,452	101,557	National, longitudinal, census-linked mortality study
Hungary	1999	2002	21,031,348	363,508	National, unlinked, cross-national mortality study
Czech Republic	1999	2003	25,759,210	344,973	National, unlinked, cross-national mortality study
Poland	2001	2003	54,883,245	717,743	National, unlinked, cross-national mortality study
Lithuania	2000	2002	5,156,703	78,399	National, unlinked, cross-national mortality study
Estonia	1998	2002	3,435,255	60,794	National, unlinked, cross-national mortality study

[a]Non-Swiss nationals are excluded.
[b]Residents of overseas territories, members of the military, and students are excluded.

years), and postsecondary (≥ 16 years). In the United States and some European countries, the lowest education category could be further divided into primary education or less (≤ 8 years of U.S. schooling) and lower secondary education (9-11 years of U.S. schooling). In these countries, supplementary analyses were performed to examine whether results based on four categories would lead to results equivalent to those based on three categories only.

Levels of education were comparable across all populations except England and Wales. For this population, census data did not appropriately distinguish individuals with lower secondary education from those with upper secondary education. Therefore, although we present data for England and Wales, rates by education level cannot be directly compared between this population and the other countries included in our study. We therefore refrain from discussing findings for England and Wales in detail in this chapter.

Statistical Analysis

All analyses were stratified by sex and education level. Age-adjusted mortality rates were first calculated based on a Poisson regression model, using the 1995 U.S. census population as a standard. While this provided an overview of mortality rates by education, directly comparing these rates is problematic because the distribution of education varies considerably across countries. Therefore, we calculated two additional measures to compare mortality related to education level across countries:

1. The population attributable fraction (PAF): this measure assumes a causal effect of education on mortality and is equivalent to the proportion of all deaths that would be avoided if exposure to a lower education level is eliminated. The size of the PAF depends on what is defined as exposure and nonexposure. For this analysis, we defined those with tertiary or higher education as the unexposed group. Thus, the PAF reflects mortality attributable to exposure to an upper secondary or lower level of education.
2. We summarized education-related disparities in mortality using the relative index of inequality (RII), a relative measure of inequality (Mackenbach and Kunst, 1997). The RII is a regression-based measure that accounts for differences in the distribution of education among countries. This measure regresses mortality on an education ranking, defined as the midpoint of the range of the cumulative distribution of education in each country (Mackenbach and Kunst, 1997). The RII can be interpreted as the ratio of mortality between

rank 1 (the lowest point of the education distribution) and rank 0 (the top end of the education distribution).

RESULTS

The Distribution of Education

The distribution of education differed dramatically across countries. Men and women in the United States reached higher levels of education than men and women in Europe (see Tables 11-2 and 11-3). While in the United States and Switzerland only 20 percent of men had lower secondary education or less (the lowest education level), the corresponding proportion was 30-50 percent in the Scandinavian countries, the Baltic countries, France,

TABLE 11-2 Mortality Rates[a] Per 100,000 Person-Years According to Education Level and Population Attributable Fraction (PAF) for Men Ages 30 to 74 in 14 European Countries and the United States

	Lower Secondary or Less		Upper Secondary		Tertiary or Higher		Total	
	Rate	%	Rate	%	Rate	%	Rate	PAF[b]
USA, all	1,840	20	1,339	54	885	26	1,379	39
USA, whites	1,779	19	1,316	54	876	27	1,334	38
USA, blacks	2,264	32	1,658	55	1,198	14	1,903	39
Finland	1,700	49	1,410	30	942	22	1,528	41
Sweden	1,151	40	953	43	706	16	1,026	33
Norway	1,498	30	1,194	48	873	22	1,272	33
Denmark	1,659	43	1,400	38	982	19	1,508	37
England/Wales[c]	1,128	83	786	7	652	10	1,074	39
Belgium	1,590	61	1,264	22	999	17	1,480	32
Switzerland	1,477	20	1,123	56	831	24	1,165	30
France	1,285	50	955	37	624	13	1,132	51
Slovenia	1,977	37	1,421	50	930	12	1,616	51
Hungary	2,614	65	1,471	21	1,029	14	2,195	58
Czech Republic	2,088	63	1,115	24	732	14	1,699	65
Poland	2,217	61	1,213	28	838	11	1,834	61
Lithuania	2,718	31	1,892	53	1,054	16	2,184	63
Estonia	2,974	32	2,393	50	1,240	17	2,480	63

[a]Rates are directly standardized to the U.S. census population of 1995.

[b]PAF = population attributable fraction. PAF calculations in this column define the "tertiary or higher education" group as the unexposed category.

[c]Education levels for England and Wales do not correspond to the International Standard Classification of Education levels. The "lower secondary or less" category include some individuals with upper secondary education as well. No further distinction was possible through census data.

TABLE 11-3 Mortality Rates[a] Per 100,000 Person-Years According to Education Level and Population Attributable Fraction (PAF) for Women Ages 30 to 74 in 14 European Countries and the United States

	Lower Secondary or Less		Upper Secondary		Tertiary or Higher		Total	
	Rate	%	Rate	%	Rate	%	Rate	PAF[b]
USA, all	1,142	20	839	61	588	19	888	36
USA, whites	1,099	18	818	62	583	20	856	34
USA, blacks	1,399	30	1,091	57	765	13	1,197	39
Finland	794	51	631	29	528	20	735	26
Sweden	657	41	534	40	402	19	589	32
Norway	801	36	616	47	484	17	697	31
Denmark	1,037	53	814	28	664	19	960	29
England/Wales[c]	670	87	472	8	394	5	652	40
Belgium	801	67	628	19	582	14	766	22
Switzerland	657	40	523	53	472	7	591	19
France	530	62	387	28	334	10	492	31
Slovenia	832	56	665	35	526	9	776	33
Hungary	1,169	64	742	26	651	11	1,061	37
Czech Republic	956	64	684	28	428	8	886	59
Poland	952	54	642	36	457	11	842	49
Lithuania	1,129	32	709	51	462	17	899	53
Estonia	1,220	29	1,000	53	592	18	1,050	50

[a]Rates are directly standardized to the U.S. census population of 1995.

[b]PAF = population attributable fraction. PAF calculations in this column define the "tertiary or higher education" group as the unexposed category.

[c]Education levels for England and Wales do not correspond to the International Standard Classification of Education levels. The "lower secondary or less" category includes some individuals with upper secondary education as well. No further distinction was possible through census data.

and Slovenia and 60-70 percent in Belgium, Hungary, the Czech Republic, and Poland. Accordingly, while 26 percent of U.S. men and 19 percent of U.S. women completed tertiary or higher education, in Europe this range was between 10 percent (England) and 24 percent (Switzerland) among men and from 5 percent (England) to 20 percent (Finland) among women. Rather than reflecting measurement problems, this variation simply reflects cross-national differences in education systems and in the overall level of educational achievements in the population. Some countries, for example the United States and Switzerland, achieved early very high levels of basic educational attainment that influenced the cohorts included in our study, while cohorts in such populations as Belgium and Hungary lagged behind in overall educational achievements in the population as a whole.

Mortality by Education Level in the United States and Europe

Among men, total mortality among U.S. black men was similar to that in Eastern European countries, which had the highest mortality rates in Europe (see Table 11-2). U.S. white men had lower rates than Eastern European countries and rates comparable to Belgium, Denmark, and Finland, which had the highest rates in Western Europe. Mortality was higher for U.S. black women than for women in any European country. U.S. white women had higher mortality rates than women in all Western European countries but Denmark, while their mortality rate was comparable to that in Eastern European countries, which had the highest rates in Europe (see Table 11-3).

Lower education level was associated with higher mortality rates in all countries. Among men and women with only primary education or less, mortality for U.S. blacks and whites was higher than in any Western European country, and comparable to mortality in Eastern European countries. Among men with tertiary education or higher, the pattern differed for whites and blacks: highly educated U.S. white men had similar rates as highly educated men in Norway or Switzerland, while highly educated U.S. black men had higher rates than any European country except Estonia. Among highly educated women, mortality in the United States was higher than in any Western European country and comparable to mortality of highly educated women in Eastern Europe. Highly educated U.S. black women had higher mortality rates than comparable women in any European country.

The proportion of mortality (PAF) attributable to exposure to an upper secondary or lower level of education is summarized in Tables 11-2 and 11-3. The PAF was 38 percent for U.S. white men and 39 percent for U.S. black men, which was comparable to that in Denmark (37 percent) or Finland (41 percent) but smaller than that in Eastern European countries, such as Estonia (63 percent) and the Czech Republic (65 percent). A similar pattern was observed for women.

Relative Index of Inequality (RII)

Figure 11-1 shows that a lower education rank was associated with a higher mortality rate in both the United States and Europe. Black and white U.S. men had intermediate levels of inequality in mortality compared with European countries. For example, the RII for U.S. white men was 2.4 (95% CI 2.2, 2.6), which was comparable to that in Norway, Switzerland, and France. Swedish men had the smallest inequalities, while men in Eastern Europe had the largest ones. U.S. white women had somewhat larger inequalities in mortality (2.2, 2.0, 2.4) than many Western European countries, but inequalities similar to Norway and France. The RII for U.S. black women (2.0, 1.6, 2.5) was similar to that in Norway or France. Women in Poland, Hungary, and Lithuania had the largest inequalities.

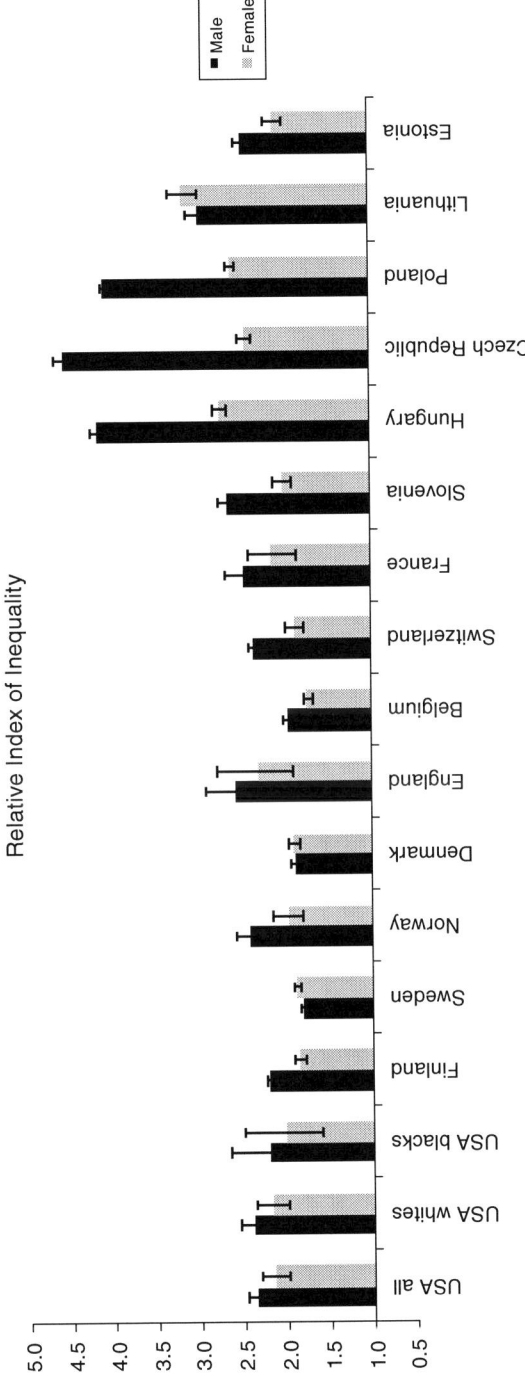

FIGURE 11-1 Relative index of inequality of mortality by education level for men and women at ages 30 to 74 in 14 European countries and the United States.

Total Mortality Rates Versus Disparities in Mortality

Figure 11-2 plots total mortality rates against the RII in each country. Although we had a limited number of observations and correlations were not significant, results generally suggest that populations with large mortality rates tend to have large relative disparities in mortality by education. Correlations were strongly driven by Eastern European countries, which had high mortality rates and large mortality disparities by education.

DISCUSSION

Previous research indicates that the United States has substantially lower life expectancy than most Western European countries. Our results partly support the hypotheses that U.S. excess mortality is to some extent attributable to larger excess mortality at lower education levels. Among women and in some cases for men, however, U.S. excess mortality is pervasive and extends across the entire education distribution. We found that inequalities in the United States are comparable to inequalities in several European countries, such as Norway and France, but smaller than inequalities in Eastern European countries.

Limitations of This Study

Some limitations of our study should be acknowledged. Despite our efforts at harmonization, comparability of data on mortality by education is imperfect. Measurement error might be larger in European countries with less well-established statistics systems, downwardly biasing associations between education and mortality. Data for most countries are longitudinal and nationally representative. However, data for some Eastern European countries are cross-sectional. Although our data mirrored previously reported international mortality patterns (World Health Organization, 2009) and comprised the best available data stratified by education, cross-national differences in mortality disparities might be partly attributable to differences in methodology and measurement error.

Data for the United States differed somewhat from data for Europe in terms of baseline measurement period, mortality follow-up, and covariate measurement. Most importantly, while European data comprised entire national census populations, data for the United States were restricted to the noninstitutionalized population. Previous reports indicate that the NHIS somewhat underestimates U.S. mortality rates, particularly for black men, and to a lesser extent for white men (Ingram, Lochner, and Cox, 2008). As indicated in the methods section, we estimated the overall underestimation of mortality in the United States to range from 9 to 14 percent. In sensitivity analyses, we found that using weights to account for this did not alter our

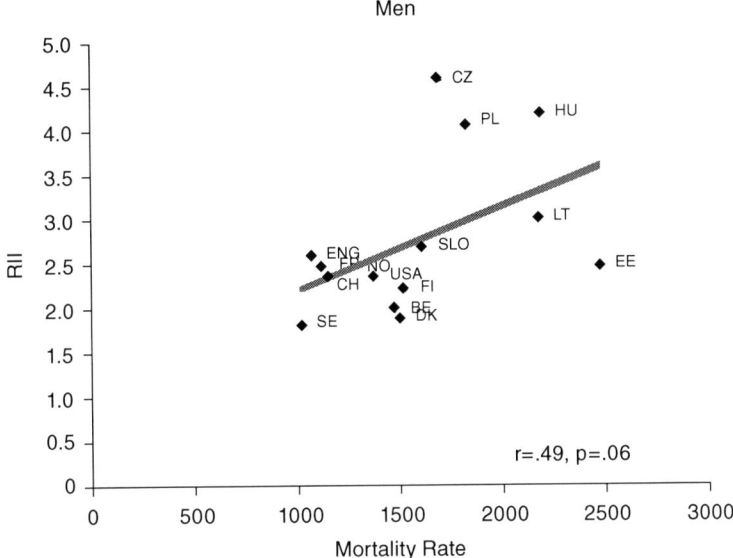

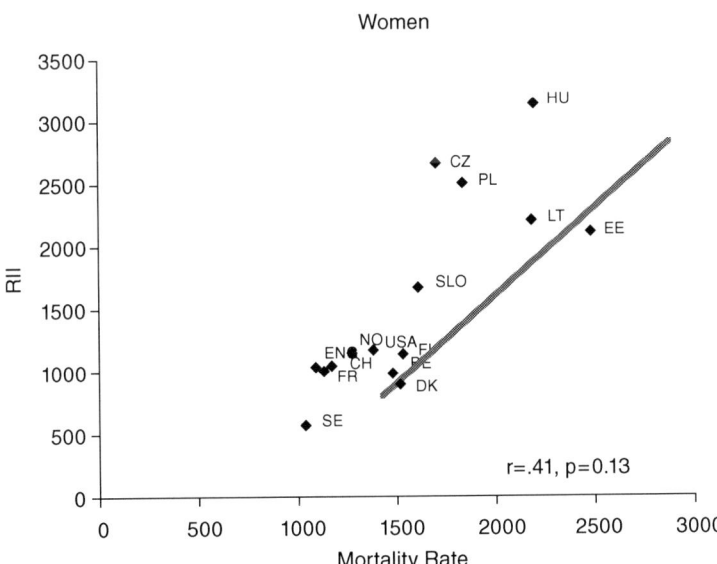

FIGURE 11-2 Pearson correlation of total mortality rates with the relative index of inequality (RII) in men and women at ages 30 to 74 in 14 European countries and the United States.
NOTES: BE = Belgium, CH = Switzerland, CZ = Czech Republic, DK = Denmark, EE = Estonia, ENG = England and Wales, FI = Finland, FR = France, HU = Hungary, LT = Lithuania, NO = Norway, PL = Poland, SE = Sweden, SLO = Slovenia, USA = United States.

overall conclusions. However, we were unable to assess whether mortality underestimation differed by education. Institutionalization rates are higher among less educated people, leading to larger exclusions of frail populations in these groups. As we observed in a previous study for morbidity (Huisman, Kunst, and Mackenbach, 2003), we may have underestimated mortality in the less educated groups in the United States, leading to underestimation of U.S. excess mortality and related disparities by education.

Despite their comprehensiveness, our data included a limited set of covariates. Other than age, our estimates were unadjusted for relevant confounders, such as parental education and early life conditions. Furthermore, our data are observational, and education might be an endogenous variable in our models. For example, personal characteristics unobserved in our study but related to both poor health and lower educational achievements (e.g., personality features, parenting styles, poor childhood nutrition) might account for at least part of the association between education and mortality. Thus, our estimates encompass both causal and noncausal effects of education on mortality. Although we calculated the reduction in mortality that would be achieved if "exposure to lower education" would be eliminated (PAF percentage), estimates are most likely to be an overestimation of the true mortality attributable to the causal effect of education. Future studies should expand our descriptive approach by examining in more detail to what extent total mortality rates are determined by the distribution of mortality by education, taking into account the issues described above.

We calculated the RII to take into account the position of individuals in the education distribution. However, this measure assumes linearity of education effects on mortality. Although there appeared to be a linear association in most countries, this assumption may not be met in all cases. We compared mortality across broad education groups to improve comparability. However, we may have ignored relevant differences, particularly among individuals in the lower end of the education distribution. In sensitivity analyses for countries with more detailed data, we found that dividing the less educated group into up to primary education and lower secondary education did not change the relative position of the United States in terms of disparities. However, it resulted in more extreme excess U.S. mortality in the bottom end of the education distribution compared with European countries (results not shown).

We have used education as a social stratification variable in our study, because it is relatively easy to measure, it is roughly comparable for men and women, and it can be made comparable across countries. In addition, although educational achievement is influenced by childhood health and other early life influences, education is less endogenous to adult health than other social stratification measures, such as income and wealth (Lleras-Muney, 2005). However, education captures only one social stratification dimension, while such measures as occupational class, income, and wealth may be more relevant social stratification measures at older ages and might be more sensitive to welfare state policies that are fundamentally different between the United States and Europe. Thus, our findings for education do not necessarily apply for effects of income, wealth, and occupation, each of which has a distinct relationship with health and mortality (Smith, 2007).

We recoded country-specific levels of education into internationally comparable education levels based on the ISCED international classification. Therefore, levels of education are in theory comparable in terms of educational achievement. However, education systems differ across countries at least in two ways: First, educational practices, curricula, quality of schooling, and other qualitative aspects of education differ dramatically among the countries included in our study. By focusing only on educational achievement, our analysis assumes that the quality and type of education is homogenous across countries. If this assumption is not met, differential effects of education will partly reflect the impact of different types and quality of education across countries, rather than only the impact of educational achievement on mortality.

Second, the distribution of education differed across countries, which makes comparisons of mortality levels by education cumbersome. Although we calculated the RII to ameliorate this problem, this approach does not fully account for the fact that overall levels of educational achievement are higher in some countries, such as the United States and Switzerland, than in Hungary, Poland, or even the Scandinavian countries. This cross-national variation probably reflects different levels of public investment in education, compulsory schooling laws, and other aspects related to education policy. Because this influences overall educational achievements and the "returns" to education, part of the cross-national differences in mortality associated with education might reflect the different value of education across countries. We did not have data to test these potential differences in the value of education or in the different mechanisms through which education relates to mortality in different countries.

Our analysis of mortality disparities by education rank were based on the RII, a relative measure of inequality. In sensitivity analysis, we calculated the slope index of inequality (SII), an equivalent measure of absolute inequalities. We found that cross-country variations in absolute differences generally mirrored variations in relative differences in mortality by education.

Interpretation

We found that excess mortality in the United States compared with some European countries is generally larger at lower levels of the education distribution. Notwithstanding possible limitations, several explanations for this finding should be considered: behavioral differences, differences in health care systems, differences in social and economic policies that particularly impair the health of Americans, and the extent to which mortality gradients by education reflect causality or selection. Although our data are not comprehensive enough to examine the role of these mechanisms, in this section we draw on evidence from other data sources to discuss the potential role of these explanations. Succinct examination of these issues should be the focus of future research.

Higher excess mortality at the bottom of the education distribution in the United States may stem from larger disparities in behavioral risk factors than in some European countries. In most of Europe and the United States, lower education is associated with higher smoking prevalence (Cavelaars et al., 2000; Zhu et al., 1996). However, the smoking epidemic started earlier and reached a higher pick in the United States (Lopez, Collishaw, and Piha, 1994), particularly among women. We used data from the Health and Retirement Survey (HRS) (Heeringa and Connor, 1995) and the Survey of Health, Ageing and Retirement in Europe (SHARE) (Borsch-Supan et al., 2005) to examine smoking prevalence across the education distribution. At ages 50-74, ever-smoking prevalence in men with lower secondary education or less was 75 percent in the United States, while in Western Europe it ranged from 51 percent in Austria to 79 percent in the Netherlands. Ever-smoking prevalence among women with lower secondary or less education was 53 percent in the United States, while in Western Europe it ranged from 13 percent in Spain to 68 percent in Denmark. These differences reflect a longer smoking history among Americans compared with most Europeans, particularly for men at the bottom of the education distribution and for women of all education levels. A similar smoking history may also explain why Danes and Americans share similar excess mortality compared with other European countries. However, some countries, such as the Netherlands and Sweden, have similar smoking prevalence but lower mortality rates than the United States, suggesting that smoking might not be the only explanation for the U.S. excess mortality.

The obesity epidemic is more advanced in the United States, where prevalence is higher than in most European countries (Avendano et al., 2009; Silventoinen et al., 2004). Lower education might be associated with more extreme levels of obesity in the United States. Data from the HRS (Heeringa and Connor, 1995) and SHARE (Borsch-Supan et al., 2005) for 2004 suggests that, at ages 50-74, prevalence of obesity among less educated men was 32 percent in the United States, while in Western Europe it ranged from 15 percent (Sweden and Switzerland) to 23 percent (Spain and Belgium). Obesity prevalence among less educated women in the United States was 36 percent, while in Europe it ranged from 16 percent (Switzerland) to

28 percent (Austria). These differences stem across the entire education distribution, suggesting that obesity might contribute to U.S. excess mortality at all levels of education. The prevalence and social patterning of excessive alcohol consumption, physical inactivity, and poor diet might also be more extreme in the United States than in some European countries, but we did not have comparable data sources to formally examine distributions across countries.

A key finding of our study is that among women and in some cases among men, U.S. excess mortality is not limited to the low end of the education distribution, but even highly educated Americans experience higher mortality than comparable Western Europeans. Smoking and obesity are more prevalent in the U.S. population as a whole and may contribute to disparities across the entire education distribution. However, particularly for women, our findings point also at specific U.S. policies that might impair the health of Americans in all education levels. Women in the United States entered the labor market earlier (Jaumotte, 2003/2) and may have been more exposed to work-related hazards than women in many European countries. U.S. work policies are also less comprehensive and less targeted to the needs of female workers compared with European policies. For example, the United States has less accessible programs of maternity benefits and related income replacement programs than most European countries. Although less educated American women are most vulnerable, the health of women of all education levels may have also been influenced by the lack of comprehensive policies.

The United States has larger income and wealth inequalities, partly as a result of lower provision of social transfers and less redistributive policies than most European countries (Organisation for Economic Co-operation and Development, 2008; Wolff, 1996). It has been hypothesized that these policies might contribute to the U.S. health disadvantage. Particularly noticeable is the large number of uninsured Americans (Adams et al., 2007; Decker and Remler, 2004; Ross and Mirowsky, 2000), which contrasts with national coverage programs in most of Western Europe. However, although disparities in the United States were larger than disparities in Sweden, they were similar to disparities in Norway and Finland. These countries have universal access to care and higher levels of welfare state intervention, social transfers, and income redistribution policies than the United States (Dahl et al., 2006; Wolff, 1996). Norway and Finland share with the United States a strong social gradient in behavioral risk factors, such as smoking and alcohol consumption. Thus, although the longer Swedish welfare state may have contributed to smaller health disparities, welfare state policies may not always counteract autonomous social behavioral patterns underlying health disparities.

Our study suggests that part of the U.S. health disadvantage is attributable to higher excess mortality among black Americans of all education levels. We did not have data on ethnicity and race for Europe, so we were unable to compare black Americans with black or other ethnic minorities in Europe. However, blacks are a larger share of the U.S. population and have a documented history of disproportionate exposure to poor socioeconomic circumstances, high prevalence of risk factors, and social exclusion. Addressing the fundamental causes of racial disparities in the United States may thus contribute to reducing overall excess mortality.

We observed much higher mortality rates and disparities in mortality by education in Eastern European countries than in Western Europe. Particularly among men, Eastern European countries have high levels of excessive alcohol consumption, which contribute strongly to the health gap between Western, Central, and Eastern Europe (Rehm et al., 2007, 2009). Eastern European countries have experienced substantial economic, social, and policy transitions during the last decades, which may have caused increased excessive alcohol consumption (Stickley et al., 2007) and mortality levels during the 1990s (Stuckler, King, and McKee, 2009). It is interesting to note that despite having much higher levels of stability and economic prosperity, women and less educated men in the United States had mortality rates comparable to their counterparts in several Eastern European countries. This suggests that improving overall economic prosperity may not be sufficient to achieve population health gains in all segments of the population.

An important finding of our study is that despite somewhat steeper gradients in the United States than in several Western European countries, the proportion of U.S. mortality attributable to exposure to low education (PAF) was comparable to that in Denmark and Sweden. This is due to the fact that the proportion of Americans with low education was much lower than in Europe, which reflects a century of aggressive U.S. government investment in education. If effects of education on mortality are causal (Lleras-Muney, 2005), we could argue that this reflects important health returns of education investment in the United States. Had a higher proportion of Americans been in the lowest education categories, mortality attributable to education would have been even larger.

The mechanisms discussed above as possible explanations of the education gradient in mortality rely on the assumption that associations observed are primarily the result of causality running from education to mortality. However, associations may also result from selection: healthier individuals (or individuals with characteristics associated with better health) are more likely to be selected into the highest education groups, while unhealthy individuals (or those with characteristics associated with poor health) are more likely to be selected into the lower education groups, generating a correlation between education and health. The role of selection in generating associations between education and health is likely to differ across countries, which may partly explain the differential effects of education on mortality.

For example, the United States and Switzerland have achieved very high overall levels of schooling in the population, so that only a relatively small proportion of individuals are being "left behind" in the lowest education categories. These individuals probably represent a selection of the weakest, resulting in a marked health disadvantage associated with low education. In contrast, selection may be less dramatic in some countries, such as Belgium, where overall educational achievements have been more modest than in the United States, so that more than half of the population is classified in the lowest education categories. In this case, selection effects would be weaker, resulting in a weaker association between education and health. Thus, differences in the effect of education in mortality observed in our study may reflect the differential role of selection mechanisms, even if education has the same causal effect on mortality in all countries. Distinguishing causation from selection mechanisms is crucial to understand our findings and should be the focus of future studies.

Implications

This chapter is a first attempt to understand U.S. excess mortality by taking into account different social groupings within countries, but further confirmation of our findings is required. If confirmed in future studies, our findings imply that efforts and policies to improve the health of socially disadvantaged populations—particularly those with low education—might moderately contribute to reduce U.S. excess mortality. However, our results also show that the U.S. health disadvantage is pervasive across all education levels, particularly among women. Therefore, policies that address the broader causes of high mortality among all Americans are essential to address the U.S. health disadvantage. Future studies should focus on studying the causes of these mortality differentials.

ACKNOWLEDGMENTS

The work on this chapter by Mauricio Avendano was supported by a grant from the Netherlands Organisation for Scientific Research (NWO, grant no. 451-07-001), a fellowship from the Erasmus University, and a David E. Bell fellowship from the Harvard Center for Population and Development Studies. The European data were collected in the Eurothine study, funded by the Public Health Program of the European Commission (grant no. 2003125).

Members of the Eurothine consortium contributed to this chapter; their comments on a previous version of this paper are gratefully acknowledged: P. Martikainen, Department of Sociology, University of Helsinki; O. Lundberg, Center for Health Equity Studies Stockholm, Stockholm University; B.H. Strand, Division of Epidemiology, Norwegian Institute of Public Health, Oslo; O. Andersen, National Institute of Public Health, Copenhagen; M. Glickman, Office of National Statistics, Newport, United Kingdom; P. Deboosere, Center of Sociology, Vrije Universiteit Brussel, Brussels; G. Desplanques, Institut National de la Statistique et des Études Économiques, Paris; B. Artnik, Department of Public Health, Faculty of Medicine, Ljubljana, Slovenia; K. Kovacs, Demographic Research Institute, Hungarian Central Statistical Office, Budapest; J. Rychtarikova, Department of Demography and Geography, Faculty of Science, Charles University, Prague; B. Wojtyniak, Department of Medical Statistics, National Institute of Hygiene, Warsaw; R. Kalediene, Kaunas University of Medicine, Kaunas, Lithuania; Department of Epidemiology and Biostatistics, National Institute for Health Development, Tallinn, Estonia.

REFERENCES

Adams, P.F., Dey, A.N., and Vickerie, J.L. (2007). Summary health statistics for the U.S. population: National Health Interview Survey, 2005. *Vital Health Statistics, 10*(233), 1-104.

Anderson, G., and Hussey, P.S. (2001). Comparing health system performance in OECD countries. *Health Affairs (Millwood), 20*(3), 219-232.

Avendano, M., Glymour, M.M., Banks, J., and Mackenbach, J.P. (2009). Health disadvantage in U.S. adults aged 50 to 74 years: A comparison of the health of rich and poor Americans with that of Europeans. *American Journal of Public Health, 99*(3), 540-548.

Banks, J., Marmot, M., Oldfield, Z., and Smith, J.P. (2006). Disease and disadvantage in the United States and in England. *Journal of the American Medical Association, 295*(17), 2037-2045.

Borsch-Supan, A., Brugiavini, A., Jürges, H., Mackenbach, J., Siegrist, J., and Weber, G. (2005). *Health, Ageing and Retirement in Europe.* Morlenbach, Germany: Strauss GmbH.

Cavelaars, A.E., Kunst, A.E., Geurts, J.J., Crialesi, R., Grotvedt, L., Helmert, U., et al. (2000). Educational differences in smoking: International comparison. *British Medical Journal, 320*(7242), 1102-1107.

Dahl, E., Fritzell, J., Lahelma, E., Martikainen, P., Kunst, A., and Mackenbach, J.P. (2006). Welfare state regimes and health inequalities. In J. Siegrist and M. Marmot (Eds.), *Social Inequalities in Health: New Evidence and Policy Implications.* London, England: Oxford University Press.

Decker, S.L., and Remler, D.K. (2004). How much might universal health insurance reduce socioeconomic disparities in health?: A comparison of the United States and Canada. *Applied Health Economics and Health Policy, 3*(4), 205-216.

Eurothine Group. (2007). *Tackling Health Inequalities in Europe: An Integrated Approach Eurothine.* Rotterdam, The Netherlands: Erasmus MC.

Heeringa, S., and Connor, J. (1995). *Technical Description of the Health and Retirement Study Sample Design.* Ann Arbor: Survey Research Center, University of Michigan.

Huisman, M., Kunst, A.E., and Mackenbach, J.P. (2003). Socioeconomic inequalities in morbidity among the elderly: A European overview. *Social Science & Medicine, 57*(5), 861-873.

Ingram, D., Lochner, K., and Cox, C. (2008). Mortality experience of the 1986-2000 National Health Interview Survey linked mortality files participants. National Center for Health Statistics. *Vital Health Statistics,* 2(147).

Jaumotte, F. (2003/2). Labour force participation of women: Empirical evidence on the role of policy and other determinants in OECD countries. *OECD Economic Studies, 37,* 51-107.

Kunst, A.E., and Mackenbach, J.P. (1994). The size of mortality differences associated with educational level in nine industrialized countries. *American Journal of Public Health, 84*(6), 932-937.

Lleras-Muney, A. (2005). The relationship between education and adult mortality in the United States. *Review of Economic Studies, 72*(1), 189-221.

Lopez, A.D., Collishaw, N., and Piha, T. (1994). A descriptive model of the cigarette epidemic in developed countries. *Tobacco Control,* 3, 242-247.

Mackenbach, J.P., and Kunst, A.E. (1997). Measuring the magnitude of socio-economic inequalities in health: An overview of available measures illustrated with two examples from Europe. *Social Science & Medicine, 44*(6), 757-771.

Mackenbach, J.P., Kunst, A.E., Groenhof, F., Borgan, J.K., Costa, G., Faggiano, F., et al. (1999). Socioeconomic inequalities in mortality among women and among men: An international study. *American Journal of Public Health, 89*(12), 1800-1806.

Mackenbach, J.P., Stirbu, I., Roskam, A.J., Schaap, M.M., Menvielle, G., Leinsalu, M., et al. (2008). Socioeconomic inequalities in health in 22 European countries. *New England Journal of Medicine, 358*(23), 2468-2481.

Massey, J.T. (1996). *Analytic and Reporting Guidelines: The Third National Health and Nutrition Examination Survey, NHANES III (1988-1994).* National Center for Health Statistics. Hyattsville, MD: U.S. Department of Health and Human Services.

Massey, J.T., Moore, T.F., Parsons, V.L., and Tadros, W. (1989). National Health Interview Survey, 1985-1994: Design and estimation. National Center for Health Statistics. *Vital Health Statistics,* 9(110).

Organisation for Economic Co-operation and Development. (2006). *Health Data 2006.* Paris: Author.

Organisation for Economic Co-operation and Development. (2008). *Growing Unequal? Income Distribution and Poverty in OECD Countries.* Paris: Author.

Rehm, J., Mathers, C., Popova, S., Thavorncharoensap, M., Teerawattananon, Y., and Patra, J. (2009). Global burden of disease and injury and economic cost attributable to alcohol use and alcohol-use disorders. *Lancet, 373*(9682), 2223-2233.

Rehm, J., Sulkowska, U., Manczuk, M., Boffetta, P., Powles, J., Popova, S., et al. (2007). Alcohol accounts for a high proportion of premature mortality in Central and Eastern Europe. *International Journal of Epidemiology, 36*(2), 458-467.

Ross, C.E., and Mirowsky, J. (2000). Does medical insurance contribute to socioeconomic differentials in health? *Milbank Quarterly, 78*(2), 291-321.

Silventoinen, K., Sans, S., Tolonen, H., Monterde, D., Kuulasmaa, K., Kesteloot, H., et al. (2004). Trends in obesity and energy supply in the WHO MONICA Project. *International Journal of Obesity and Related Metabolic Disorders, 28*(5), 710-718.

Smith, J.P. (2007). The impact of socioeconomic status on health over the life-course. *Journal of Human Resources, 42*(4), 739-764.

Stickley, A., Leinsalu, M., Andreev, E., Razvodovsky, Y., Vagero, D., and McKee, M. (2007). Alcohol poisoning in Russia and the countries in the European part of the former Soviet Union, 1970-2002. *European Journal of Public Health, 17*(5), 444-449.

Stuckler, D., King, L., and McKee, M. (2009). Mass privatisation and the post-Communist mortality crisis: A cross-national analysis. *Lancet, 373*(9661), 399-407.

Wolff, E.N. (1996). International comparisons of wealth inequalities. *Review of Income and Wealth, 42*(4), 433-451.

World Health Organization. (2009). *WHO Statistical Information System*. Geneva, Switzerland: Author. Available: http://apps.who.int/whosis/data/ [accessed August 2009].

World Health Organization Regional Office for Europe. (2010). *European Health for All Database (HFA-DB)*. Geneva, Switzerland: Author. Available: http://data.euro.who.int/hfadb/ [accessed February 2010].

Zhu, B.P., Giovino, G.A., Mowery, P.D., and Eriksen, M.P. (1996). The relationship between cigarette smoking and education revisited: Implications for categorizing persons' educational status. *American Journal of Public Health*, 86(11), 1582-1589.

12

Geographic Differences in Life Expectancy at Age 50 in the United States Compared with Other High-Income Countries

John R. Wilmoth, Carl Boe, and Magali Barbieri

INTRODUCTION

Just as mortality differs across countries, it also differs geographically within countries. In the United States, for example, the range of life expectancy at birth (e_0) for the years 1999-2001 extended from 72.3 for the District of Columbia (lowest) and 73.6 for Mississippi (second lowest) to 79.0 for Minnesota (second highest) and 79.7 for Hawaii (highest).[1] Life expectancy at age 50 (e_{50}) for the same years reflected a similar hierarchy: from 28.0 for both the District of Columbia and Mississippi to 31.4 for Minnesota and 32.4 for Hawaii. These ranges are smaller than those found across a broad group of high- and middle-income countries in 2000 (see Table 12-1). They are, however, larger once we exclude countries of Eastern Europe and the former Soviet Union from the comparison set.

The geographic variation of life expectancy at age 50 in the United States is illustrated here in Figure 12-1, which shows results separated by sex (men and women) and by administrative unit (states and counties). The broad pattern of geographic variation is similar across the four panels of Figure 12-1: relatively low values of e_{50} in the District of Columbia and across a large area of the Southeast, extending northward into Appalachia and to a lesser extent into parts of the Great Lakes region; and relatively high values of e_{50} across the far north central region of the country, extending into the mountain states as well.

Despite an increasing trend in life expectancy during the latter half

---

[1] Estimates of life expectancy in 1999-2001 for states of the United States were computed by the authors using vital registration and census data (see Annex A regarding data sources).

TABLE 12-1 Life Expectancy at Birth and at Age 50 in States of the United States and Two Sets of Comparison Countries (in 2000)

Areas	Life Expectancy at Birth (in years)			Life Expectancy at Age 50 (in years)		
	Min	Max	Range	Min	Max	Range
States of the United States	72.3	79.7	7.4	28.0	32.4	4.4
All comparison countries	65.4	81.4	16.0	23.0	33.2	10.2
Selected high-income countries	76.7	81.4	4.7	29.1	33.2	4.1

NOTES: The full set of comparison countries includes Australia, Austria, Belarus, Belgium, Bulgaria, Canada, Chile, the Czech Republic, Denmark, Estonia, Finland, France, Germany, Hungary, Iceland, Ireland, Israel, Italy, Japan, Latvia, Lithuania, Luxembourg, the Netherlands, New Zealand, Norway, Poland, Portugal, Russia, Slovakia, Slovenia, Spain, Sweden, Switzerland, Taiwan, Ukraine, the United Kingdom, and the United States.

The selected set of countries includes all of the above except Chile, Israel, and Taiwan plus countries of Eastern Europe and the former Soviet Union (Belarus, Bulgaria, the Czech Republic, Estonia, Hungary, Latvia, Lithuania, Poland, Russia, Slovakia, Slovenia, and Ukraine).
SOURCE: Data from the Human Mortality Database (see http://www.mortality.org [accessed July 26, 2009]).

of the 20th century at all ages and for all states (plus the District of Columbia), the rankings of the various states or regions in this geographic hierarchy have changed rather little over this time period (National Center for Health Statistics, 1975, 1998). Moreover, in a recent investigation at the county level, Ezzati and colleagues uncovered an even greater range of disparities in life expectancy at birth in the United States, of around 13 years for women and 18 years for men in 1999 (Ezzati et al., 2008). The authors point out that, whereas geographic variability diminished during the 1960s and 1970s, the distribution of e_0 by county in the United States started to diverge from the early 1980s onward. They demonstrated that this divergence—which was more pronounced for women than for men—was due to disparate trends affecting the more and the less advantaged areas of the country, as the former experienced a continuous rise in longevity while the latter experienced stagnation and, in the most extreme cases, a partial reversal of gains achieved in previous decades.

The divergence of the geographic distribution of mean longevity in the United States during the last two decades of the 20th century coincided with a rapid fall in the country's position in international rankings with respect to various measures of mortality or longevity. The deterioration of the U.S. position is well documented with regard to infant mortality (for a recent discussion on this topic, see in particular MacDorman and Mathews, 2008) but appears to be less well known regarding mortality at older ages.

In 1980, among the full set of comparison countries used here,[2] values of life expectancy at age 50 extended from 24.2 for Hungary and the Czech Republic to 29.6 for Iceland, and the United States ranked 10th out of 33 with an e_{50} of 28.0 (Human Mortality Database, see http://www.mortality.org [accessed November 13, 2009]).[3] By 2006, the level of e_{50} for the United States had risen to 31.3, a gain of 3.3 years. Over the same period, however, other countries experienced an even faster pace of improvement. Japan, with an e_{50} of 34.4 in 2006, had moved into the top position by gaining 5.5 years since 1980. As a result of its relatively poor performance during these years, the position of the United States fell to 20th among the 34 comparison countries with data available in 2006. In fact, only Taiwan, Denmark, and the 12 countries of Eastern Europe and the former Soviet Union fared worse than the United States at that time.

Figure 12-2 illustrates the change in international ranking for e_{50} among a more limited collection of comparison countries (excluding countries of Eastern Europe and the former Soviet Union, where mortality trends have been consistently less favorable than in the United States since 1980). The figure shows that, whereas until 1994 the United States was positioned among the upper 50 percent of the countries (not weighted by population size) with a rank that fluctuated between 9th and 12th, it lost position rapidly thereafter, falling to 13th in 1996, 14th in 1997, 18th in 1999, and 20th in 2005 and 2006 (just above Denmark in the list of 21 countries with data available for the most recent years).[4] Although the difference in e_{50} between the United States and the highest-ranking country was just 1.6 years in 1980, it grew to 2.2 years in 1995, 3.0 years in 2000, and 3.1 years in 2006.

Like the geographic divergence in the United States, the loss of position by the country in these rankings has been much more severe for women than for men. From 1980 to 2006, the ranking of U.S. women in terms of e_{50} fell from 11th to 20th (out of 21 countries) and for U.S. men from 10th to 15th.[5] Among all 21 countries on Figure 12-2, only Danish women had shorter lives, on average, after age 50 than U.S. women in 2006. Furthermore, the gap that separates the United States from other high-income countries is growing: whereas in 1980 women in the United States lived an average of

---

[2]The set includes Western Europe (see the notes to Table 12-1) and other high-income countries (Australia, Canada, Japan, New Zealand, and Taiwan), plus certain countries of Eastern Europe and the former Soviet Union (Belarus, Bulgaria, the Czech Republic, Estonia, East Germany, Hungary, Latvia, Lithuania, Poland, Russia, Slovakia, and Ukraine).
[3]The country with the highest life expectancy is ranked first.
[4]See the notes to Table 12-1 for a list of the countries included in the comparison.
[5]If we include Taiwan and countries of Eastern Europe and the former Soviet Union in this comparison, the ranking of U.S. women fell from 11th (out of 33) to 22nd (out of 34) and for U.S. men from 10th to 15th.

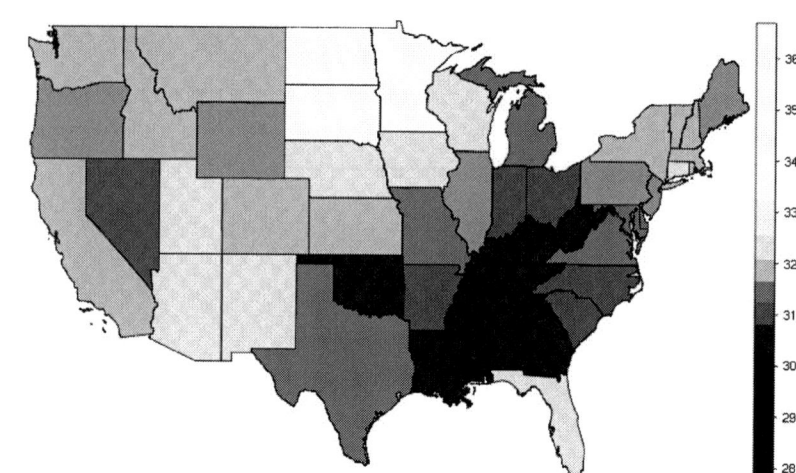

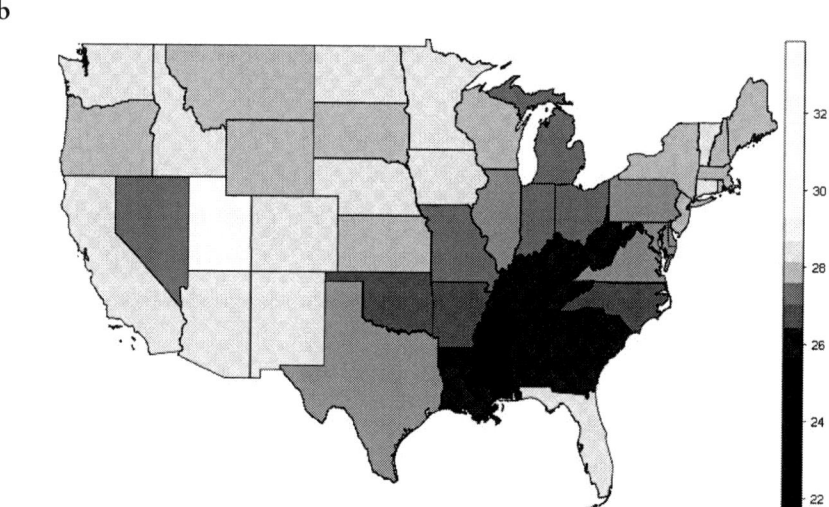

FIGURE 12-1 Geographic variation in life expectancy at age 50 in the contiguous United States, 2000.
(a) Female life expectancy at age 50 (e_{50}) by state
(b) Male life expectancy at age 50 (e_{50}) by state
(c) Female life expectancy at age 50 (e_{50}) by county
(d) Male life expectancy at age 50 (e_{50}) by county
NOTES: Both state and county data are centered on the year 2000. State data refer to years 1999-2001; county data, to years 1998-2002.

GEOGRAPHIC DIFFERENCES IN LIFE EXPECTANCY AT AGE 50   337

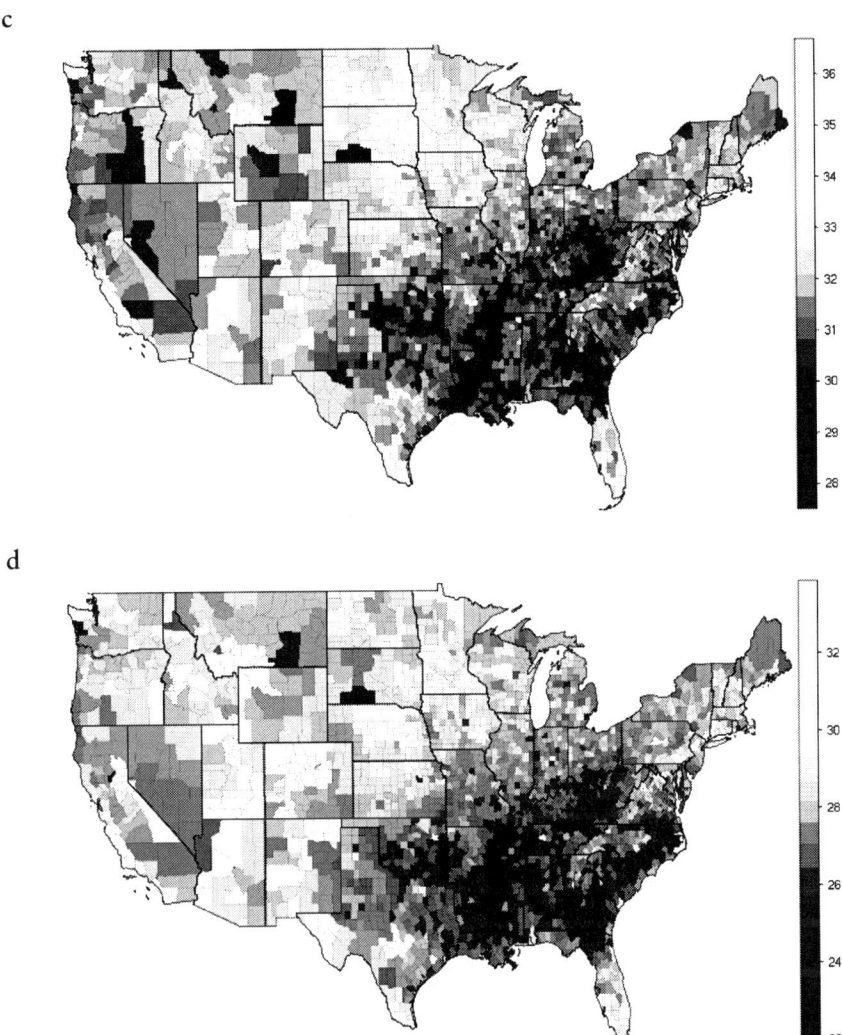

Many of the 3,141 counties in the United States are too small for reliable estimation of mortality. The 2,068 "counties" used here consist of 1,439 individual counties and 629 merged county units (thus, an average of 2.7 counties per merged unit).
SOURCES: For (a) and (b), authors' calculations based on data for 1999, 2000, and 2001 from the National Center for Health Statistics and the U.S. Census Bureau (from data files provided by Andrew Fenelon); for (c) and (d), Ezzati et al. (2008) (from updated data files provided by Sandeep Kulkarni).

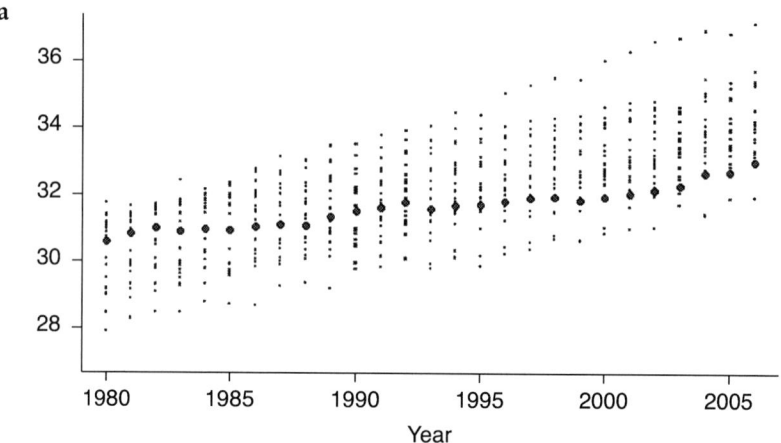

FIGURE 12-2 U.S. rankings for life expectancy at age 50 (e_{50}) among selected high-income countries, 1980-2006.
(a) Women
(b) Men
NOTES: The full set of comparison countries includes Australia, Austria, Belarus, Belgium, Bulgaria, Canada, Chile, the Czech Republic, Denmark, Estonia, Finland, France, Germany, Hungary, Iceland, Ireland, Israel, Italy, Japan, Latvia, Lithuania, Luxembourg, the Netherlands, New Zealand, Norway, Poland, Portugal, Russia, Slovakia, Slovenia, Spain, Sweden, Switzerland, Taiwan, Ukraine, the United

just 1.1 years less on average than women in Iceland (who had the highest value of e_{50} at that time), in 2006 they lived 4.1 years less than women in Japan. Men in the United States are doing better in international rankings and have also been more successful than women at progressively narrowing the gap that separates them from the top-ranking countries (Iceland in 1980, Australia in 2006) in terms of e_{50}, reducing this difference from 2.5 years in 1980 to 1.3 years in 2006.

Given the coincidence of timing (from the early 1980s until recently) and the shared characteristic of a greater impact on women, it is natural to inquire whether the increasing geographic disparity observed by Ezzati and colleagues is related in some causal fashion to the reduced pace of increase in values of life expectancy for the United States and thus to the country's loss of position in international rankings for this key indicator of population health. In the simple model of change proposed here (see the section on Methods), narrowing the gap between the most and the least advantaged

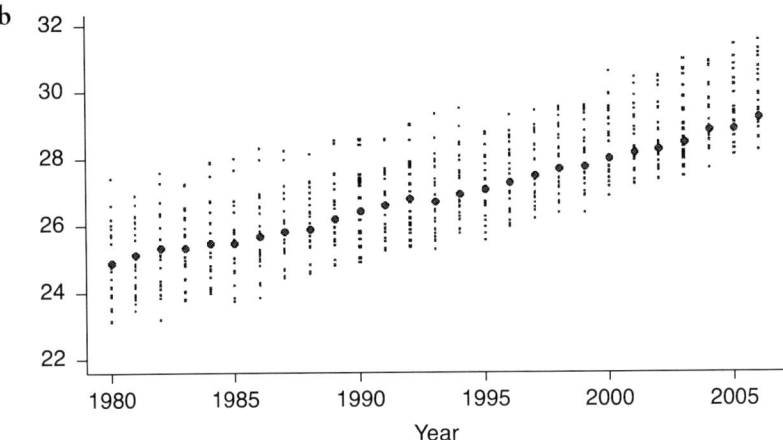

Kingdom, and the United States.

The selected set of countries includes all of the above except Chile, Israel, and Taiwan plus countries of Eastern Europe and the former Soviet Union (Belarus, Bulgaria, the Czech Republic, Estonia, Hungary, Latvia, Lithuania, Poland, Russia, Slovakia, Slovenia, and Ukraine).

Annual data were available from 1980 for all countries included here; data series end in 2006 for all countries except Austria (2005) and New Zealand (2003).
SOURCE: Data from the Human Mortality Database (see http://www.mortality.org [accessed July 2009]).

---

areas of a country tends to accelerate a rise in longevity, whereas widening this gap tends to slow down and may even halt or reverse an increasing trend.

In this chapter we compare levels and trends in the variability of life expectancy at age 50 in the United States and four other countries (Canada, France, Germany, and Japan) and across an aggregate of countries or subnational areas of Western Europe. Our main purpose is to determine whether the increasing disparity in values of life expectancy in the United States may have contributed in a mechanical or otherwise causal fashion to the country's deteriorating position in international comparisons.

THEORETICAL FRAMEWORK

Although social and economic inequality is often cited as an explanation for the poor ranking of the United States in international comparisons of mortality or longevity, the exact nature of the connection is by no means obvious. In some studies, mortality or longevity is viewed as a response variable that can be expressed as a function of a stimulus variable, such as income.[6] In this framework, an important question is whether variability in income (or some other stimulus) is negatively associated with levels of average longevity: in other words, can one attribute a lower level of life expectancy for some population to its higher level of income inequality? The correct answer is not necessarily "yes." In fact, if the functional relationship between stimulus and response is linear, a symmetrical increase of variability in the stimulus induces no change in the response, as gains in longevity for those at the top of the income distribution are balanced exactly by losses for those at the bottom (see Duleep, 1995; Rodgers, 1979).

In the specific case of income, however, the functional relationship with longevity is distinctly nonlinear: as demonstrated using both aggregate- and individual-level data, gains in longevity decelerate sharply as income rises (Preston, 2007; Preston and Taubman, 1994; Antonovsky, 1967). In general, if a positive relationship between stimulus and response becomes weaker at higher levels of the stimulus, a symmetrical increase of inequality in the stimulus leads necessarily to a decrease of the mean response: in our example, gains in longevity by those at the top of the distribution have less impact on the mean longevity of the population than losses by those at the bottom.[7]

The problem posed here, however, is somewhat different, as we are studying the relationship between trends in the mean and the variance of a single variable, with no model of stimulus and response. In this situation, quantifying the contribution of changes in variance to changes in mean requires choosing a reference group in the population, which could be the highest-ranking half, third, fifth, etc., in terms of the variable of interest (here, life expectancy at age 50). By thus identifying a "leading group" in the population, we develop in the next section a simple means of quantifying the contribution of changes in the geographic distribution of longevity in a population to changes in mean longevity.

In this way we are able to obtain some key insights about the role of changing geographic disparities in e_{50} to trends in e_{50} itself for the United States and other high-income countries. Using this framework, convergence of subnational levels of e_{50} helps to accelerate the national trend, as the less

---

[6]It is well known that the direction of this causal relationship is more complex than depicted here (e.g., Smith, 1999). Nevertheless, we limit our discussion to this simplistic example in order to focus attention on other topics.

[7]Substituting either "negative" for "positive" or "stronger" for "weaker" reverses the conclusion. Changing both at the same time leaves the conclusion unchanged.

advantaged locations catch up to the leaders;[8] conversely, divergence slows down the national increase, as the laggards fall farther and farther behind the more advantaged locations.

Although we are focusing here on the variation of mean longevity across geographically delimited population groups, it is also possible to analyze levels and trends of inequality among individual members of a population. Studies of the "compression of mortality" or "rectangularization of the survival curve" address the issue of internal variability for a given population as described by the distribution of deaths in a life table (Wilmoth and Horiuchi, 1999; Edwards and Tuljapurkar, 2005): we may call this *intra*population variability. In contrast, the approach we are following here consists of studying inequality across countries or their geographic subunits: *inter*population variability. Both of these notions of variability or inequality of longevity are valid, and a more comprehensive analysis of the effects of changes in inequality on changes in mean longevity would take both perspectives into account. In this chapter, however, we focus on aggregate geographic differences as a means of gaining some preliminary insights into this matter.

DATA

Mortality indicators for selected years from 1950 to 2006 were collected for the United States, Canada, Japan, and 19 national or large subnational areas of Western Europe, namely Austria, Belgium, Denmark, England and Wales, Finland, France, West Germany, Iceland, Republic of Ireland, Northern Ireland, Italy, Luxembourg, the Netherlands, Norway, Portugal, Scotland, Spain, Sweden, and Switzerland. These estimates were obtained from the Human Mortality Database (see http://www.mortality.org [accessed July 26, 2009]) and are based on information from vital registration, censuses, and when available, population registers. These data series begin in 1950 or earlier for all except two countries, West Germany (1956) and Luxembourg (1960).

We gathered regional data on mortality and longevity for five countries for which such information was readily available to us; in addition to the United States, this group includes Canada, France, Germany, and Japan. Whenever possible, we collected full life tables from the available published sources. However, in some cases we collected only values for the expectation of life, as this is the main indicator used for this analysis. Annex A contains a detailed accounting of the data sources used.

---

[8]Although in theory the deterioration of a country's international position could equally be achieved by a convergence resulting from the more advantaged locations regressing to the level of the less advantaged ones, this situation is not observed in the data presented here.

The size of basic geographic units varies enormously by country, as does presumably their heterogeneity, reflecting national traditions with regard to administrative divisions and political functions. Thus, we obtained data for states and counties of the United States, for prefectures of Japan, for departments of France, for provinces of Canada, and for federal states of Germany. The underlying idea was that counties of the United States could be compared with relatively smaller administrative units in other countries, whereas states of the United States could be compared with larger administrative units within countries and with countries of Western Europe.

At one level of aggregation, the United States is composed of 50 states plus the District of Columbia, with an average population (in 2000) of 5.5 million persons and an average surface area of 189 square kilometers. At another level the country can be divided into 3,141 counties; however, since many of these counties are too small for reliable mortality estimation, we have adopted the practice of Ezzati and colleagues by analyzing data for 2,068 individual counties or merged county aggregates, with an average population (in 2000) of 136,000 people and an average surface area of around 5 square kilometers.

For two of the comparison countries, the internal geographic divisions used here are relatively detailed and thus similar in some respects to U.S. counties. The 47 prefectures of Japan and the 96 departments of France are roughly similar in physical size although much more populous on average than U.S. counties (see Table 12-2). For the other two comparison countries, available data refer to much larger geographic subunits. In terms of average population, the 10 provinces of Canada and the 15 federal states of Germany resemble states of the United States (see Table 12-2).

In many cases the estimates of life expectancy used here refer to multiyear time periods rather than a single calendar year. To simplify the exposition, we often refer to multiyear estimates in terms of the middle year. For states of the United States, data refer to 3-year time periods around census years: 1939-1941, 1949-1951, ..., 1999-2001. Note that for 1939-1941 and 1949-1951, the life table values are available only for whites and for nonwhites separately and for men and women separately as well. The life tables for 1959-1961 include estimates for the total population with sexes combined, but not separately by sex. Using various assumptions (see Annex A), we have approximated some missing pieces of information for purposes of this analysis. For U.S. counties, data refer to 5-year intervals around single calendar years from 1961 to 2003. Thus, it should be understood that when we cite estimates of life expectancy for states or counties in, say, 1990, the data refer to 1989-1991 for states and 1988-1992 for counties. Some of the data for French departments also refer to multiyear time periods.

TABLE 12-2 Summary of Data on Geographic Variation in Mortality in Five Countries and Across Countries of Western Europe

Country	Geographic Division	Number of Subunits	Date Range of Data Used Here	In 2000: Population (Millions)	Surface Area, sq km (1,000s)	Average Population (1,000s)	Average Area, sq km (1,000s)
Canada	Provinces	10	1921-2005	31	9,971	3,100	997
France	Departments	91-96	1922-1999	59	552	614	6
Germany	States + Berlin	16-17	1990-2007	82	357	5,125	22
Japan	Prefectures	46-47	1965-2005	125	378	2,660	8
United States	States + DC	49-51	1940-2000	282	9,629	5,529	189
	counties	2068	1961-2003	282	9,629	136	5
Western Europe	Mostly countries	17-19	1950-2005	362	3,470	19,053	183

NOTES: Many of the 3,141 counties in the United States are too small for reliable estimation of mortality. The 2,068 "counties" used here consist of 1,439 individual counties and 629 merged county units (thus, an average of 2.7 counties per merged unit).

Western Europe is not a country but rather a statistical conglomeration that consists of the following countries and subnational areas: Austria, Belgium, Denmark, England and Wales, Finland, France, Iceland, Republic of Ireland, Northern Ireland, Italy, Luxembourg, the Netherlands, Norway, Portugal, Scotland, Spain, Sweden, Switzerland, and West Germany. All data are from the Human Mortality Database (see http://www.mortality.org [accessed July 26, 2009]). Data for 1950 are unavailable for West Germany and Luxembourg.

Some data used here refer to multiyear time periods. Such information is identified here by the middle year of the time period. For a more complete description of data and sources, see Annex A.

SOURCE: For population size, data from the Human Mortality Database (see http://www.mortality.org [accessed July 2009]); for surface area, data from the *Demographic Yearbook 2000* (see http://unstats.un.org [accessed July 2009]).

METHODS

The analysis of geographic variability presented here is based entirely on period values of life expectancy at age 50, e_{50}, measured at both national and subnational levels. Life expectancy at age 50 was chosen as the main indicator of mortality at older ages to comport with the other studies in this volume. Some of our methods of presenting and manipulating this measure of mean longevity are standard and require no explanation. For example, Figure 12-3 presents the level of female versus male e_{50} by state in 1950 and 2000 in the form of a simple scatter plot. Other methods are somewhat less traditional and require additional documentation.

The ellipses of Figure 12-4 were derived by the method of principal components. As explained in more detail in Annex B, the axes of each ellipse are aligned with the first and second principal components of the bivariate distribution of male and female e_{50} for a given population and time period. The size of the ellipse is the minimum required in order to include at least 90 percent of the data points. The method is similar though not identical to that used by Coale and colleagues in their historical analysis of the decline of fertility in Europe (Coale and Treadway, 1986).

As a global measure of the geographic variability of life expectancy in a population, we computed the standard deviation across N population subunits, taking into account their relative sizes. For each population and time period, the weighted standard deviation of e_{50} was computed as follows:

$$SD = \sqrt{\frac{\sum_{i=1}^{N} w_i (x_i - \bar{x})^2}{1 - \sum_{i=1}^{N} w_i^2}},$$

where $x_1, x_2, \ldots, x_N$ represent the values of e_{50} across N subunits, and $w_1, w_2, \ldots, w_N$ are weights proportional to population size (scaled so that $\sum_{i=1}^{N} w_i = 1$, and $\bar{x} = \sum_{i=1}^{N} w_i x_i$ is a weighted mean.[9] Trends in this measure of variability are presented in Figure 12-5.

Both the quintile trends of Figures 12-6 and 12-7 and the analysis of convergence effects in Table 12-3 and 12-4 require the computation of percentiles for empirical distributions of e_{50} across geographic space. The input for such calculations includes not only the value of e_{50} but also the associ-

---

[9]The denominator of the formula for the weighted standard deviation ensures an unbiased estimate under standard statistical assumptions. Note that if $w_i = \frac{1}{N}$ for all observations, this formula reduces to the usual one with $N - 1$ in the denominator.

ated population size for all geographic subunits. Using the same notation as above but specifying that the values of e_{50} for population subunits $(x_1, x_2, \ldots, x_N)$ are in increasing order, the value of the $100p$-th percentile of e_{50} equals x_k, where k is the smallest integer (between 1 and N) such that

$$\sum_{i=1}^{k} w_i \geq p.$$

In standard usage, the term "quintile" may refer either to the value of cut points located at the 20th, 40th, 60th, and 80th percentiles or to each of five equal-sized groups of ordered observations (where some observations are split in appropriate proportions across adjacent groups). For this analysis, a quintile has the latter meaning. A key set of results (see Figures 12-6 and 12-7) consists of trends in the average value of e_{50} within the five quintiles of a given population.[10]

The results presented in Tables 12-3 and 12-4 involve dividing the various populations into two equal-sized groups of ordered observations and, as before, computing the average value of e_{50} for each half in (or around) the years 1980 and 2000.[11] The focus of this analysis is the mean change in values of e_{50} between these 2 calendar years (in years per annum) for the population as a whole and for the two halves, as described in columns (a), (b), and (c) of Table 12-3. The mean change for the entire population is the average of mean changes for the two halves.[12]

We define a convergence effect to be the difference between the mean changes for the total population and for the upper half of the geographic distribution, as shown in column (d) of Table 12-3; this effect also equals one-half the difference between the mean changes for the lower and upper halves of the distribution. So defined, the convergence effect represents the increased rate of change for the total population that is attributable to faster change in the lower half of the geographic distribution compared with the upper half. If change is faster in the upper half, the value is negative and thus represents a divergence effect. Finally, column (e) of Table 12-3 gives the magnitude of the convergence effect as a fraction of the total change.

---

[10]Similar results could be obtained using tertiles, quartiles, deciles, etc. After some experimentation, we concluded that quintiles offer an adequate level of detail without making the graph so cluttered that it becomes difficult to read.

[11]Note that a given subpopulation may be included in different halves of the geographic distribution in 1980 and 2000.

[12]One complication encountered here arises from the fact that e_{50} for the total population does not equal the weighted average of e_{50} for geographic subunits. Since it is typically quite small, we ignore this difference in practice and express our results in terms of the weighted average of e_{50} for the population subunits.

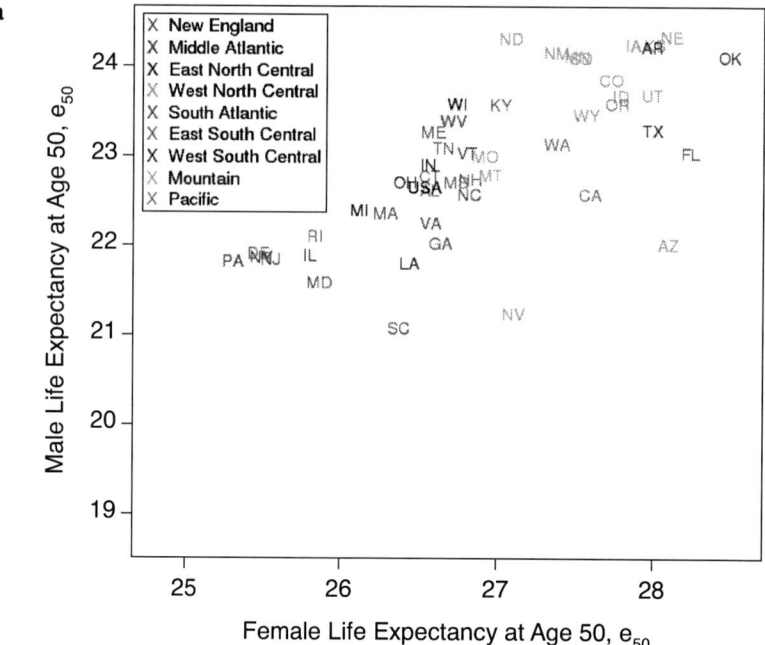

FIGURE 12-3 Levels of life expectancy at age 50 (e_{50}) by sex and state, United States 1950 and 2000.
(a) 1950
(b) 2000

The values of Table 12-4, which are derived directly from those of Table 12-3, indicate how the differential pace of increase in e_{50} from 1980 to 2000 (for the United States compared with the other populations in the study) can be apportioned to each of three components. A slower pace of improvement for the United States can result from (1) a difference in the trends of e_{50} for the upper 50 percent of the geographic distribution in the United States versus the upper 50 percent of the geographic distribution for the comparison population, (2) a divergence between the lower and the upper 50 percent of the geographic distribution for the United States,

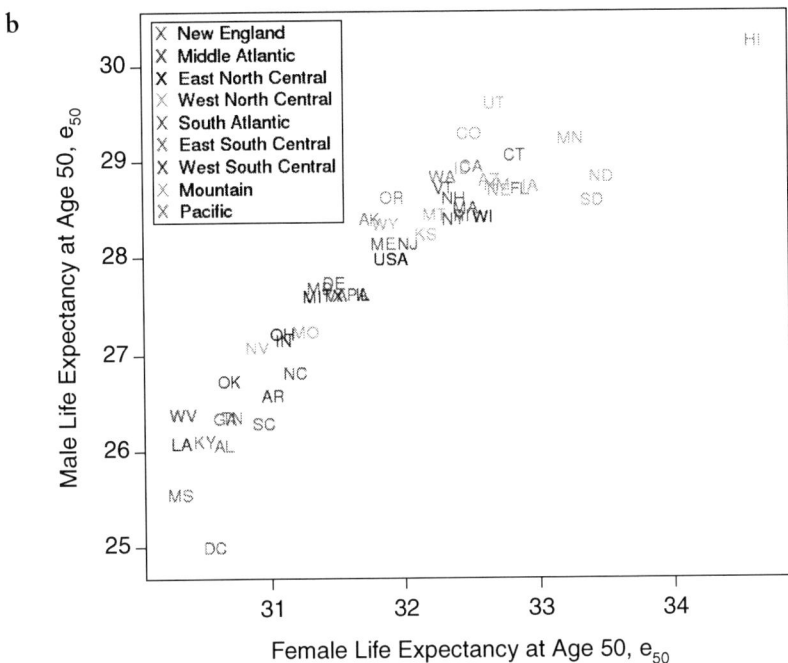

SOURCES: Data for 1950, from National Office of Vital Statistics, *State and Regional Life Tables: 1949-51*; for 2000, authors' calculations based on data for 1999, 2000, and 2001, from the National Center for Health Statistics and the U.S. Census Bureau (from data files provided by Andrew Fenelon).

and (3) a convergence between the lower and the upper 50 percent of the geographic distribution in the comparison area. The first component can be interpreted as the portion of the differential increase that is attributable to factors affecting all states (or counties) of the United States in a similar fashion, whereas the second and third components measure the portions attributable to increasing geographic variability in the United States or declining variability in the comparison population. The sum of the second and third components represents the portion of the differential increase due to different trends in geographic variability.

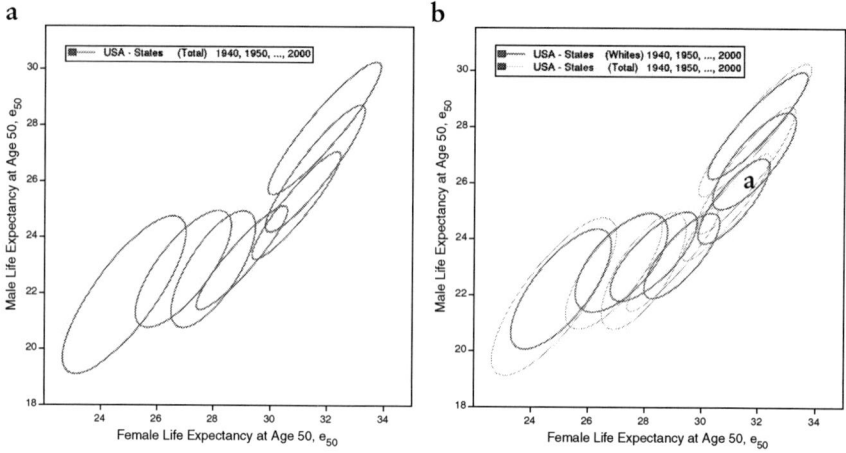

FIGURE 12-4 Changes in life expectancy at age 50 (e_{50}) by sex, race, and state, United States 1940-2000.
(a) Total, by state
(b) Total and whites, by state
(c) Blacks and whites, by state
(d) Total, by state and county
NOTES: For each ellipse, the axes are aligned with the first and second principal components of the relationship between male and female life expectancy for a given population and year; the size is the minimum required in order to include at least 90 percent of the data points. See Annex B for technical details.

RESULTS

In this section we first describe trends in U.S. life expectancy at age 50 by sex and race as well as changes in the degree of geographic variation, at both state and county levels. We then describe changes in regional disparities among the other high-income countries in the study before presenting the results of our analysis relating changes in regional variability within countries to changes in variability between countries.

Geographic Disparities in the United States

The geographic variability of mortality levels at older ages in the United States has been and continues to be quite large. In 1950, the difference in e_{50} between the best- and the worst-ranking state was 4.5 years. By 2000, this value had declined only slightly, to 4.4 years.

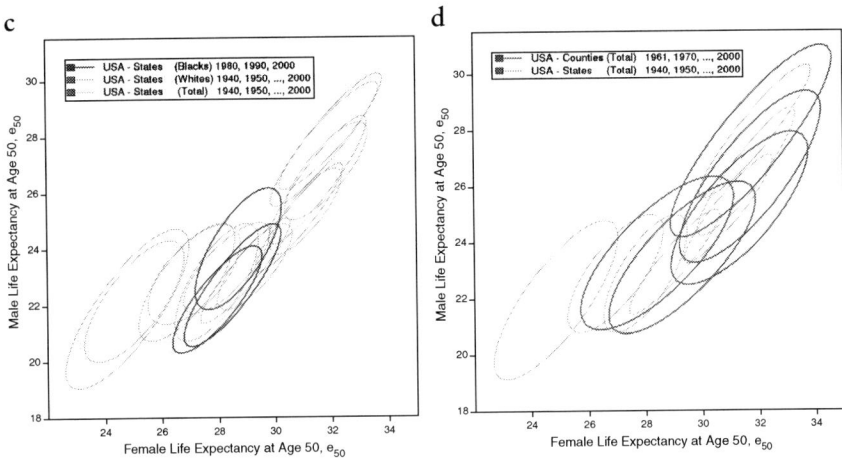

The series of ellipses based on state data for the total or white population refer to 3-year periods centered on 1940, 1950, ..., 2000. The series based on state data for the black population refers to 3-year periods centered on 1980, ..., 2000. The series based on county data refers to 5-year periods centered on 1961, 1970, ..., 2000.
SOURCES: Authors' analysis of data from various sources: for states from 1940 to 1990, National Center for Health Statistics and predecessors, state life table publications; for states in 2000, authors' calculations based on data for 1999, 2000, and 2001, from the National Center for Health Statistics and the U.S. Census Bureau (from data files provided by Andrew Fenelon); for counties, Ezzati et al. (2008) (from updated data files provided by Sandeep Kulkarni).

These results for the total population mask the different experiences of men and women. Geographic disparities in mortality at older ages have been and continue to be larger for men than for women (with ranges of e_{50} equaling 5.5 versus 3.6 years in 1950 and 5.3 versus 4.3 years in 2000), even though women have a considerably longer length of life after age 50 than men. However, whereas the range of geographic variability for men has narrowed slightly, it has increased considerably for women, to the point that women in the worst-off counties of the United States now live fewer years, on average, after age 50 than men in the best-off counties. It is thus possible that the future range of geographic variability of life expectancy in the United States may become more similar for the two sexes.

For both men and women, the geographic pattern of disparity in e_{50} across states of the United States has remained relatively stable since 1950 (see Figure 12-3). In 1950 as in 2000, several states in the southeastern

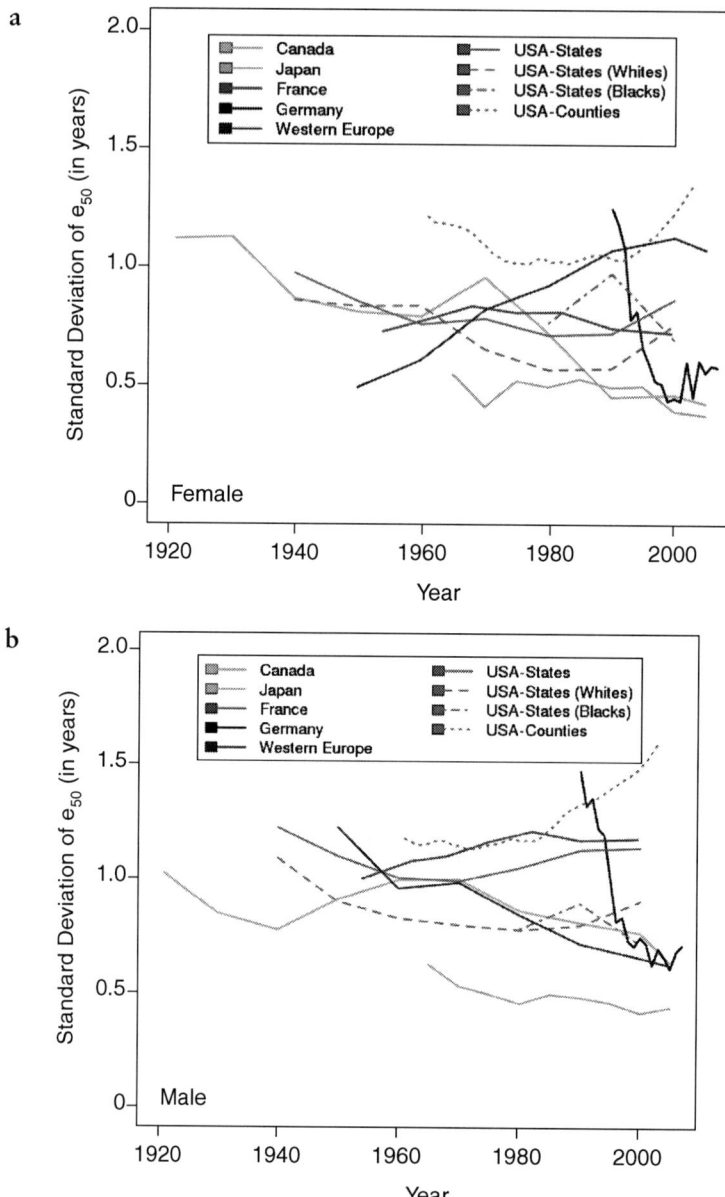

FIGURE 12-5 Trends in the standard deviation of e_{50} across geographic subunits, five countries plus Western Europe, 1921-2007.
(a) Female
(b) Male
SOURCE: Author's calculations using data from various sources (see Annex A).

TABLE 12-3 Annual Rates of Change in Life Expectancy at Age 50 (e_{50}), Plus Convergence Effects Due to Faster Change in Lower 50 Percent of Geographic Distribution, for Five Countries Plus Western Europe as a Whole, 1980-2000

	Average Annual Increase in e_{50} (in years/annum)			Convergence Effect	
	For Total Population	For Upper 50%	For Lower 50%	Value	As a Fraction of Total Change
	(a) = [(b) + (c)] / 2	(b)	(c)	(d) = (a) − (b) = [(c) − (b)] / 2	(e) = (d) / (a)
Women:					
Canada	0.107	0.098	0.117	0.009	0.084
France	0.168	0.165	0.170	0.003	0.018
Germany	0.215	0.179	0.251	0.036	0.167
Japan	0.247	0.244	0.250	0.003	0.012
United States					
—by state	0.057	0.064	0.050	−0.007	−0.123
—by county	0.053	0.061	0.044	−0.009	−0.151
Western Europe	0.158	0.168	0.149	−0.010	−0.063
Men:					
Canada	0.176	0.172	0.180	0.004	0.023
France	0.187	0.182	0.191	0.005	0.027
Germany	0.242	0.214	0.270	0.028	0.116
Japan	0.157	0.153	0.162	0.005	0.025
United States					
—by state	0.145	0.154	0.136	−0.009	−0.062
—by county	0.150	0.163	0.137	−0.013	−0.087
Western Europe	0.180	0.176	0.184	0.004	0.022

NOTES: Data for most countries or populations were available for periods centered on 1980 and 2000. The exceptions are France (from 1982 to 1999) and Germany (from 1990 to 2000).

The annual rate of change in e_{50} for the total population equals the average of the annual rates of change for the upper and lower 50 percent of each geographic distribution.

The convergence effect represents the increased rate of change for the total population that is attributable to a more rapid increase in the lower 50 percent of the geographic distribution compared with the upper 50 percent. If the pace of change is faster in the upper 50 percent, the value is negative and thus represents a divergence effect.

SOURCE: Authors' calculations based on data from various sources (see Annex A).

quadrant of the country (including the District of Columbia), plus Nevada, have experienced relatively low values of life expectancy at age 50, whereas many states of the north central and mountain regions, plus Hawaii in 2000, have had greater longevity at older ages. Some state rankings appear implausible and may reflect flaws in the data, especially for earlier years.

TABLE 12-4 Differences in Rate of Increase of Life Expectancy at Age 50 (e_{50}) Between the United States and Four Countries Plus Western Europe as a Whole, and Portions of Each Difference Due to Three Components, 1980-2000

Population	Difference in Average Annual Change of e_{50} from 1980 to 2000			
		Portion of Difference (in %) due to:		
	Total Difference (in years/annum)	Difference of Trends for Upper 50% (of geographic distributions)	Divergence in the U.S. (between lower and upper 50%)	Convergence in Comparison Area (between lower and upper 50%)
Women				
Canada	0.052	66.7	15.2	18.1
France	0.113	90.7	7.1	2.3
Germany	0.160	72.4	5.0	22.6
Japan	0.192	94.2	4.2	1.6
Western Europe	0.104	101.6	7.7	−9.3
Men				
Canada	0.029	47.8	37.7	14.5
France	0.039	60.6	27.6	11.8
Germany	0.094	58.7	11.5	29.8
Japan	0.009	−62.0	114.4	47.5
Western Europe	0.033	55.0	33.0	12.1

NOTES: Using the column notation of Table 12-2, the partitioning of differential rates of change shown here can be expressed as follows: Comparison(a) − U.S.(a) = [Comparison(b) − U.S.(b)] − U.S.(d) + Comparison(d). Values of (a), (b), and (d) for the United States used in this calculation were the mean of state and county values, which differ slightly.

Data for most countries or populations were available for periods centered on 1980 and 2000. The exceptions are France (from 1982 to 1999) and Germany (from 1990 to 2000).
SOURCE: Authors' calculations based on data from Table 12-3.

In particular, the favorable positions of Arkansas, Oklahoma, and Texas in 1950 seem inconsistent with the socioeconomic position of that region and are strongly contradicted by data from later years. Together with Nevada, these three states were the last to be admitted by the U.S. Census Bureau, then in charge of the vital statistics system, to the death registration area of the United States due to coverage issues (Hetzel, 1997). Admission was granted only when at least 90 percent of deaths were registered. Arkansas was admitted in 1927, Oklahoma in 1928, and Texas in 1933. It is possible that a significant proportion of unregistered deaths remained in the early 1950s, inducing artificially high levels of expectation of life at birth and at older ages in these states. The only major change of state rankings in e_{50} that seems plausible (i.e., not spurious due to changes in data quality) is the rising position of New Jersey, New York, and Pennsylvania over the latter half of the 20th century. Our results at the state level are consistent with those at the county level of Ezzati and colleagues (2008), who also showed a pattern of regional stability over a somewhat shorter time interval.

Using ellipses to summarize scatter plots (see Methods section), Figure 12-4 illustrates the simultaneous rise of female and male e_{50} from 1940 to 2000 across states and counties of the United States. On average across all population subgroups, people who survived to age 50 were expected to live over 8 years longer in 2000 than in 1940, corresponding to an increase in e_{50} from 23 years in 1940 to 31.3 years in 2006, or an average rise of 1.3 years per decade. This increase was particularly rapid between 1940 and 1950 (+1.7 years) and between 1970 and 1980 (+1.8 years) and relatively slow between 1950 and 1970 (less than 1 year for each of the two decades, 1950-1960 and 1960-1970).

However, the pace as well as the timing of improvement varied by subgroup of the population. For example, when comparing men with women, it is apparent not only that women already lived longer than men after age 50 in 1940 (24.3 versus 21.6 years), but also that they have experienced a faster pace of improvement, with a gain of 8.6 versus 7.7 years between 1940 and 2006. Whereas for women most of the increase (70 percent) took place before 1980, for men most of it (60 percent) occurred between 1980 and 2006. Consequently, the sex gap in e_{50} was largest in the second half of the 1970s, when it exceeded 5.8 years compared with 2.8 years in 1940 and 3.8 years in 2006. This differential trend is well illustrated by Figure 12-4a, which shows an initial movement of the ellipses away from a diagonal line toward the right, followed by a later movement back toward the diagonal line. Variations by race are illustrated in Figures 12-4b and 12-4c; however, the information is limited by the fact that e_{50} is available for blacks only since 1980 and that similar information for other racial or ethnic groups is not currently available.

Figure 12-4d illustrates the changing values of female and male e_{50} by state and by county from 1940 until 2000. Since counties are both more homogeneous and far more numerous than states, it is not surprising that regional variations are larger at the county than at the state level, as illustrated here by the larger area covered by the series of ellipses representing the counties than by those representing the states (see also Figure 12-1).

Comparison with Other High-Income Countries

Figure 12-5 shows trends in the (weighted) standard deviation of e_{50} across geographic subunits in five countries, as well as among the countries of Western Europe, from 1921 to 2007. For the countries with available data, it appears that the level of regional variability in e_{50} fell somewhat dur-

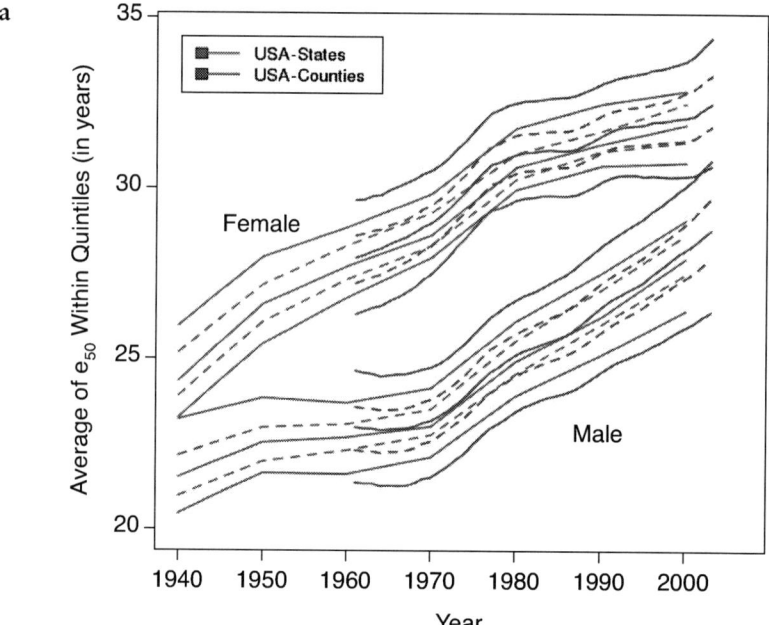

FIGURE 12-6 Trends in the average value of e_{50} within quintiles of state or county distributions, United States (total, white, and black populations), 1940-2003.
(a) Total, by state and county
(b) Blacks and whites, by state
SOURCES: Authors' analysis of data from various sources: for states from 1940 to

ing the first half of the 20th century but then tended to stabilize or increase slightly after 1950. An exception is Germany, which experienced a sharp drop in the regional variability of e_{50} following reunification in 1990.

The figure also shows substantial differences in levels of geographic variability in e_{50} by population and by sex. For women (Figure 12-5a), Canada is the only population for which regional disparities have mostly declined over time, at least from 1921 to 1990, with only a short increase in the 1960s. By contrast, France and Japan exhibited a relatively stable level of internal disparity throughout the observation period (1954-1999 and 1965-2005, respectively), as did Germany beginning about 10 years after reunification. Western Europe as a whole shows a continuous and steep increase in regional variability attributable to the differential pace of growth in female life expectancy among the various countries. Women in the United States experienced a small but continuous decline in regional dis-

GEOGRAPHIC DIFFERENCES IN LIFE EXPECTANCY AT AGE 50   355

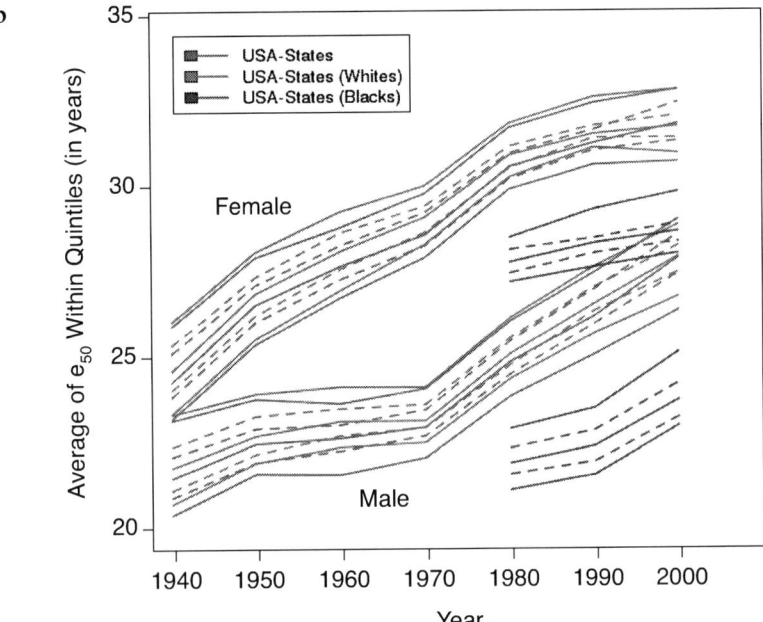

1990, National Center for Health Statistics and predecessors, state life table publications; for states in 2000, authors' calculations based on data for 1999, 2000, and 2001, from the National Center for Health Statistics and the U.S. Census Bureau (from data files provided by Andrew Fenelon); for counties, Ezzati et al. (2008) (from updated data files provided by Sandeep Kulkarni).

parities (whether looking at states or counties) up to 1980 but a significant increase afterward, especially between 1990 and 2000.

For men (Figure 12-5b), the picture is quite different: variability declined everywhere between 1960 and 1980 and either continued its decline (in Canada, Western Europe as a whole, and Germany in particular) or remained stable (in Japan) between 1980 and 2000, except for France and the United States, where variability has increased since the 1950s and 1970s, respectively. For both men and women, Figure 12-5 suggests that trends in geographic variability may have been somewhat different by race during the last two decades of the 20th century. However, the meaning of such differences should not be exaggerated, as they could result at least partly from changes in racial classification over time.

Overall, geographic variability was greater in the United States than in other high-income countries during 1980-2000 but similar to levels of vari-

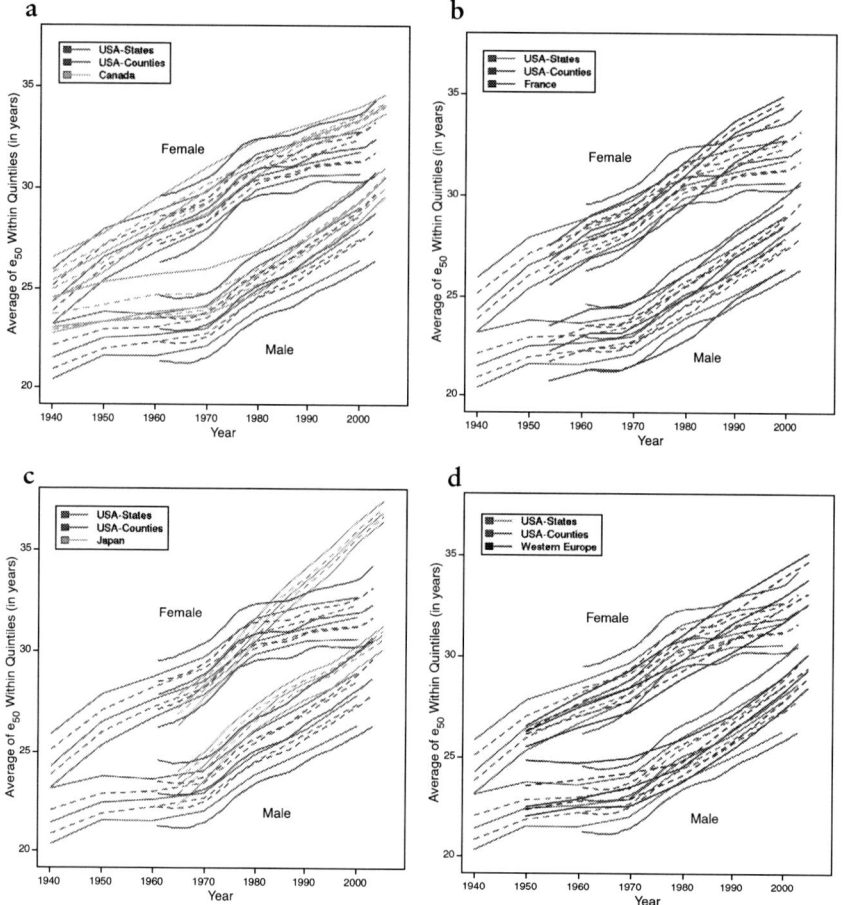

FIGURE 12-7 Trends in the average value of e_{50} within quintiles of geographic distributions, United States compared with Canada, France, Japan, and Western Europe, 1940-2005.
(a) United States and Canada
(b) United States and France
(c) United States and Japan
(d) United States and Western Europe
SOURCES: Authors' analysis of data from various sources: for Canada, Canadian Human Mortality Database (see http://www.bdlc.umontreal.ca/CHMD [accessed March 2009]); for France, Daguet, 2006 (from data files provided by France Meslé and Jacques Vallin); for Japan, Ministry of Health, Labour, and Welfare, various years (from data files provided by Futoshi Ishii); for Western Europe, Human Mortality Database (see http://www.mortality.org [accessed July 2009]). See Annex A for further details.

ability across Western Europe as a whole, especially for women. Notably, the United States is the only population examined here for which geographic disparities increased over the last two decades of the 20th century for *both* men and women.

The Contribution of Increasing Geographic Variation to Deterioration of the U.S. Position in International Rankings

Table 12-3 presents the average change in e_{50} (in years per annum) for each population as a whole and for the upper and lower 50 percent of its geographic distribution between 1980 and 2000, as well as the value of the convergence effect (see the section on Methods), both in absolute level and as a fraction of the total change over this time period. The table shows that between 1980 and 2000 all areas in the study improved their level of e_{50} and that, except for Japan, men benefited more than women from the decline in mortality at older ages (Table 12-3, column (a)). Table 12-3 also shows that the United States exhibited the smallest progress in e_{50} compared with the other countries in the study. Although the intercountry gap was relatively small for men, it was quite sizeable for women, with average annual gains of less than 3 additional weeks of life in the United States compared with more than 1 month in Canada, nearly 2 months in Western Europe as a whole, 3 in Germany, and 4 in Japan. Male e_{50} increased by somewhat less than 2 months per calendar year in the United States, which is not far from the gains achieved in the other areas (with the exception of Germany, following reunification, which gained nearly 3 months per year on average during the 1990s).

More to the point, regional inequalities in longevity above age 50 increased in the United States for both men and women from 1980 to 2000 while declining everywhere else, except for women in Western Europe as a whole (Table 12-3, column (d)). Following the political reunification that occurred in 1990, Germany was especially successful in reducing regional disparities for both men and women; a more modest geographic convergence of e_{50} occurred in Canada, France, Germany, and Japan after 1980.

How much of the growing mortality disadvantage of the United States compared with other high-income countries can be explained by its growing geographic inequality? Figures 12-6 and 12-7 present our findings in a graphical way. Like Figure 12-5, Figure 12-6a shows that trends in regional variability in the United States are quite similar whether looking at states or at counties (even though the measured level of variability is, not surprisingly, greater when using smaller geographic units). Figure 12-6b shows that improvements in e_{50} for whites and blacks are similar though somewhat less favorable for white compared with black women.

The key point that emerges from a comparison of the data presented in Figures 12-6 and 12-7 is that the expectation of life at age 50 has exhibited relatively unfavorable trends even in the most advantaged areas of the United States (whether states or counties) since 1980. A faster pace of increase for the various comparison populations has yielded geographic distributions of e_{50} that barely overlap in some cases. For example, the lowest quintile of life expectancy at age 50 for women across Japanese prefectures has been above the highest quintile for U.S. states continuously since the mid-1980s (see Figure 12-7c). For U.S. counties, the cross-over occurred a few years later (around 1990). Comparisons of U.S. trends with those for Canada, France, and Western Europe as a whole (Figures 12-7a, 12-7b, and 12-7d) yield a smaller though still noticeable pattern of temporal divergence for women; similar though less extreme patterns are observed for men.

Although the results of the analysis presented in Tables 12-3 and 12-4 vary somewhat depending on the choice of comparison area, some general findings apply in all instances. In particular, it is clear that increasing regional variability in the United States, combined with decreasing variability in all comparison populations (except women in Western Europe), contributed to a growing U.S. disadvantage in life expectancy at age 50 from 1980 to 2000. However, the share attributable to different patterns of geographic convergence or divergence differs strongly by sex. For men, for whom the differential increase during this period was modest, up to 50 percent is attributable to different trends in geographic disparities. (Note that the breakdown of the difference between the United States and Japan in Table 12-4 is essentially meaningless in the case of men due to the very small differential trend.) Divergence in the United States is the main driving force rather than convergence in the comparison area, except in Germany. Over 30 percent of the difference in the average annual change of e_{50} between the United States and Western Europe on one hand, Canada on the other, is attributable to increasing regional variability in the former and only 12 and 14 percent, respectively, to declining regional variability in the latter.

For women, the portion of differential increase due to trends in geographic variability is around 30 percent when comparing the United States with Canada or Germany but less than 10 percent when comparing the United States with France, Japan, or Western Europe as a whole. The latter comparisons seem more pertinent, since the German example is atypical because of reunification while the Canadian data are severely limited by the small number and uneven size of the geographic subunits. Thus, we conclude that the role of changing geographic variability for explaining differential trends in e_{50} is nonnegligible for both sexes though rather small in the case of women, for whom the largest differential trends are observed.

DISCUSSION

To summarize our main results, every population in our study experienced gains in e_{50} from 1980 to 2000 at a pace of at least half a year per decade. In general, improvements in longevity during this period benefited men more than women, so that the gender gap has been progressively closing. The United States has made smaller progress than all the other populations with, for women, a gain of 1.1 years between 1980 and 2000 compared with 2.1 years in Canada, 3.2 in Western Europe, 3.4 in France, 4.3 in Germany, and 4.9 in Japan, and for men, a gain of 3.0 years compared with 3.5 years in Canada, 3.6 in Western Europe, 3.7 in France, 4.8 in Germany, and 3.1 in Japan. A substantial drop in the U.S. position in international rankings of e_{50} reflects this relatively slow improvement.

Our analysis has demonstrated that the slower progress achieved by the United States is partially due to its increasing regional variability compared with other high-income countries. Indeed, whereas internal disparities in the United States, whether measured at the state or at the county level, tended to decline up to the early 1980s, they have increased since then, in contrast to most other populations in the study (with the notable exception of women in Western Europe taken as a whole), which have experienced stability or an ongoing decline of geographic variability. For men, the difference of trends in regional disparities explains up to 50 percent of the relatively slower pace of increase in e_{50} for the United States compared with three of the four countries examined here (as noted earlier, this comparison is not meaningful in the case of Japan, since the pace of change in male e_{50} was nearly the same as in the United States over this time period). For women, however, rather little (under 10 percent in the most relevant cases) of the slow progress recorded by the United States in e_{50} compared with other countries can be attributed to differential trends in regional disparities. Indeed, the difference between the United States and the other countries in the number of years of life gained after age 50 over the last 20 years of the 20th century was not much different when comparing only the better-off 50 percent of each population than when comparing the worse-off 50 percent.

Thus, although the relatively less favorable trend in life expectancy at age 50 for the United States was due in part to increasing geographic disparities in the country during 1980-2000, combined with a general reduction of such disparities in the other countries examined, most of the slower pace of improvement must be attributed to policies, practices, and behaviors that are characteristic of the nation as a whole. This conclusion is consistent with the findings by Banks and colleagues (Banks et al., 2006), who showed that, even within similar income strata, the English are in much better health than their U.S. counterparts with regard to seven key health indicators (diabetes, hypertension, heart disease, myocardial infarctions, strokes, diseases of the lung, and cancer). These researchers also found that the gradient of mortality differentials by socioeconomic status (measured by years of education and household income) is substantial in both countries but steeper in the United States. They noted that neither individual behaviors, such as smoking, alcohol consumption or diet, nor access to medical care, measured by whether respondents had health insurance, explained much of the difference between the two countries.

In conclusion, we think that this analysis helps to rule out an increase in geographic disparities as a dominant explanation for the deteriorating position of the United States in international rankings of life expectancy, especially for women. Any proposed explanation of the divergence in levels and trends of life expectancy observed among high-income countries in recent decades needs to acknowledge that even the most advantaged areas of the United States (at the state or county level) have been falling behind in international comparisons.

ACKNOWLEDGMENTS

This project received financial support from the National Institute on Aging, grants no. R01-AG011552 and 2P30AG012839, and from the Institut National d'Études Démographiques, INED research project no. P05-3-7.

REFERENCES

Antonovsky, A. (1967). Social class, life expectancy, and overall mortality. *The Milbank Memorial Fund Quarterly, 45*(2 pt. 1), 31-73.

Banks, J., Marmot, M., Oldfield, Z., and Smith, J.P. (2006). Disease and disadvantage in the United States and in England. *Journal of the American Medical Association, 295*(17), 2037-2045.

Canadian Human Mortality Database. *Introduction.* Department of Demography, Université de Montréal (Canada). Available http://www.demo.umontreal.ca/chmd/ [accessed March 2009].

Coale, A.J., and Treadway, R. (1986). A summary of the changing distribution of overall fertility, marital fertility, and the proportion married in the provinces of Europe. In A.J. Coale and S.C. Watkins (Eds.), *The Decline of Fertility in Europe* (pp. 31-181). Princeton, NJ: Princeton University Press.

Daguet, F. (2006). Espérance de vie à certains âges par département et région. Données de démographie régionale 1954-1999. *Insee Résultats Société* n° 49, décembre 2005.

Duleep, H.O. (1995). Mortality and income inequality among economically developed countries. *Social Security Bulletin, 58*(2), 34-50.

Edwards, R.D., and Tuljapurkar, S. (2005). Inequality in life spans and a new perspective on mortality convergence across industrialized countries. *Population and Development Review, 31*(4), 645-674.

Ezzati, M., Friedman, A.B., Kulkarni, S.C., and Murray, C.J.L. (2008). The reversal of fortunes: Trends in county mortality and cross-county mortality disparities in the United States. *PloS Medicine, 5*(4), 0557-0568.

Federal Statistical Office, Germany. *Death Counts by Age and Year of Birth by Federal States (Table S09),* various years.

Federal Statistical Office, Germany. *Population as of 31st December by Age and Year of Year of Birth (Table B15),* various years.

Hetzel, A.M. (1997). *History and Organization of the Vital Statistics System.* Hyattsville, MD: National Center for Health Statistics.

Human Mortality Database. *Overview.* University of California, Berkeley (USA), and Max Planck Institute for Demographic Research (Germany). Available: http://www.mortality.org/ or http://www.humanmortality.de/ [accessed June 2010].

MacDorman, M.F., and Mathews, M.S. (2008). *Recent Trends in Infant Mortality in the United States.* NCHS Data Brief 9.

Ministry of Health, Labour and Welfare (Japan). *Prefectural Life Tables,* various years.

National Center for Health Statistics. (1966). *State Life Tables: 1959-1961.* Vol. 2, Nos. 1-51. PHS Publication HRA 1252. Washington, DC: U.S. Department of Health, Education, and Welfare, Public Health Service. Available: http://www.cdc.gov/nchs/data/lifetables/life59_2_1-26.pdf or http://www.cdc.gov/nchs/data/lifetables/life59_2_27-51.pdf [accessed June 2010].

National Center for Health Statistics. (1975). *State Life Tables: 1969-1971.* Vol. II, Nos. 1-51. DHEW Publication HRA 75-1151-1. Rockville, MD: U.S. Department of Health, Education, and Welfare, Public Health Service. Available: http://www.cdc.gov/nchs/data/lifetables/life69_2_12-6.pdf or http://www.cdc.gov/nchs/data/lifetables/life69_2_27-51.pdf [accessed June 2010].

National Center for Health Statistics. (1986). *U.S. Decennial Life Tables for 1979-1981.* Vol. II, Nos. 1-51. DHHS Publication PHS 86-1151-1-1. Hyattsville, MD: U.S. Department of Health, Education, and Welfare, Public Health Service. Available: http://www.cdc.gov/nchs/products/life_tables.htm [accessed June 2010].

National Center for Health Statistics. (1998). *U.S. Decennial Life Tables for 1989-1991.* Vol. II, State Life Tables 1-51. DHHS Publication PHS-98-1151-1. Hyattsville, MD: U.S. Department of Health, Education, and Welfare, Public Health Service.

National Office of Vital Statistics. (1948). *State and Regional Life Tables: 1939-41. Life Tables for the White Population of the United States, Each State, and Certain Groups of States, by Sex.* Washington, DC: U.S. Federal Security Agency, Public Health Service. Available: http://www.cdc.gov/nchs/data/lifetables/life39-41.pdf [accessed June 2010].

National Office of Vital Statistics. (1956). *State and Regional Life Tables: 1949-1951. Life Tables for the White Population of Each State, and for the Nonwhite Population of 16 Southern States and the District of Columbia.* Vital Statistics-Special Reports Vol. 41, Supplement. Washington, DC: U.S. Department of Health, Education, and Welfare, Public Health Service. Available: http://www.cdc.gov/nchs/data/lifetables/life49-51_41supp.pdf [accessed June 2010].

Preston, S.H. (2007). The changing relation between mortality and level of economic development. *International Journal of Epidemiology, 36*(3), 484-490.

Preston, S.H., and Taubman, P. (1994). Socioeconomic differences in adult mortality and health status. In National Research Council, L.G. Martin and S.H. Preston (eds.), Committee on Population. Division of Behavioral and Social Sciences and Education. *Demography of Aging* (pp. 279-318). Washington, DC: National Academy Press.

Rodgers, G.B. (1979). Income and inequality as determinants of mortality: An international cross-section analysis. *Population Studies, 33*(2), 343-351.

Smith, J.P. (1999). Healthy bodies and thick wallets: the dual relation between health and economic status. *Journal of Economic Perspectives, 13*(2), 144-166.

Statistics Bureau (Japan), Ministry of Internal Affairs and Communications. *Population Census of Japan,* various years.

Wilmoth, J.R., and Horiuchi, S. (1999). Rectangularization revisited: Variability of age at death within human populations. *Demography, 36*(4), 475-495.

ANNEX 12A

DOCUMENTATION OF DATA SOURCES

All mortality data at the national level were obtained from the Human Mortality Database (see http://www.mortality.org [accessed July 26, 2009]). Regional data come from a variety of sources and present different issues depending on the country involved, as explained below.

United States

States

For 1940-1990, mortality statistics for the individual states of the United States and the District of Columbia come from the decennial life tables that are published each decade by the National Center for Health Statistics (NCHS 1966, 1975, 1986, 1998) and its predecessor, the National Office of Vital Statistics (NOVS 1948, 1956). The full series in PDF format is available at the Centers for Disease Control and Prevention/NCHS website, see http://www.cdc.gov. Only the recent 1989-1991 tables have been digitized by NCHS, and therefore we have keypunched the q_x values (conditional probabilities of dying between ages x and $x + 1$) from the facsimiles and constructed life tables based on these probabilities.

Before 1960, the collection includes no tables for sexes combined. Therefore, we computed life tables for both sexes combined in 1940 and 1950 as a weighted average of sex-specific values, $q_x^{tot} = (q_x^f l_x^f + q_x^m l_x^m) / (l_x^f + l_x^m)$, where l_x is the proportion surviving to age x. In addition, tables are lacking in this period for the total population with all races combined (indeed, for many states the only tables available refer to the white population). To impute values of e_{50} for the total U.S. population, we applied to the 1940 and 1950 data for whites an adjustment factor equal to the average ratio (by sex and state) of e_{50} for the total population to that of whites over all subsequent decades (1960 through 2000).

In the life tables for 1959-1961, data by race are available only for men and women separately. Therefore, as for the preceding decades, we computed weighted averages of sex-specific q_x values to obtain race-specific life tables for both sexes combined. Life tables by state in this period are available for all races combined but only for men and women together. Since data by sex in this period are available for whites in all states, we computed sex-specific life tables for all races combined in this period by assuming that age-specific ratios of q_x for the total versus white populations were the same by sex as for the sexes combined.

As of March 2010, NCHS had published a decennial life table for 1999-2001 for the country as a whole but had not yet released tables for the individual states. Andy Fenelon, at the University of Pennsylvania, provided us with death counts by state for the years 1999, 2000, and 2001 (from multiple cause of death data files available from NCHS) and matching state population counts from census tabulations in 2000. Following standard practice, the life tables for 1999-2001 used in this analysis were computed using deaths by place of residence.

Counties

Life expectancy at birth at the U.S. county level for 1961-1999 was obtained from the *PloS* supplemental website for the Ezzati and colleagues (2008) paper. These data include Federal Information Processing Standards (FIPS) county identifiers for 3,150 counties as well as a mapping of how these counties were merged for sampling reasons into 2,048 regions. Sandeep Kulkarni, one of the coauthors of the above paper, provided us with more detailed data through 2003, namely life expectancies by age (including age 50) and county-specific population counts. More information about the method of combining the least populous counties into larger aggregates is available in the original paper.

France

Data by department for France, centered on the years 1954, 1962, 1968, 1975, 1982, 1990, and 1999, were obtained from Daguet (2006). Population estimates by age and sex come from Table 1, and life expectancies by age (e_x) from Table 3.5 of that publication. These data were given to us by France Meslé and Jacques Vallin of the Institut National d'Études Démographiques in Paris.

Germany

Death counts (Table S09) and population counts (Table B15) for 1990-2007 for the German States come from the Federal Statistical Office of Germany. Eva Kibele, of the Max Planck Institute for Demographic Research in Rostock, Germany, computed annual life tables for federal states using these underlying vital statistics and provided all life-table and population data for Germany used in this analysis.

Canada

Regional data for 10 Canadian provinces during 1921-2005 were obtained from the Canadian Human Mortality Database, (see http://www.bdlc.umontreal.ca/chmd [accessed March 2009]).

Japan

Spreadsheets with full life table data for 47 prefectures in 1995, 2000, and 2005 were provided by Futoshi Ishii of the National Institute of Population and Social Security Research in Japan. The data collection for 2005 includes retrospective information for key indicators (including life expectancy by sex at age 50) at 5-year intervals back to 1965. For 1995, we used the adjusted life tables that remove the effect of earthquake mortality in Hanshin/Kobe prefecture. The underlying source for the life tables is Ministry of Health, Labour and Welfare (various years). Population data for the prefectures come from the census (Statistics Bureau, Japan, various years).

ANNEX 12B

USE OF PRINCIPAL COMPONENTS FOR CREATING GRAPHICAL ELLIPSES

As illustrated here in Figures 12-3 and 12-4, male and female values of life expectancy at age 50 for a given time period have a strong positive correlation across states and counties of the United States An efficient means of characterizing the two-dimensional distribution of male-female values is to draw ellipses that contain most or all of the data points. A simple method for creating such ellipses in a different application was described by Coale and Treadway (1986). Here, we employ an alternative approach based on principal components analysis (PCA).

In words, we begin by centering the data points around their mean values, identifying their two principal axes and projecting the points onto the new basis (i.e., computing coordinates of the data points in relation to their principal axes), and then rescaling each point using standard deviations of projected abscissa and ordinate values. This series of calculations turns the original ellipsoidal scatterplot into a circular collection of points centered on the origin. To reduce the influence of outliers, we approximate the circular distribution while ignoring the outer 10 percent of data points; that is, we find a minimum radius r such that a circle with this radius (centered on the origin) contains 90 percent of the observed points. This centering, projecting, and scaling process is then reversed, so that the points on the circle with radius r are remapped (i.e., scaled, projected, and centered) so that they are comparable to the original values of male and female life expectancy, forming an ellipsoid that contains 90 percent of the data points.

In formulas, let $\mathbf{x}_1 = (x_{11}, x_{21}, \ldots, x_{n1})^T$ and $\mathbf{x}_2 = (x_{12}, x_{22}, \ldots, x_{n2})^T$ be column vectors containing male and female values of life expectancy at age 50 by state or country for a given year, and let $\mathbf{x} = (\mathbf{x}_1, \mathbf{x}_2)$ be an n by 2 matrix. Suppose that μ_1 and μ_2 are the mean values of $\mathbf{x}_1$ and $\mathbf{x}_2$, and let $\mathbf{Y} = (\mathbf{x}_1 - \mu_1, (\mu_1, \mathbf{x}_2), \mathbf{x}_2 - \mu_2)$ be an n by 2 matrix whose columns contain the recentered values of male and female life expectancy. The sample covariance matrix, $S^2 = \frac{1}{n}\mathbf{Y}^T\mathbf{Y}$, can be decomposed using PCA by invoking the spectral decomposition theorem (Mardia, Kent, and Bibby, 1979, pp. 213ff, 469): $S^2 = \frac{1}{n}\mathbf{Y}^T\mathbf{Y} = \mathbf{U}\Lambda\mathbf{U}^T$, where the columns of $\mathbf{U} = [\mathbf{u}_1, \mathbf{u}_2]$ comprise an orthonormal basis, and $\Lambda = \text{diag}(\lambda_1, \lambda_2)$ is a diagonal matrix with positive elements $\lambda_1 > \lambda_2 > 0$. By computing $\mathbf{Z} = \mathbf{Y}\mathbf{U}\Lambda^{-\frac{1}{2}}$, we project the original data points onto the span of $\mathbf{u}_1$ and $\mathbf{u}_2$ and simultaneously rescale them so that the variation along each axis is now unity: $\frac{1}{n}Z^TZ = I$. Note that the matrix, Z, like X and Y previously, contains two column vectors, $z_1 = (z_{11}, z_{21}, \ldots, z_{n1})^T$ and $z_2 = (z_{12}, z_{22}, \ldots, z_{n2})^T$, both of length n.

Let $C_r = \{(z_{i1}, z_{i2}) : z_{i1}^2 + z_{i2}^2 = r^2 \text{ for all } i\}$ be a set of points that lie on a circle of radius r centered on the origin, and let $Z = [z_1, z_2]$ be a matrix containing these points (the number of points is arbitrary and can be adjusted upward or downward to obtain any desired level of precision for drawing the circle or corresponding ellipse). We find the minimum radius r such that 90 percent of the transformed data points lie inside the circle. Computing $Y = Z(U\Lambda^{\frac{1}{2}})^T = Z\Lambda^{\frac{1}{2}}U^T$ and $X = (y_1 + \mu_1, y_2 + \mu_2)$, where y_1 and y_2 are the columns of Y, each point in the circle is mapped back onto the original basis. The points corresponding to rows of X form an ellipse that encloses 90 percent of the original data points.

Part V

International Case Studies

13

Renewed Progress in Life Expectancy: The Case of the Netherlands

Johan Mackenbach and Joop Garssen

During the 1980s and 1990s a complete stagnation of mortality decline in older age groups has occurred in the Netherlands, while other high-income countries continued their rapid mortality declines. At first, the stagnation of old-age mortality decline was misinterpreted as a (hopeful) sign of the "rectangularization" of the survival curve as predicted by Fries (Nusselder and Mackenbach, 1996, 1997). Later comparative analyses of old-age mortality developments in a range of high-income countries made clear, however, that the Netherlands is an exception to the rule of continuing old-age mortality decline (Janssen, Mackenbach, and Kunst, 2004). Analyses of cause-of-death patterns showed that the stagnation of old-age mortality decline in the Netherlands could partly be attributed to smoking-related causes of death. The evidence also showed a contribution of ill-defined causes of death, which are typical for old age (e.g., mental and neurological disorders) (Janssen et al., 2003).

A stagnation of mortality decline among the elderly has also been observed in a small number of other countries, particularly the United States and Denmark (Meslé and Vallin, 2006; Glei, Meslé, and Vallin, Chapter 2, in this volume). Interestingly, however, progress in mortality decline among the elderly resumed in Denmark around 1995 (Juel, Bjerregaard, and Madsen, 2000) and in the Netherlands around 2002. The reversal of stagnation into renewed decline in the Netherlands was first noted by Statistics Netherlands in 2002, when the final count of the absolute annual number of deaths in 2001 was slightly lower than the number of deaths in 2000, despite the fact that the proportion of elderly in the population continued to rise. In the first press releases by Statistics Netherlands this was tentatively ascribed to climatic factors (mild winters, cool summers). When the period of continuous mortality decline became longer, however, it became more and more unlikely that it would be due solely to milder temperatures (Garssen and van der Meulen, 2007).

As Figure 13-1 shows, from 2002 to 2008 life expectancy at birth increased by almost 2 years (from 76.0 to 78.3 years among men and from 80.7 to 82.3 years among women). A substantial part of this increase of life expectancy at birth is due to advances at higher ages, as is evident from the fact that life expectancy at age 65 has increased by more than a year (from 15.6 to 17.3 years among men and from 19.3 to 20.5 years among women). The sharpest upturn in life-expectancy trends is seen at age 85, for which 2002 marked a reversal from almost complete stagnation to a period of rapid increases.

No systematic analysis of possible determinants of this remarkable development has been made until now. This chapter aims to assess the possible causes of the reversal from stagnation to renewed decline of old-age mortality in the Netherlands. After an analysis of patterns of decline by age, gender, and cause of death, we review all main groups of determinants: biological factors, factors in the physical and social environment, lifestyle factors, and health care factors. We used readily available data to assess whether changes in these factors have occurred preceding or coinciding with the changes in mortality that could plausibly explain the change in old-age mortality trend.

DATA AND METHODS

Mortality data were extracted from the registry kept at Statistics Netherlands, which is derived from the municipal population registries in the Netherlands. Underlying causes of death were coded according to the International Classification of Diseases (9th and 10th revisions). No changes in coding occurred around 2002. In order to calculate the cause-specific contributions to the gain in life expectancy, we calculated, for both periods, the number of life-years that would be gained if only the observed age-specific mortality risk for a specified cause changed during the period, keeping all other age- and cause-specific mortality risks constant.

Data on determinants of mortality were extracted from various registries and surveys kept at Statistics Netherlands, which are mostly available online at http://statline.cbs.nl/statweb/ [accessed June 8, 2010]. Data on self-reported health problems, lifestyles, and medical care utilization were collected in a multipurpose survey (Permanent Onderzoek Leef Situatie) that is conducted on a continuous basis among a representative sample of the noninstitutionalized population.

Data on clinical incidence (i.e., incidence of the first clinical episode for

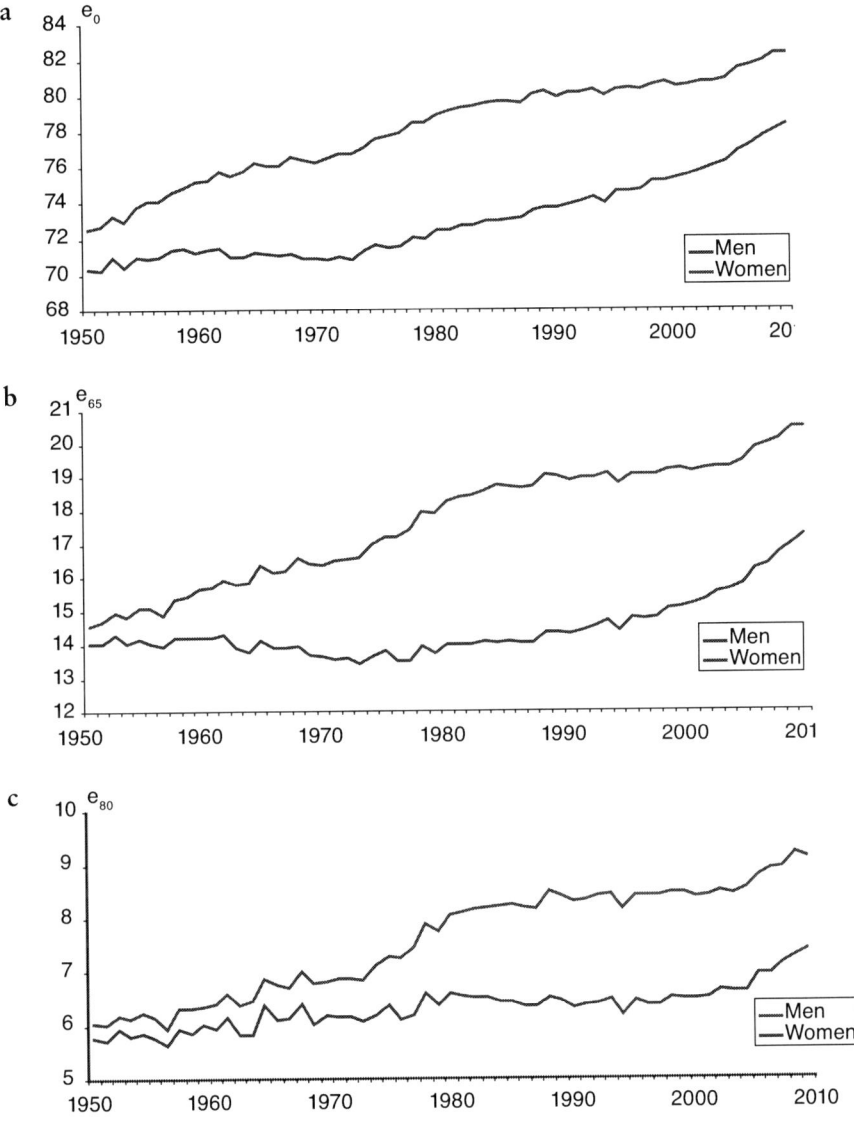

FIGURE 13-1 Life expectancy at birth, age 65 and age 80, by gender, the Netherlands, 1950-2008.
(a) At birth
(b) At age 65
(c) At age 80
SOURCE: Data from Statistics Netherlands (see http://statline.cbs.nl/statweb/ [accessed June 2010]).

a particular disease) and case fatality (i.e., 1-year mortality after the first clinical episode for a particular disease) of specific conditions were extracted from a database constructed by Statistics Netherlands. To construct this database, a linkage has been made between the population registry and the national registry of hospital admissions, which covers more than 90 percent of the Dutch population. This linkage was used to eliminate readmissions of the same individual for the same condition, and to estimate case-fatality rates in a 1-year follow-up period of individuals admitted for a particular condition. Results of these linkages are available for the period 2000-2005 only. The registry of hospital admissions includes clinical as well as day care admissions.

Detailed cost-of-illness studies have been performed by the National Institute for Public Health and the Environment of the Netherlands for the years 1999, 2003, and 2007. These studies are based on a wide range of administrative data covering all health care sectors. Age- and gender-specific patterns of health care expenditure have been determined for 2003 (Slobbe et al., 2006), and data from the 1999 and 2007 studies have been reanalyzed for this chapter to determine time trends of health care expenditure by age and gender.

RESULTS

Mortality Decline

The exact turning point in the mortality trend is difficult to establish because of year-to-year fluctuations in the number of deaths, which are partly determined by climatic conditions (cold winters, hot summers) and influenza epidemics. Around the year 2000 there were several such events: large winter peaks in mortality in early 1999 (around 2,000 additional deaths due to influenza) and early 2000 (around 2,000 additional deaths due to cold), and large summer peaks in mortality in 2003 (between 1,000 and 2,000 additional deaths due the large European heat wave) and in 2006 (two heat waves causing more than 1,000 additional deaths). These events may have partly obscured the starting point of an "underlying" mortality decline.

A simple look at the absolute number of deaths shows that an almost uninterrupted decline in mortality started in 2003. The total numbers of deaths were 140,487 in 1999, 140,527 in 2000, 140,377 in 2001, 142,355 in 2002, 141,936 in 2003, 136,553 in 2004, 136,402 in 2005, 135,372 in 2006, and 133,022 in 2007 (see http://statline.cbs.nl/statweb/ [accessed June 8, 2010]). Despite the 2003 heat wave, the number of deaths in that year was already lower than in 2002, and a year-to-year decline in the absolute number of deaths continued into 2007. The exceptionally large decline from 2003 to 2004 can probably be explained by the fact that an already declining mortality trend was partly obscured by a temporary rise in mortality due to the 2003 heat wave.

After 2002, mortality declined in all age groups. In younger age groups this represented a continuation of preexisting trends, but in older age groups it reflected a reversal from stable to declining mortality rates. Figure 13-2 shows that this reversal occurred for men in all age groups above age 85, and for women in all age groups above age 65. The simultaneous acceleration of mortality trends in a wide range of age groups also indicates that this was a period rather than a cohort effect.

Many causes of death have contributed to the rise in life expectancy at age 65 after 2002, as shown in Figure 13-3. As expected, cardiovascular disease is the main contributor (more than 0.8 years among men, more than 0.6 years among women), but this disease group does not account for most of the trend reversal, because it contributed only slightly less to the rise in life expectancy at age 65 between 1995 and 2002 than to that between 2002 and 2008. The main contributors to the *acceleration* of the rise in life expectancy at age 65 are causes of death for which the trends were distinctly more favorable in the second as compared with the first period. These include symptoms and ill-defined conditions (mortality from this cause of death category increased during the earlier period and declined during the second period), stroke, diabetes, dementia, and pneumonia. Figure 13-4 illustrates some of the striking changes in trends.

Changes in Determinants

Reviewing trends in a wide range of determinants of mortality, we did not find favorable trends among the elderly in health status indicators paralleling the trend in mortality, which suggests that declining mortality in this period cannot be attributed to improved biological conditions. Table 13-1 shows a few examples. The prevalence of self-reported health problems among the elderly shows a stable or increasing trend, both for generic indicators, like functional limitations, and for specific indicators, like diabetes and hypertension. The clinical incidence of specific diseases has also mostly increased, although there has been a 9 percent decline in the clinical incidence of acute myocardial infarction.

The physical and social environments of the elderly also have not substantially improved in the period under consideration (see Table 13-1). Environmental protection measures have gradually reduced emissions of a number of air pollutants. The main air pollutant which is still contributing to a large number of deaths in the Netherlands is fine dust (PM10), for which emissions have been reduced by about 10 percent, following more rapid declines in the 1990s. Due to climate change, winters are gradually becom-

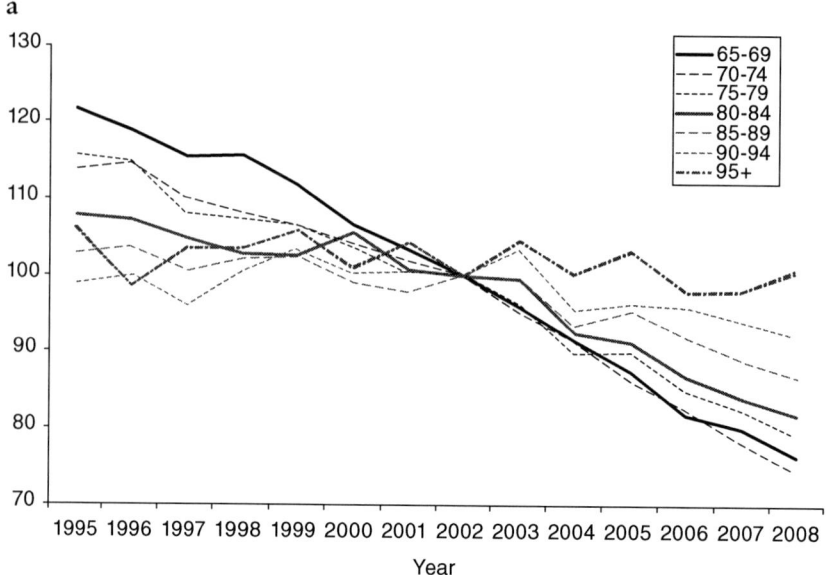
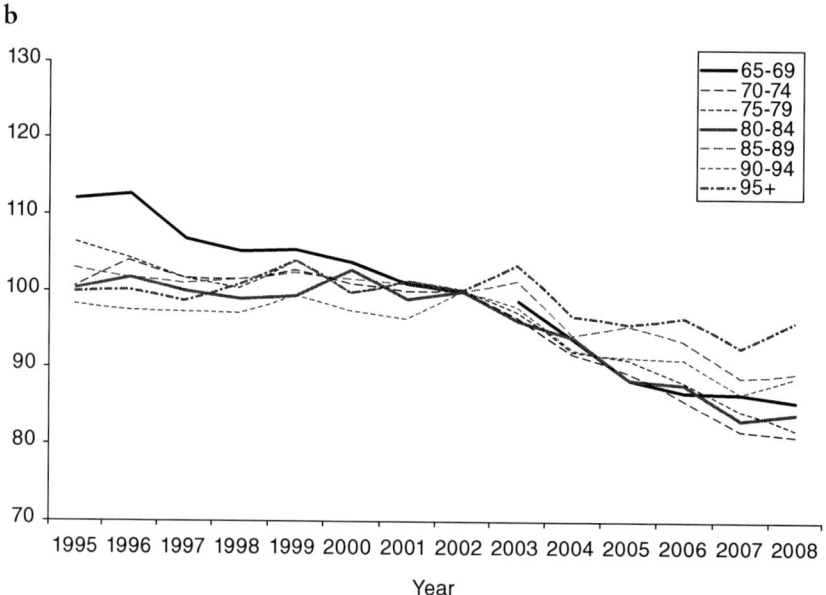

FIGURE 13-2 Age-specific mortality trends, by gender, the Netherlands, 1995-2008.
(a) Men
(b) Women
SOURCE: Authors' analyses of data available at Statistics Netherlands.

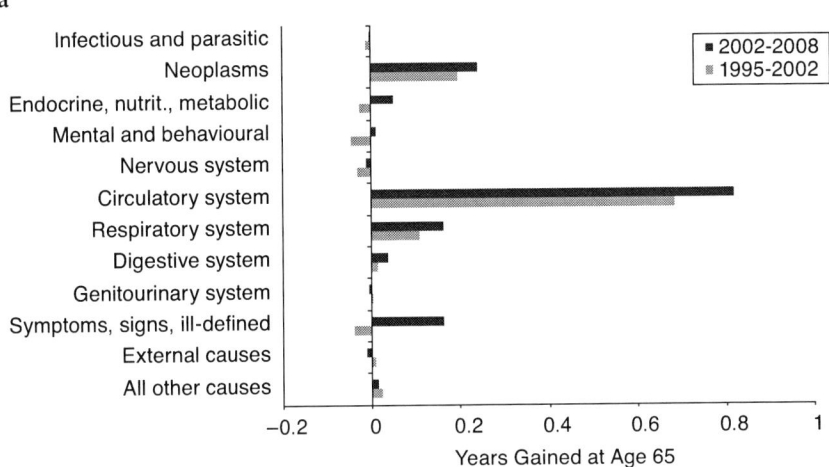

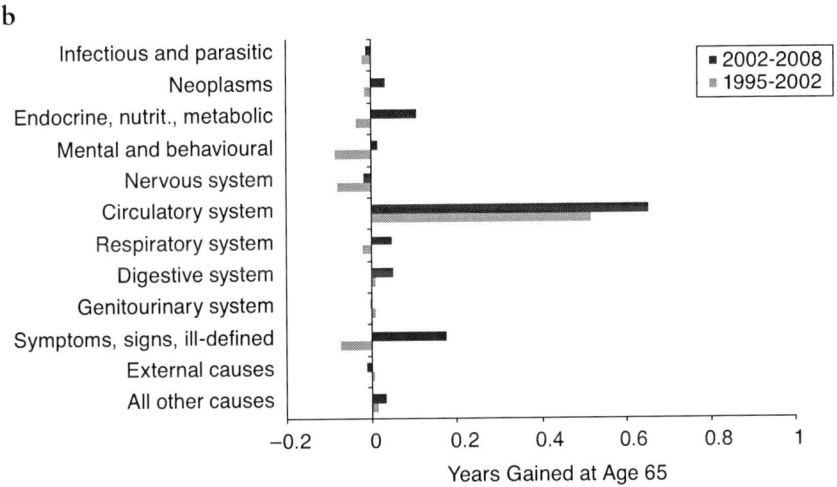

FIGURE 13-3 Cause-specific contributions to life-expectancy gains at age 65, by gender, 1995-2002 and 2002-2008.
(a) Men
(b) Women
SOURCE: Authors' analyses of data available at Statistics Netherlands.

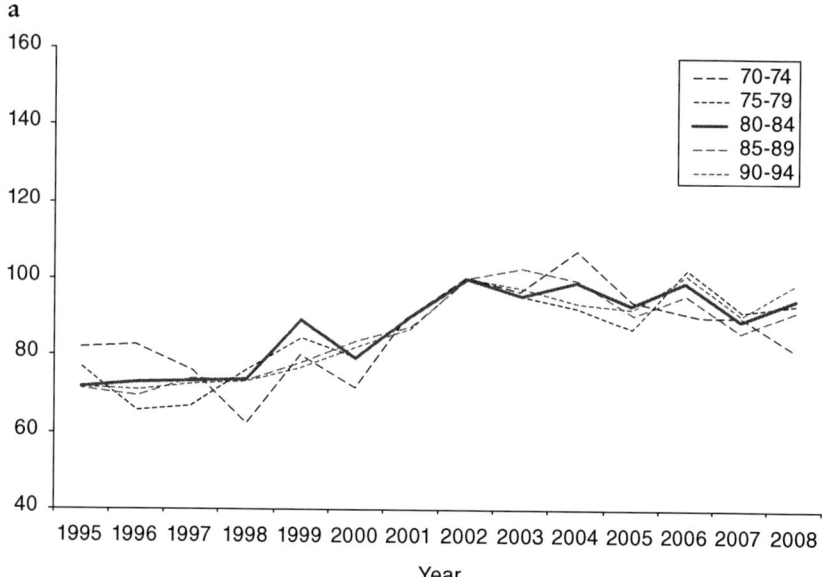
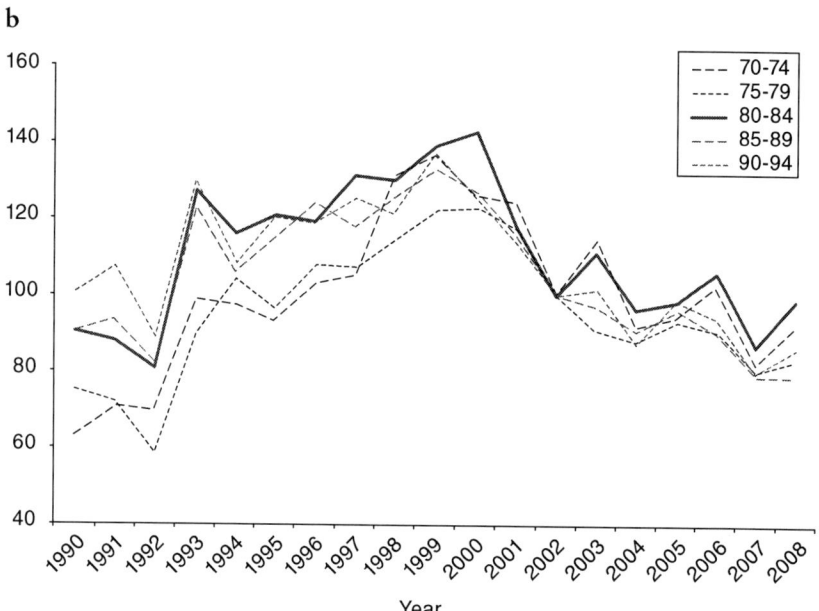

FIGURE 13-4 Selected cause-specific mortality trends, by age, women, the Netherlands.
(a) Mental disorders, 1995-2008
(b) Pneumonia, 1990-2008
SOURCE: Authors' analyses of data available at Statistics Netherlands.

ing warmer, but this started far before the turn of the century, and winters were not significantly warmer after 2002 than during the 1990s. There have not been very favorable trends for social determinants, either. For example, poverty rates among the elderly have been more or less stable.

Health-related lifestyles also have not substantially improved during this period (see Table 13-1). Smoking rates among the elderly have been stable since the turn of the century. Historical data show that the prevalence of smoking among women ages 65 and above has hovered between 10 and 15 percent since 1980, and among men it has come down substantially during the 1980s and 1990s (Stivoro, 2009). This may partly explain the divergence of old-age mortality trends between men and women during the 1980s and 1990s, but, assuming a time-lag between smoking trends and mortality trends, this divergence cannot account for the reversal among women since 2002. Excessive alcohol consumption and regular exercise among the elderly have been stable as well, while obesity has increased.

The only category of determinants for which substantial changes were seen since the turn of the century are health care factors (see Table 13-1). Modest increases occurred in the proportion of elderly vaccinated against influenza (about 5 percentage points, after more rapid rises during the 1990s), the proportion of elderly seeing a medical specialist (about 3 percentage points), and the proportion of elderly using prescribed drugs (an increase of about 5 percentage points). More substantial increases occurred in the hospital admission rate. In the Netherlands, hospital admission rates rose slowly during the 1990s, but the rate of increase suddenly accelerated after 2001. This acceleration was seen for all age groups, but the strongest acceleration occurred among the elderly (see Table 13-1). This acceleration was seen for many disease groups, including cancer, diseases of the nervous system, cardiovascular diseases, and injuries.

At the same time, mortality within 1 year after hospital admission declined for many conditions (see Table 13-1). Although declines in case fatality were larger for younger people, they were substantial for elderly patients as well. Among those ages 80 and over, the average decline (for all conditions combined) was about 14 percent (from 26 to 22 percent). This decline occurred for many conditions, including coronary heart disease (for which 1-year case fatality declined from 34 to 28 percent) and stroke (for which 1-year case fatality declined from 52 to 45 percent).

More About the Changes in Health Care

The acceleration of the hospital admission trend coincided with a clear-cut change in growth of health care expenditure in the Netherlands. Long-term trends in health care spending in the Netherlands show a very distinct pattern, characterized by rapid growth in the 1960s and 1970s, relatively

TABLE 13-1 Determinants of Mortality, the Netherlands, 1991-2007

Biological Factors	Unit	Age	1991	1995
Diabetes (self-reported)	%	65+		
Hypertension (self-reported)	%	65+		
One or more OECD limitations (self-reported)	%	65+		
One or more ADL limitations (self-reported)	%	65+		
Clinical incidence of acute myocardial infarction	per 10,000 py	80-84		
Clinical incidence of stroke	per 10,000 py	80-84		
Clinical incidence of pneumonia	per 10,000 py	80-84		

Environmental Factors	Unit	Age	1991	1995
Emission of PM10 particles	Mkg	all	81.0	61.0
Average winter temperature in De Bilt	°C	n.a.	2.2	5.3
First-generation immigrants	%	65+		0.9
Married	%	65+		54.0
Income inequality	Gini	all		
Poverty (> 1 year at less than 120% of social minimum)	%	65		

Lifestyle Factors	Unit	Age	1991	1995
Current smoking (self-reported)	%	65+		
Heavy drinking (self-reported)	%	65+		
Regular exercise (self-reported)	%	65+		
Obese (based on self-reported height and weight)	%	65+		

Health Care	Unit	Age	1991	1995
Vaccinated against influenza (self-reported)	%	75+	31.9	47.7
Contact with general practitioner in 1 year (self-reported)	%	65+	86.6	86.7
Contact with specialist in 1 year (self-reported)	%	65+	54.8	58.7
Use of prescribed drugs	%	65+	70.1	74.4
Hospital admission (total)	per 10,000 py	80-84		3672
Hospital admission (cardiovascular disease)	per 10,000 py	80-84		798
1-year mortality after first admission for any disease	%	80+		
1-year mortality after first admission for coronary heart disease	%	80+		
1-year mortality after first admission for stroke	%	80+		
Health care expenditure	BEuro	n.a.	33.5	37.3
Health care expenditure per capita	Euro per head	n.a.	1907	2274
Health care expenditure as % of gross domestic product	%	n.a.	11.2	11.5

NOTE: ADL = activities of daily living, na = not applicable, OECD = Organisation for Economic Co-operation and Development, py = person-year.

1999	2000	2001	2002	2003	2004	2005	2006	2007
		11.4	10.5	10.4	13.0	12.6	13.2	14.1
		24.5	29.9	31.3	31.6	32.8	35.5	34.9
	31.6	33.6	30.6	31.3	35.5	32.7	31.2	30.0
	18.1	19.2	18.6	17.0	21.6	20.9	17.5	18.9
	68.3	68.9	71.3	67.5	65.8	62.1	58.0	59.3
	101.7	103.8	106.0	111.4	115.4	118.2	115.7	113.7
	57.2	52.4	57.6	64.5	67.7	79.5	83.6	84.6

1999	2000	2001	2002	2003	2004	2005	2006	2007
	51.0	50.0	49.0	46.0	46.0	45.0	45.0	45.0
4.4	5.0	4.1	4.8	2.4	4.1	3.6	2.8	6.5
1.1	1.2	1.4	1.5	1.7	1.9	2.0	2.2	2.3
55.0	55.0	55.0	55.0	56.0	56.0	56.0	57.0	57.0
	0.28	0.27	0.27	0.27	0.27	0.27	0.26	0.27
	22.6	22.9	22.0	21.5	20.8	19.6	19.4	19.0

1999	2000	2001	2002	2003	2004	2005	2006	2007
		18.0	17.2	17.0	17.3	17.6	19.6	16.8
	3.0	4.3	4.1	3.1	5.0	3.4	4.5	4.3
		58.0	59.0	59.0	57.0	58.0	58.0	58.0
	12.0	12.8	10.8	13.4	12.6	13.7	14.4	14.0

1999	2000	2001	2002	2003	2004	2005	2006	2007
77.9	80.1	84.2	87.5	81.5	81.3	82.6	84.7	85.4
86.4	88.7	88.7	85.7	86.7	85.6	85.8	85.8	84.9
59.1	58.4	61.5	59.3	60.6	63.0	64.4	62.9	64.8
74.5	74.4	74.6	75.3	77.1	78.1	79.2	79.8	80.4
3854	3892	3962	4273	4592	4899	5196	5452	5731
788	771	796	827	855	899	933	957	980
		25.8	25.2	24.7	24.0	23.1	22.3	
		34.3	33.1	33.8	32.0	30.3	28.2	
		52.2	51.3	50.7	48.1	47.1	44.6	
42.1	43.6	46.0	48.0	50.0	51.7	53.1	54.5	56.2
2774	2949	3276	3639	3910	4026	4155	4316	4524
11.4	11.2	11.7	12.6	13.3	13.3	13.2	13.1	13.1

SOURCE: Data from Statistics Netherlands (see http://statline.cbs.nl/statweb/ [accessed June 2010]).

slow growth in the 1980s and 1990s, and rapid growth again in the first years of the new millennium. The growth of health care expenditure (in constant prices, i.e., adjusted for inflation and compared to the year before) was exceptionally high in 2001, 2002, and 2003. It was 3.1 percent in 1999, 3.6 percent in 2000, 5.4 percent in 2001, 4.4 percent in 2002, 4.3 percent in 2003, 3.2 percent in 2004, 2.9 percent in 2005, 2.6 percent in 2006, and 3.1 percent in 2007. A similar acceleration in 2001 and subsequent years was seen for health care expenditure per capita (see Table 13-1).

Detailed studies of health care expenditure by age and health care sector have been performed for 1999, 2003, and 2007 (see Figure 13-5). Between 1999 and 2003 health care expenditure per head of population (in nominal prices) rose by more than 40 percent. In relative terms, the increase was shared among all age groups, including the old and very old, and benefited most health care sectors, including hospital care and care for the elderly. For men above age 85, health care expenditure rose from €17,128 per person per year in 1999 to €23,331 per person per year in 2003, representing a rise of 36 percent, or more than €6000. The corresponding figures for women above age 85 were €21,638 and €30,446, representing a rise of 41 percent, or almost €9000 per person per year.

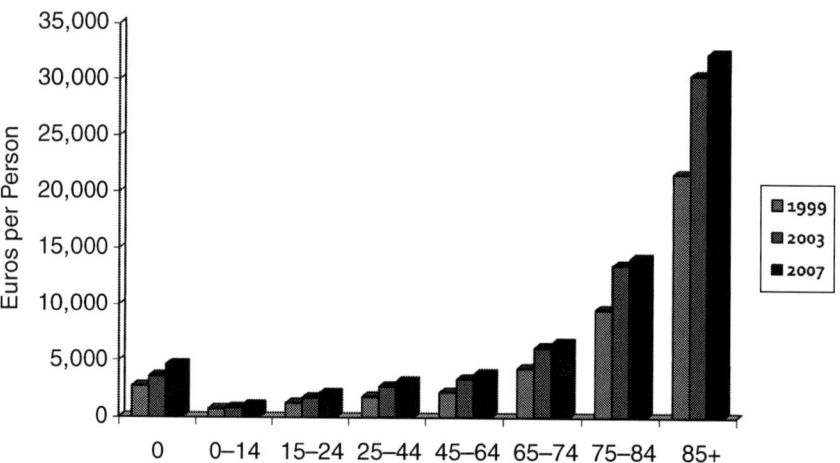

FIGURE 13-5 Health care expenditure by age, women, the Netherlands, nominal prices in Euros per person, 1999-2007.
SOURCE: L.C.J. Slobbe (personal communication, National Institute for Public Health and the Environment, 2009). Data collected and analyzed by the National Institute for Public Health and the Environment.

DISCUSSION

The reversal from stagnation to renewed decline of old-age mortality in the Netherlands shows some very distinct patterns. It was abrupt and shared by a wide range of age groups (particularly among women), suggesting that the causal factor or factors acted immediately rather than with a long delay, and pointing at a period rather than a cohort effect.

The pattern of cause-of-death contributions to this renewed decline is also rather striking. While the stagnation of old-age mortality during the 1980s and 1990s was partly due to smoking-related causes, the decline of old-age mortality after 2002 is not. Striking accelerations or even reversals of mortality trends are seen for causes like stroke, pneumonia, dementia, and symptoms and ill-defined conditions.

Of the four categories of determinants that we reviewed, health care factors seems the best candidate to explain the reversal of mortality trends among the elderly. There have been no sudden changes in health status among the elderly, in their physical or social environment or in their lifestyles that could explain this reversal. Most of these factors have been stable, and some have even deteriorated. When they have changed for the better, as in the case of fine dust air pollution, the cause-of-death pattern of mortality decline does not suggest a causal connection.

By contrast, health care for the elderly, particularly in the hospital sector, has grown rapidly. The timing of these changes roughly corresponds to the timing of the renewal of mortality decline. Substantial and sustained mortality decline started in 2003, and if one assumes a certain delay between improved treatment and reduced death rates, the improvements in treatment should have started slightly earlier. This may indeed have been the case: the most rapid increases in health care expenditure occurred in 2001, 2002, and 2003, and the most rapid increases in hospitalization rates occurred in 2002, 2003, and 2004.

That a more liberal administration to elderly patients of life-saving treatments in hospital has played a role in mortality decline is consistent with the decline in 1-year case fatality that we have observed, although this should be interpreted with care because of the possibility that the increase in admission rates has brought milder cases of disease into the hospital after 2001. Some real declines in case fatality must have occurred as well, because case fatality for coronary heart disease among the elderly has declined along with a decline in the clinical incidence of myocardial infarction (see Table 13-1). In the case of stroke, a plausible explanation for the acceleration of mortality decline and the decline of the 1-year case fatality rate is more rapid and more aggressive treatment for stroke in specialized stroke units, which were implemented on a large scale from about 2000 onward (van Exel et al., 2005).

In the case of pneumonia, dementia, and symptoms and ill-defined conditions, too, a more active approach toward the treatment of seriously ill elderly patients may have played a role in mortality decline. Changes in mortality from these conditions are often regarded as indicative of "artifacts" of certification or coding, but if the rules have not changed, systematic changes as observed here must have a deeper explanation. Both pneumonia and dementia are often considered to be problematic "underlying" causes of death. Among elderly patients with one or more serious chronic diseases, pneumonia will often act as the direct cause of death, but should not be certified as the underlying cause. If the death is certified as being caused by pneumonia, then this can be interpreted as a decision by the physician not to search for a better diagnosis, or if a better diagnosis is available not to treat the patient for this disease, but to let him or her die from what has been called the "old man's friend." Among elderly patients, deaths from pneumonia can therefore often be seen as the outcome of a conscious or unconscious nontreatment decision. The same applies to dementia, which as long as its complications are adequately treated will in itself not lead to death. If a death is being certified as caused by dementia, the physician actually acknowledges that he or she has decided that further treatment is ineffective. For this very reason, dementia has long not been accepted as a possible underlying cause of death (Van der Meulen and Keij-Deerenberg, 2003).

A more active approach toward the treatment of seriously ill elderly patients is also suggested by the decreasing proportion of deaths in which treatment was withheld or withdrawn. In the Netherlands, data on the frequency of end-of-life practices were collected in four surveys in 1990, 1995, 2001, and 2005. The overall frequency of end-of-life decisions rose from 39 to 43 percent during the first half of the 1990s and remained stable thereafter. The frequency of specific end-of-life practices, however, showed some important changes coinciding with the reversal of old-age mortality trends. From 2001 to 2005 the frequency of euthanasia, assisted suicide, and withholding or withdrawing life-prolonging treatment declined, while the frequency of intensified alleviation of symptoms increased (Van der Heide et al., 2007).

The sudden rise in health care expenditure after 2001, which seems to have facilitated the increase in health care for the elderly, was due to a conscious decision by the Dutch government to relax the budgetary restraints of the 1980s and 1990s. During these two decades, the Dutch government had successfully limited the growth of health care expenditure, first by a strict regulation of supply (hospital beds, expensive equipment, specialized personnel, etc.), then by imposing budget constraints for in-patient care. As a result, the proportion of gross domestic product spent on health care in the Netherlands rose less than in other high-income countries. By 2001 public dissatisfaction with waiting lists and other problems of access to the health care system had become so massive that the government decided to remove budgetary restraints. In the plan *"Zorg verzekerd"*—"Care insured (or ensured)"—the government promised that all necessary treatments would be eligible for reimbursement (Actieplan Zorg Verzekerd, 2000). As a result, health care costs exploded, until new but less tight restrictions were reimposed around 2004.

As is often the case with trends in aggregate population health, it is difficult to produce direct evidence on cause-effect relationships. The evidence presented here for a role of health care utilization in the reversal of old-age mortality trends in the Netherlands is only circumstantial. It is partly by exclusion that we have arrived at health care factors as the most plausible candidate, and it is mainly on the basis of consistency of most of the descriptive findings with this interpretation that we feel confident in proposing this as a hypothesis—but it is currently not much more than that.

Sometimes international comparisons can help to test such hypotheses, but in this case these will not bring us very far. There are only three countries with similar histories of stagnation of old-age mortality decline, Denmark, the Netherlands, and the United States. While stagnation started around the same time in these three countries, suggesting similar explanations, the reversal from stagnation to progress differs strongly in timing. Denmark's renewed decline already started in 1995, and in the United States it has not yet started at all. On one hand, for Denmark, improvements in lifestyle as well as in medical and surgical treatment have been suggested as explanations (Chapter 14, in this volume), which is partly similar to what we have proposed. On the other hand, the United States has a much higher level of health care expenditure than Denmark and the Netherlands, which reduces the likelihood that a reversal of life expectancy trends there can be expected to occur when health care expenditure would rise even further.

In conclusion, although important questions remain, the most plausible hypothesis for explaining the sudden reversal of old-age mortality trends in the Netherlands is more health care for the elderly, facilitated by a sudden relaxation of budgetary restraints.

ACKNOWLEDGMENTS

Lany Slobbe of the National Institute for Public Health and the Environment provided the data in Figure 13-5. Agnes de Bruin helped with collecting data for Table 13-1. Agnes van der Heide provided useful comments on the trend in end-of-life practices in the Netherlands.

REFERENCES

Actieplan Zorg Verzekerd. (2000, November). *The Hague: Ministerie van Volksgezondheid, Welzijn en Sport.* Available: http://www.minvws.nl/artikelen/staf/actieplan_zorg_verzekerd.asp [accessed June 2010].

Garssen, J., and van der Meulen, A. (2007). Overlijdensrisico's naar herkomstgroep: Daling en afnemende verschillen. *Bevolkingstrends, 55*(4), 56-72.

Janssen, F., Nusselder, W.J., Looman, C.W.N., Mackenbach, J.P., and Kunst, A.E. (2003). Stagnation in mortality decline among elders in the Netherlands. *Gerontologist, 43,* 722-734.

Janssen, F., Mackenbach, J.P., and Kunst, A.E. (2004). Trends in old-age mortality in seven European countries, 1950-1999. *Journal of Clinical Epidemiology, 57,* 203-216.

Juel, K., Bjerregaard, P., and Madsen, M. (2000). Mortality and life expectancy in Denmark and other European countries. What is happening to middle-aged Danes? *European Journal of Public Health, 10,* 93-100.

Löfmark, R., Nilston, T., Cartwright, C., Fischer, S., van der Heide, A., Mortier, F., et al. (2008). Physicians' experiences with end-of-life decision-making: Survey in 6 European countries and Australia. *BMC Medicine, 6,* 4.

Meslé, F., and Vallin, J. (2006). Diverging trends in female old-age mortality: The United States and the Netherlands versus France and Japan. *Population and Development Review, 31,* 123-145.

Nusselder, W.J., and Mackenbach, J.P. (1996). Rectangularization of the survival curve in the Netherlands, 1950-1992. *Gerontologist, 36,* 773-782.

Nusselder, W.J., and Mackenbach, J.P. (1997). Rectangularization of the survival curve in the Netherlands: An analysis of underlying causes of death. *Journals of Gerontology Series B: Psychological Sciences and Social Sciences, 52,* S145-S154.

Nusselder, W.J., and Mackenbach, J.P. (2000). Lack of improvement of life expectancy at advanced ages in the Netherlands. *International Journal of Epidemiology, 29,* 140-148.

Polder, J.J. (2009). De zorguitgaven als januskop. Trends in getallen en gezichtspunten. In J.P. Mackenbach (Ed.), *Trends in Volksgezondheid en Gezondheidszorg.* Maarssen, Netherlands: Elsevier.

Slobbe, L.C.J., Kommer, G.J., Smit, J.M., Groen, J., Meerding, W.J., and Polder, J.J. (2006). *Kosten van Ziekten in Nederland 2003* [Costs of Illnesses in The Netherlands 2003]. Bilthoven, Netherlands: National Institute for Public Health and the Environment [in Dutch].

Stivoro. (2009). *Feiten en Cijfers [Facts and figures].* Available: http://www.stivoro.nl/Voor_professionals/Feiten___Cijfers.aspx?mId=9929&rId=77 [accessed June 2010].

Van der Heide, A., Onwuteaka-Philipsen, B., Rurup, M.L., Buiting, H.M., van Delden, J.J.M., Hanssen-de Wolff, J.E., et al. (2007). End-of-life practices in the Netherlands under the Euthanasia Act. *New England Journal of Medicine, 356,* 1957-1965.

Van der Meulen, A., and Keij-Deerenberg, I. (2003). Sterfte aan dementie. *Bevolkingstrends, 51*(3), 24-28.

Van Exel, N.J.A., Koopmanschap, M.A., Scholte op Reimer, W., Niessen, L.W., and Huijsman, R. (2005). Cost-effectiveness of integrated stroke services. *Quarterly Journal of Medicine, 98*(6), 415-425.

14

The Divergent Life-Expectancy Trends in Denmark and Sweden— and Some Potential Explanations

Kaare Christensen, Michael Davidsen, Knud Juel, Laust Mortensen, Roland Rau, and James W. Vaupel

INTRODUCTION

A priori it could be expected that Denmark was among the countries with the longest life expectancy in the world for both men and women due to the fact that other Nordic countries are among the world's leaders in life expectancy. In the period 1950-1980, life expectancy in Denmark was indeed among the highest in the world, but at the beginning of the new millennium its relative position in the world with regard to life expectancy had changed. In 2000, a life-expectancy chart for 20 Organisation for Economic Co-operation and Development (OECD) countries put Denmark close to the bottom. In particular, the difference between Denmark and its Nordic neighbor, Sweden, countries separated by only a few miles of water, is intriguing. Sweden maintained its position among the world leaders in life expectancy throughout the 20th century and made significant gains in comparison to Denmark. The life-expectancy difference between Sweden and Denmark grew from marginal in the 1950s to 3 years in the early 1990s (Juel, 2008). Starting in the mid-1990s, life expectancy in Denmark (as well as in Sweden) increased annually at a rate corresponding to that of the best-performing countries, although Denmark has been unable to catch up.

This chapter describes the trends in overall mortality and cause-specific mortality, suggests some underlying determinants of reduced life span in Denmark, and compares Denmark with other countries, in particular Sweden. The chapter consists of two parts: a descriptive section with data describing the secular trends and a discussion section that provides a number of possible explanations for the Danish trajectory, which shows improvement-stagnation-improvement but no catch-up for life expectancy at birth and at age 65.

SECULAR TRENDS

Life Expectancy in Denmark

In the 1950s, Denmark was a world leader in life expectancy for both men and women, along with Sweden and the Netherlands, which are usually considered to be very similar to Denmark in many aspects of society. A parallel increase in life expectancy for these three countries, most pronounced for women, was seen during the three decades leading up to 1980, which marked the beginning of a stagnation period of 10-15 years in Denmark (see Figure 14-1a). The Netherlands experienced a later and shorter stagnation period, and Sweden continued with positive development throughout the 20th century. From the mid-1990s, Denmark experienced an annual increase in life expectancy corresponding to that of the best-performing countries, but Danish longevity has not been able to catch up with Sweden. Denmark's trajectory—improvement-stagnation-improvement but no catch-up—is found also for life expectancy at age 65 (see Figure 14-1b) and at age 80 for men. For women at age 80, however, the trajectory is not so clear (see Figure 14-1c). This development over the second half of the 20th century means that Denmark's position in life expectancy dropped from rank 3 among 20 OECD countries in the 1950s to rank 17 for men and 20 for women in 2000, while Sweden maintained its position near the top, especially for men (see Figure 14-2) (Juel, 2008).

Another informative way to illustrate this development is by looking at the annual increase in life expectancy. Oeppen and Vaupel (2002) show that "best-practice" life expectancy, that is, the highest value recorded in a single country in a given year, rose by about 2.5 years every decade (2.43 years) for women, starting in 1840. Male life-expectancy improvements occurred at the slightly slower pace of 2.22 years per decade. A comparison of Denmark's life-expectancy improvement increases with these best-practice increases (see Figure 14-3a) shows that, in the middle and at the end of the 20th century, Denmark had attained best-practice life-expectancy increases for women, while for men best-practice increases were only seen at the end of the period. In the late 1980s and the early 1990s, Denmark's life-expectancy improvement rates were close to zero. The pattern at age 65 is similar to the patterns described above but less pronounced and are even less so at age 80 (see Figures 14-3b and 14-3c).

In Sweden, life expectancy at birth for women in 2007 reached 83 years; for women who survived to age 83, remaining life expectancy was 7.5 additional years. Life disparity can be measured as the average remaining life expectancy at the ages when death occurs: in Sweden, a female death shortly after birth would contribute 83 years, whereas a death at age 83 would contribute 7.5 years. The average of such values, weighted by the number of deaths at each age, gives a life disparity of 9 (Zhang and Vaupel, 2009). Zhang and Vaupel (unpublished) performed analyses of the correlation between life disparity in a specific year and life expectancy in that year for men and women in 33 countries and regions. They found that during the 168 years from 1840 to 2007, 113 holders of record life expectancy also had the lowest life disparity. Countries with long life expectancy tend to have low life disparity because these countries have been successful in reducing premature deaths—doing so increases life expectancy and reduces life disparity. That is, efforts to avert deaths that occur at ages well below the life expectancy of a population appear to be especially effective in increasing life expectancy—and, simultaneously, reducing life disparity. Analyses of life disparity in Denmark show that a slowing of progress in reducing differentials in life spans occurred at about the same time as the slowing of progress in increasing life expectancy (see Figures 14-4a and 14-4b).

Cause-Specific Mortality in Denmark

Analyses of cause-specific mortality for men and women in Denmark show that mortality rates from major causes of death, such as heart disease, have declined since the 1970s. However, lung cancer mortality increased for women throughout the second half of the 20th century. For men the increase was more pronounced until around 1980, when the rate stabilized. For alcohol-related mortality, an increase is seen from 1970 onward for both genders, again most pronounced for men. Denmark is now among the countries with the highest tobacco- and alcohol-related mortality rates in 20 OECD countries (see Figures 14-5a and 14-5b), when alcohol-related deaths are calculated from alcohol-related diagnoses from death certificates and tobacco-related deaths are calculated from the method of Peto et al. (1992).

These cause-specific mortality rates correspond to the trend in the incidence of major underlying diseases. Figure 14-6 shows the dramatic increase in lung cancer among women in Denmark compared with other countries in the same time period. Figure 14-7 shows the dramatic decline in heart disease mortality in all the study countries, with Denmark, however, still having the highest mortality among women at the end of the period.

Peto et al. (1992) developed a method that uses absolute age- and sex-specific lung cancer rates to indicate the approximate proportions of deaths due to tobacco not only from lung cancer itself but also, indirectly, from vascular disease and various other categories of disease. This method was applied by Brønnum-Hansen and Juel (2000) to Danish data from the early

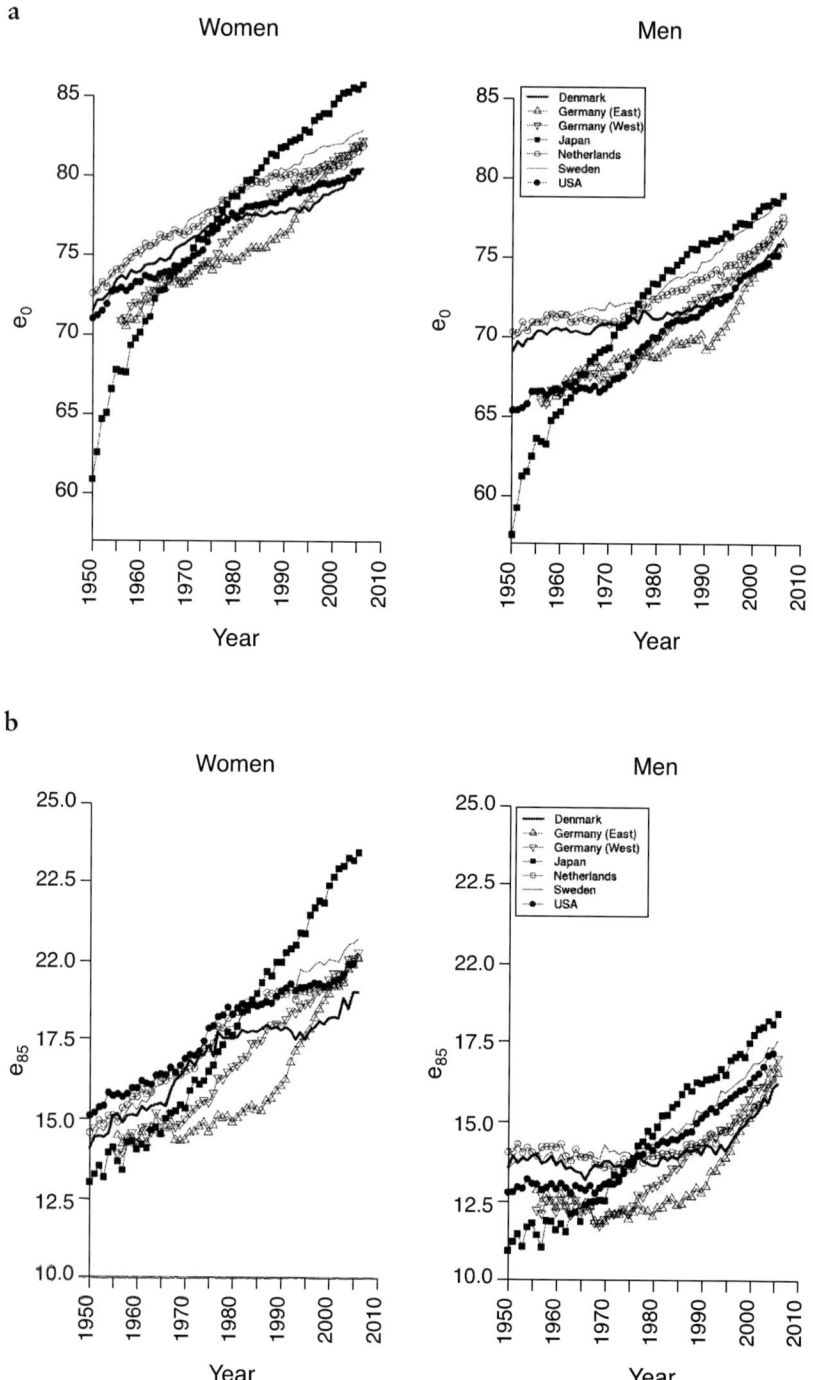

DIVERGENT LIFE EXPECTANCY TRENDS IN DENMARK AND SWEDEN 389

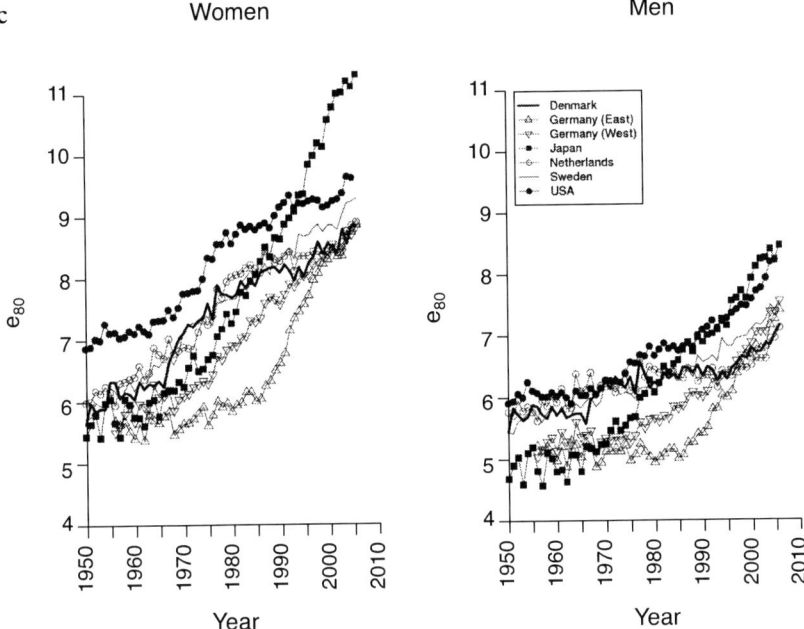

FIGURE 14-1 Life expectancy in Denmark and other high-income countries.
(a) At birth
(b) At age 65
(c) At age 80

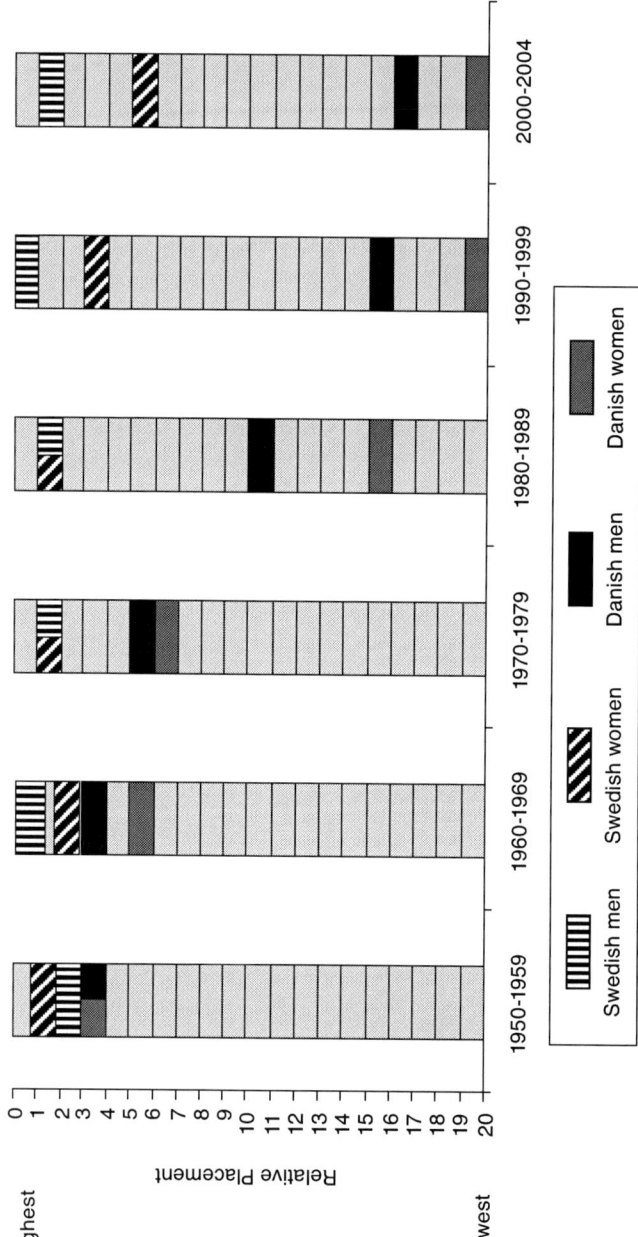

FIGURE 14-2 Denmark's and Sweden's rank in life expectancy at birth among 20 OECD countries.

1990s, and it shows that 35 percent of deaths among men and 25 percent of deaths among women were attributable to cigarette smoking. Brønnum-Hansen and Juel (2000) also applied a simulation model (Prevent), in which a multifactorial generalization of the etiological fraction is used, including information on several diseases and time dimensions simultaneously. The two methods are fundamentally different, but they give approximately the same results. The Prevent model estimated that 33 percent of deaths among men and 23 percent of deaths among women in the early 1990s were from chronic bronchitis, emphysema, ischemic heart disease, lung cancer, and stroke caused by cigarette smoking.

Life Expectancy in Denmark and Sweden

A comparison of life expectancy in Denmark and Sweden is particularly interesting due to their differences (their very divergent life-expectancy trends) and their similarities (close geographical and cultural proximity, both being Scandinavian welfare state countries, and having quite similar languages). In fact, Sweden is called *broderfolket* ("the brother people") in Denmark, and the two countries are separated by only a few miles of water (see Figure 14-8). The divergent trend of the two countries is illustrated in the OECD rankings in Figure 14-2 and in Lexis surface diagrams (Andreev, 2002). The surface diagrams show that, since 1980, Sweden has had lower or equal mortality at practically all ages for all cohorts. For children and teenagers, the Swedish advantages go back to the 1960s and 1970s. For Danish women, a clear cohort effect is seen with very high mortality, especially after age 40, for women born between the two world wars compared with similar Swedish women.

Juel (2008) estimated how much smoking- and alcohol-related mortality could explain the differences in life expectancy and mortality patterns in Denmark and Sweden. Smoking-related mortality was estimated by the Peto et al. (1992) method, and alcohol-related mortality was estimated by selecting deaths for which the diagnosis was related to alcohol (alcohol intoxication, alcoholism, cirrhosis of the liver, and pancreatitis).

Based on data from 1997-2001, Juel shows that smoking- and alcohol-related mortality could explain nearly all the difference between Danish and Swedish men and approximately three-quarters of the difference between Danish and Swedish women.

Distribution of Lifestyle Risk Factors

National comparable survey data are available for the period when Denmark went from stagnating to increasing in life expectancy. Four nationally representative health interview surveys among adult Danes were

392   INTERNATIONAL DIFFERENCES IN MORTALITY AT OLDER AGES

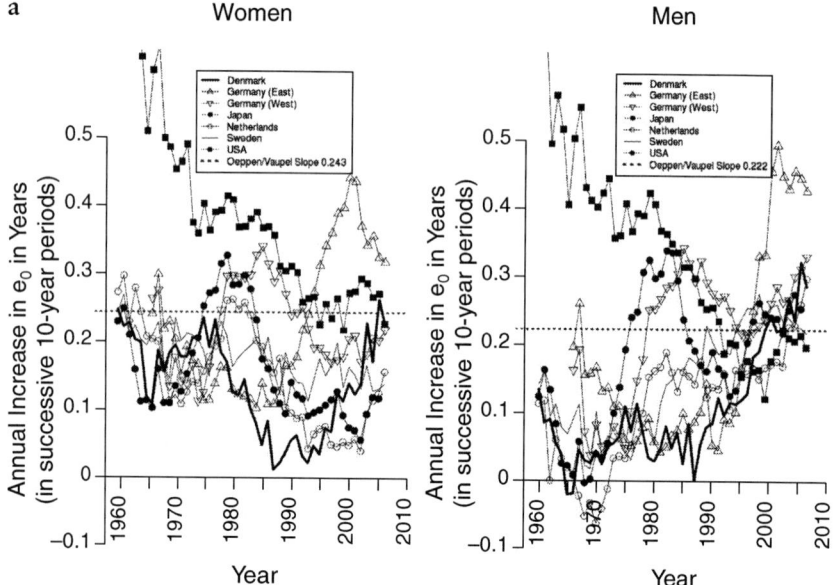

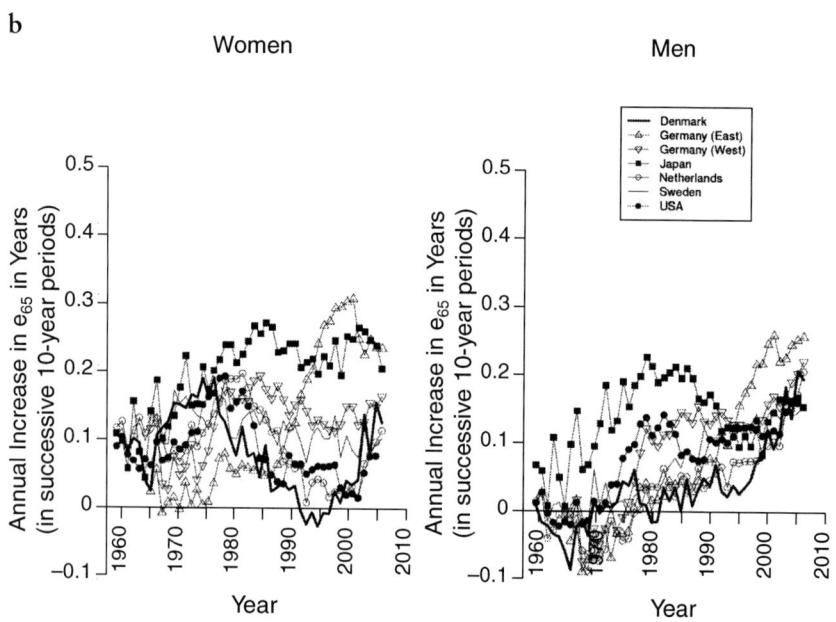

DIVERGENT LIFE EXPECTANCY TRENDS IN DENMARK AND SWEDEN

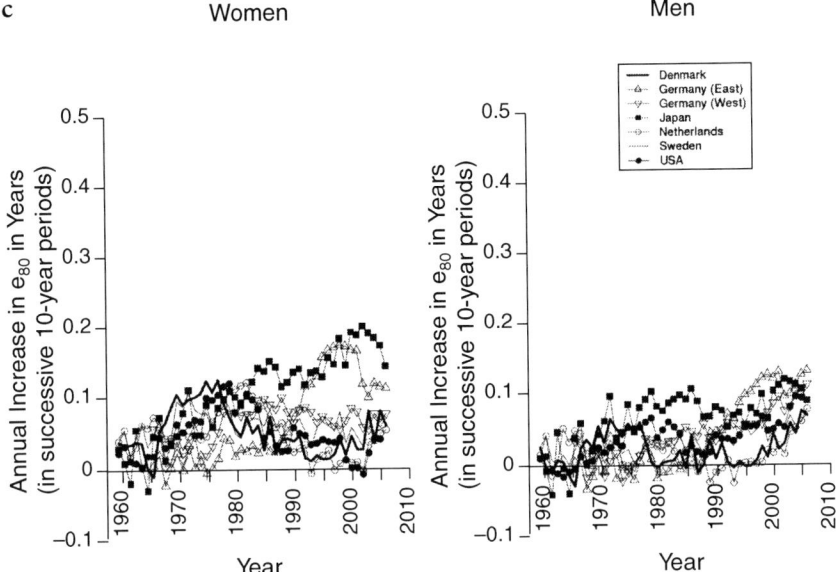

FIGURE 14-3 Annual increase in life expectancy.
(a) At birth
(b) At age 65
(c) At age 80

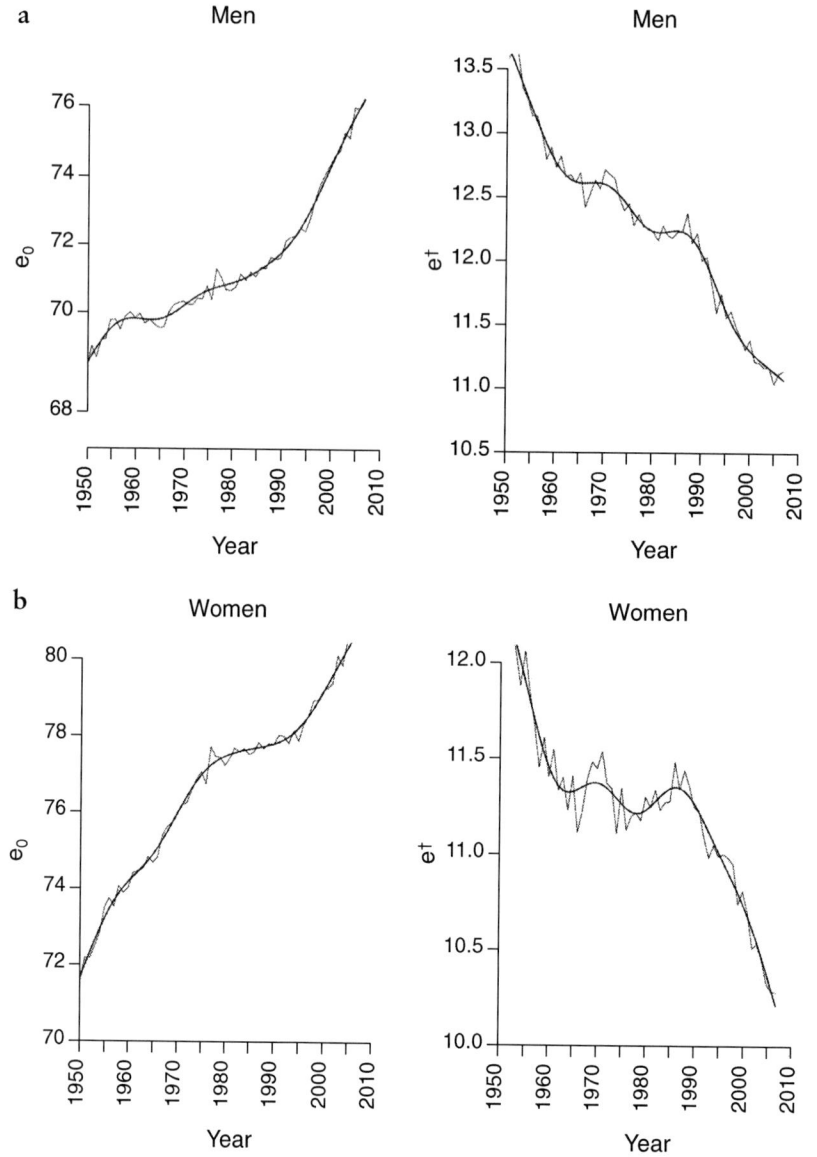

FIGURE 14-4 Life expectancy (e_0) and life disparity ($e^†$) over time for Danish women and men.
(a) Men
(b) Women
NOTE: Life disparity is a measure of discrepancies in life spans; it is calculated as the average remaining life expectancy at the ages of death (Zhang and Vaupel, 2009). Note the inverse relationship between life expectancy and life disparity: in years when life expectancy increases rapidly, life disparity decreases rapidly.

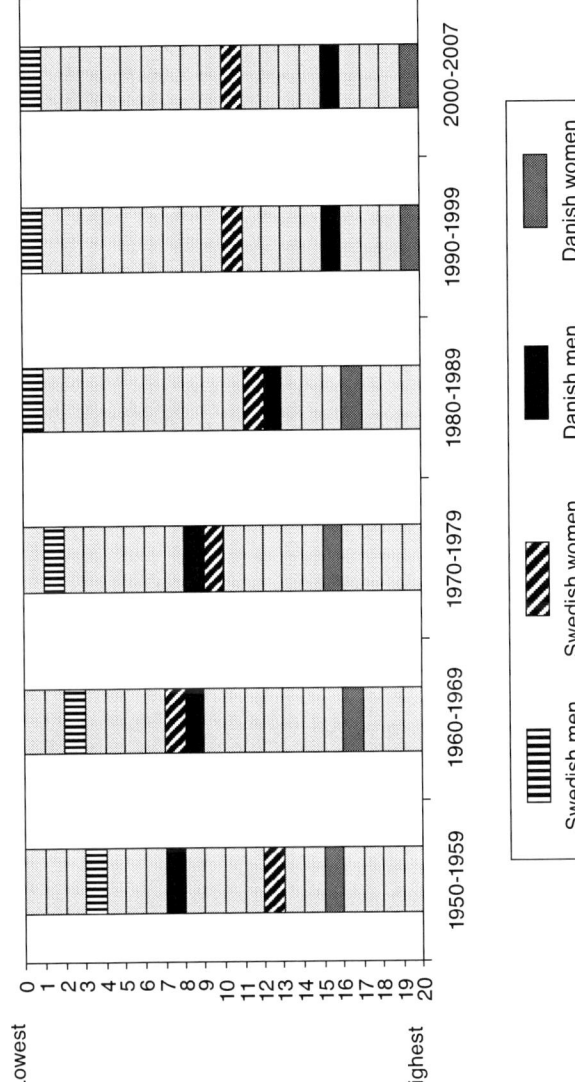

FIGURE 14-5 Denmark's rank among the 20 OECD countries for (a) tobacco-related mortality and (b) liver cirrhosis.
(a) Tobacco-related mortality
(b) Liver cirrhosis

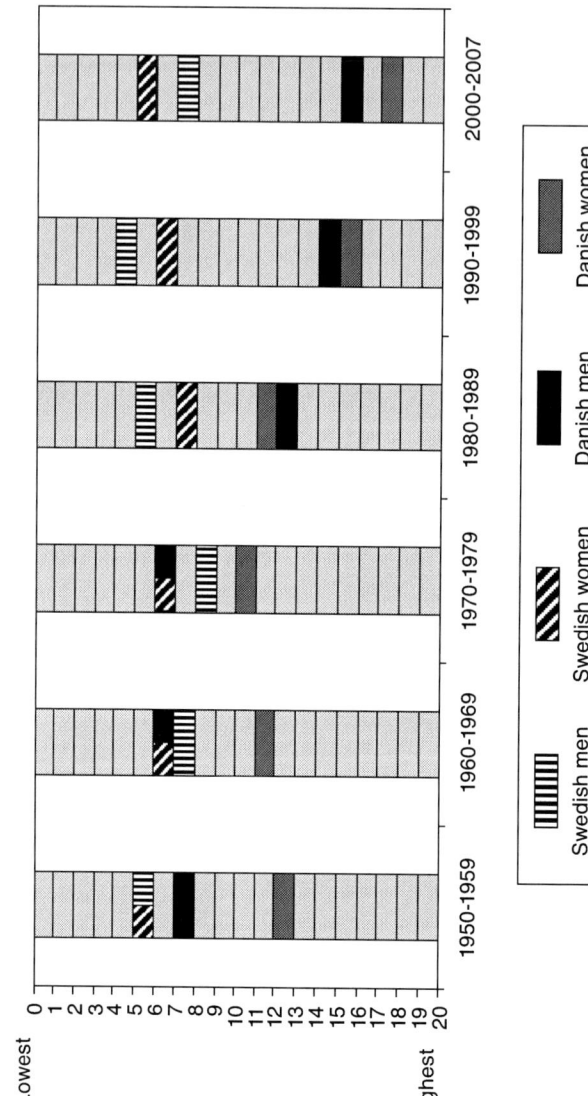

FIGURE 14-5 Continued.

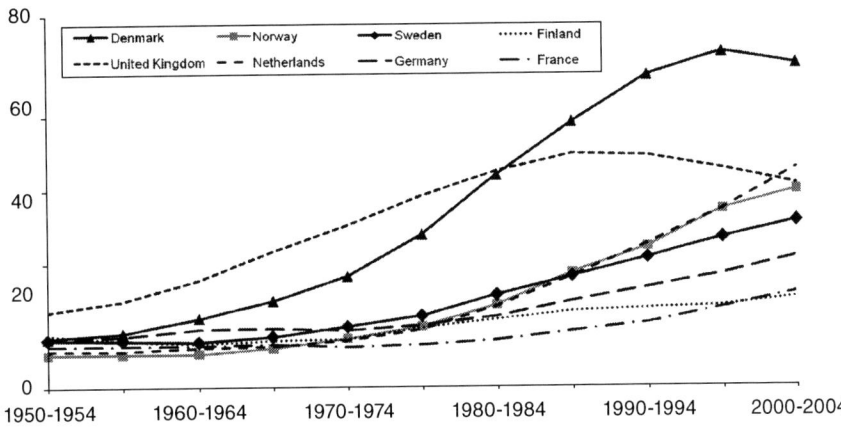

FIGURE 14-6 Lung cancer mortality for women ages 35-74 (age-standardized rates).

conducted in 1987, 1994, 2000, and 2005 (Ekholm et al., 2009). Individuals were sampled from the centralized civil register (CRS) (Pedersen et al., 2006). The CRS, which has existed in Denmark for more than 40 years, is a nationwide civil register whose purposes are to administrate the unique personal identification number system, to administer general personal data reported from national registration offices to the CRS, and to forward personal data in a technically/economically suitable manner in accordance with the Register's Act and other legislation governing civil registration. Each cohort of Danes in the health interview surveys consists of a nationally representative sample, with oversampling of some counties. For each cohort, information was collected by face-to-face home interviews in three waves. A detailed description is provided in Ekholm et al. (2009).

The analyses presented here are based on Danish men and women between the ages of 35 and 64. After the age of 35, most individuals have finished their education, and before the age of 65, most are still labor force participants. The participation rates were 80 percent, 78 percent, 74 percent, and 67 percent in the four cohorts, respectively. Behavioral variables included were alcohol consumption, smoking behavior, physical activity, and body mass index (BMI). Smoking habits were defined as "never smoker," "former smoker," "light smoker," and "heavy smoker" (≥ 15 cigarettes a day). Alcohol consumption was defined on the basis of a combination of number of drinks the last weekday and number of drinks the last weekend.

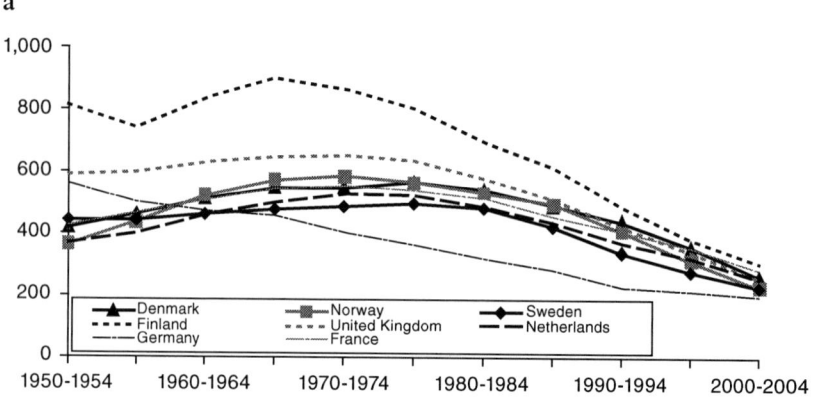
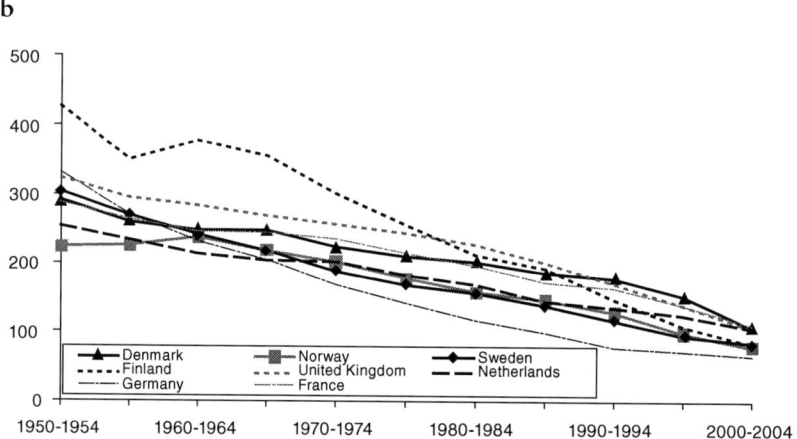

FIGURE 14-7 Heart disease mortality at ages 35-74 (age-standardized rates).
(a) Men
(b) Women

High alcohol consumption is defined as drinking above moderate drinking limits (21 units of alcohol for men and 14 for women per week). Physical activity during leisure time was categorized as none (sedentary), little (light exercise), and moderate/heavy (regular exercise more than 4 hours per week or competitive sport). From self-reported information on body weight and body height, the BMI was calculated as weight in kilograms divided by the square of height in meters. BMI was categorized as "underweight" (BMI < 18.5), "normal weight" (18.5 ≤ BMI < 25), "overweight" (25 ≤ BMI < 30),

DIVERGENT LIFE EXPECTANCY TRENDS IN DENMARK AND SWEDEN 399

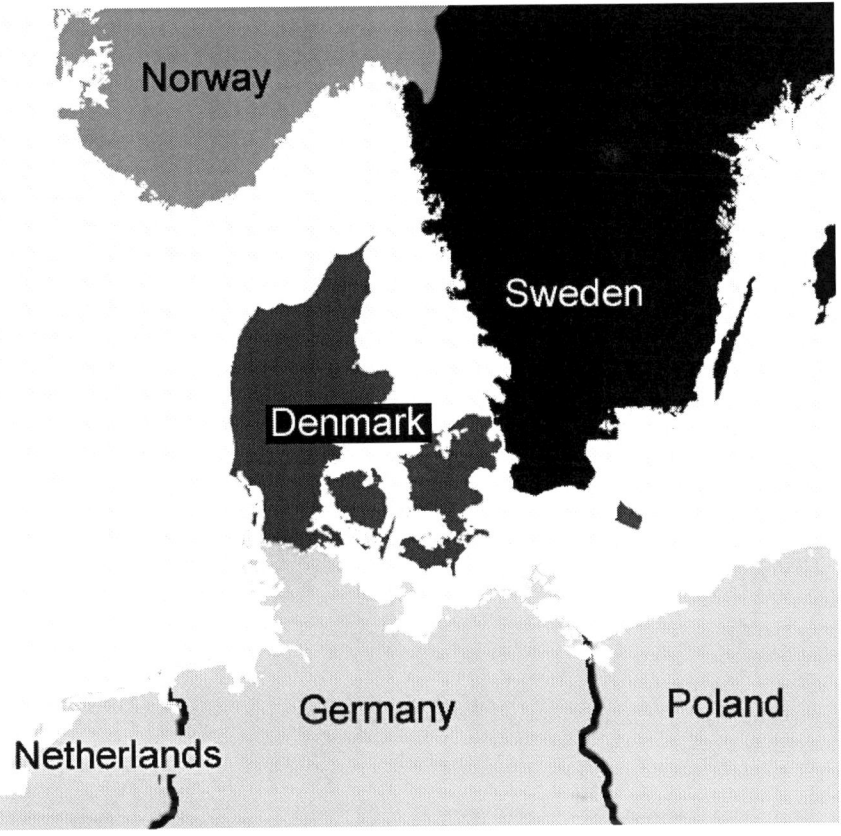

FIGURE 14-8 Neighboring Nordic countries with a 3-year difference in life expectancy: A few miles of water separate Denmark and Sweden.

and "obese" (BMI ≥ 30). The development from 1987 to 2005 is shown in Figures 14-9 through 14-12. The figures show that the improvement in Danish life expectancy that occurred in the mid-1990s co-occurs with a decrease in three mortality risk factors: smoking, alcohol consumption, and sedentary lifestyle, while one risk factor, the obesity rate, goes up, albeit to a low level compared with, for example, the United States (see Chapter 6, in this volume). A recent study shows the great impact of these risk factors on Danish life expectancy (Juel, Sorensen, and Bronnum-Hansen, 2008).

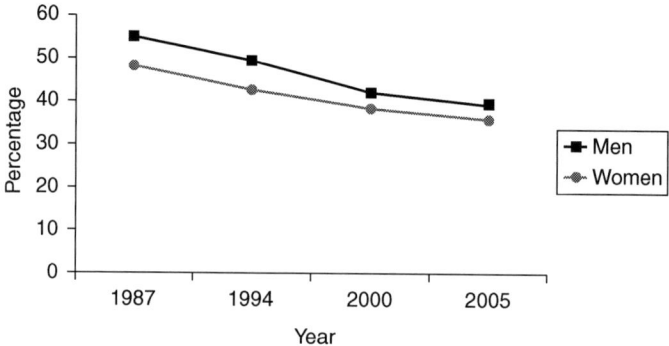

FIGURE 14-9 Proportion (%) of smokers in Denmark among men and women ages 35-64.
SOURCE: National Institute of Public Health, Copenhagen. Figures from the National Health Interview Surveys (2009).

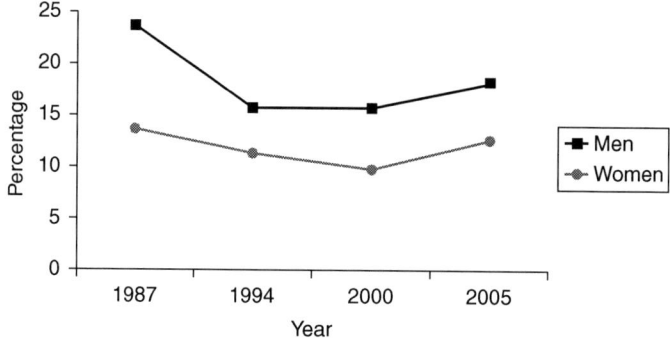

FIGURE 14-10 Alcohol consumption in Denmark among men and women ages 35-64.
NOTE: Proportion (%) drinking over moderate drinking limits. Alcohol consumption was defined on the basis of a combination of the number of drinks consumed the last weekday and the number of drinks consumed the last weekend. High alcohol consumption is defined as drinking above moderate drinking limits: 21 units of alcohol for men and 14 for women per week.

The Health Care System

There has been a long-standing debate concerning the extent to which the level of investment in the Danish health care system could account for part of the difference in life expectancy in Denmark and Sweden. Both countries base their health care policy on the Scandinavian universal welfare state model, with free and equal access to health care. Using the OECD

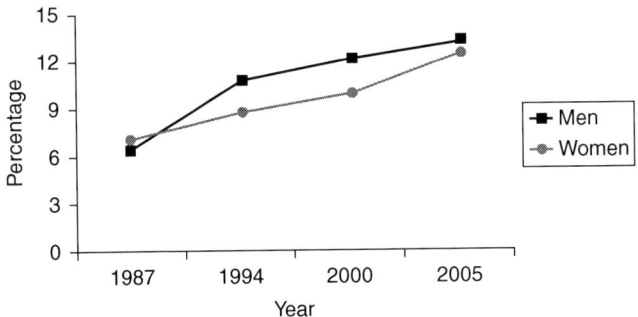

FIGURE 14-11 Proportion (%) of obese persons in Denmark among men and women ages 35-64.
NOTES: From self-reported information on body weight and body height, the BMI was calculated as weight in kilograms divided by the square of height in meters. BMI was categorized as "underweight" (BMI < 18.5), "normal weight" (18.5 ≤ BMI < 25), "overweight" (25 ≤ BMI < 30) and "obese" (BMI ≥ 30).

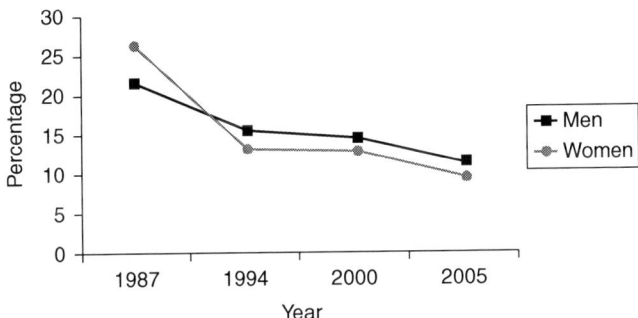

FIGURE 14-12 Proportion (%) of sedentary persons in Denmark among men and women ages 35-64.
NOTE: Physical activity during leisure time was categorized as none (sedentary), little (light exercise), and moderate/heavy (regular exercise more than 4 hours per week or participating in a competitive sport).

figures for health care expenditures (see http://www.oecd.org [accessed June 8, 2010]), Denmark and Sweden have very similar expenditures when measured as a percentage of each nation's gross domestic product (GDP). It has been argued, however, that in Denmark, unlike Sweden and many other countries, elder care (nursing homes and municipal support) is part of the official health care budget and thus raises health care expenditures by its inclusion (Søgaard, 2008). Considering that elder care is very well developed in Denmark, this entails substantial expenditures. It has been argued that if elder care were subtracted out, the real investment in more traditional health care, including hospitals, would result in a much lower figure for Denmark's health care expenditures as a percentage of GDP (Søgaard, 2008). The difference in, for example, case fatality rates for acute myocardial infarction among men ages 35-74, which is higher in Denmark (see Figure 14-13), could be due to a poorer performance of the Danish health care system, a system that might perform better with more investment. But it could also be due to the higher smoking and alcohol use in Denmark compared with Sweden, as both smoking and alcohol are known to worsen the prognosis for a wide variety of diseases.

To avoid the impact of patient lifestyle factors on the outcome, we studied neonatal mortality. Of course, maternal lifestyle factors influence neonatal mortality, but that influence is likely to be smaller than the impact of lifestyle on the individual herself. Neonatal survival chances are highly dependent on specialized medical care, which is typically administered by neonatal intensive care units, in which technologies, such as continuous positive airway pressure and surfactant therapy, have pushed the limit of viability downward (Goldenberg and Rouse, 1998). Using comparable data from the Danish, Norwegian, and Swedish national birth registries (Petersen et al., 2008), we studied neonatal mortality—defined as death within the first 28 days of life among live births, using comparable definitions in all three data sets, stratified for gestational age—and found an intriguing pattern (see Figure 14-14).

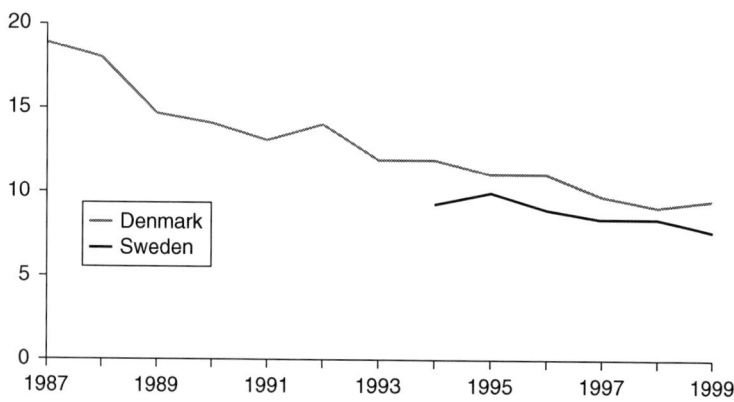

FIGURE 14-13 Health care indicator: Case-fatality rates on days 1-28 for acute myocardial infarction among men ages 35-74 in Denmark and Sweden, 1987-1999.

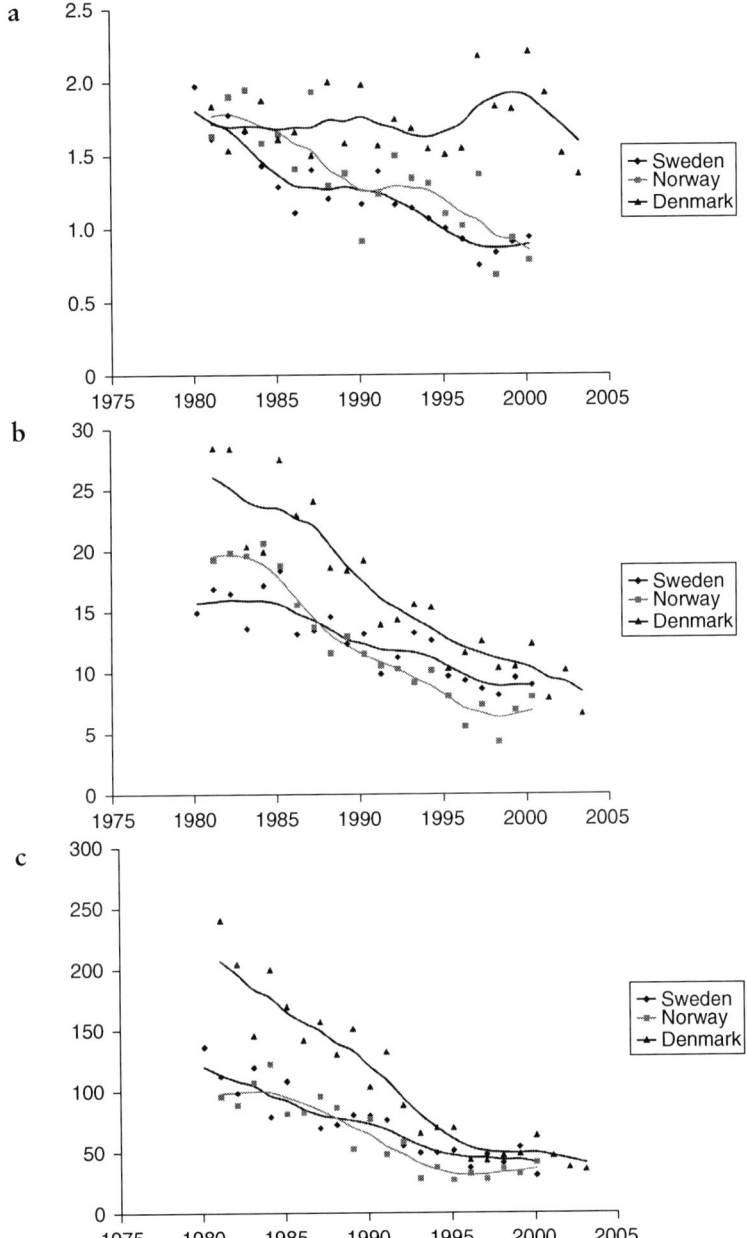

FIGURE 14-14 Neonatal mortality (0-28 days) per 1,000 births.
(a) Term newborns (37-42 weeks)
(b) Moderately preterm (33-36 wccks)
(c) Very preterm (28-32 weeks)

For children born at term, there were similar mortality rates in the three Scandinavian countries in the 1980s. In Denmark, the neonatal mortality has remained practically unchanged since that period, whereas there has been a decline in the other two Scandinavian countries. Among moderately preterm births (at 33-36 weeks), Denmark had higher mortality throughout the period but experienced a decline of a similar magnitude as the other two Scandinavian countries. Finally, for the very preterm births (at 28-32 weeks), Denmark had substantially higher mortality in the 1980s than the other two countries but caught up in the late 1990s. The result for the newborns born at term and the moderately preterm are compatible with a scenario suggesting that there is less effective health care in Denmark than in Sweden (or Norway), although a spillover of maternal effect (e.g., smoking) in Denmark cannot be excluded. However, the pattern of very preterm mortality in Denmark is not in accordance with that scenario, although it must be considered that the choice of intensity in the treatment of very preterm babies is not only a question of resources but also of ethical considerations and evaluation of the prognosis (EXPRESS Group, 2009). Apart from the effect of medical intervention following preterm birth, some of the change in association between gestational age and neonatal mortality might be due to elective termination of pregnancies, such as after screening early in pregnancy (Liu et al., 2002). However, the proportion of babies born before week 32 is similar in Sweden and Denmark (Petersen et al., 2009).

DISCUSSION

Smoking—The Major Explanation

The data presented above on cause-of-death trajectories, the disease incidence pattern, and the fractions of death estimated to be attributable to smoking using fundamentally different methods all suggest that smoking is the major explanation for the divergent Danish life expectancy trend compared with Sweden. This is in line with the work of Wang and Preston (2009) showing that cohort differences in smoking account for important anomalies in the recent age-sex pattern of mortality change in the United States.

An important question is: Why do Danes smoke more than people in comparable countries? An unusual explanation was suggested by Kesteloot (2001): "Halting of the decline in mortality occurred about 5 years after the ascension to the throne of Denmark by Queen Margrethe II. The queen is very popular in Denmark and a known cigarette smoker. As a role model for women, the Queen's example could offer an explanation for the unusual mortality in Danish women." However, the excess mortality for

Danish women born between the two world wars had previously been extensively studied (Jacobsen et al., 2000, 2001, 2004, 2006; Juel, 2000; Juel, Bjernegaard, and Madsen, 2000), and studies document that the stagnation started well before the queen took the throne. A more likely explanation is the liberal Danish tobacco policy; it was not until 2007 that smoking was prohibited in restaurants, and there are still exceptions (smoking is allowed in small restaurants).

Lifestyle and Health Care—Other Likely Contributors

The increase in alcohol-related deaths in Denmark and fractions of death estimated to be attributable to alcohol use suggest an important role also for alcohol, especially when comparing Denmark and Sweden. There are also some indications that investment in health care is lower in Denmark than in Sweden. The prognosis for both heart disease and cancer (see Figure 14-13 and Specht and Lundberg, 2001) is poorer, although it cannot be ruled out that the higher smoking prevalence and alcohol consumption, as well as other lifestyle factors, play a role in this development. Finally, analyses of life disparity (i.e., differences in life span) in Denmark suggest a slowing of progress in reducing life disparity occurring at roughly the same time as the slowing of progress in increasing life expectancy. That is, Danish life expectancy may have stagnated, at least in part, because the Danes did not continue to reduce inequalities in the length of life in the 1970s and 1980s.

What Caused the Change in Life Expectancy in Denmark?

The change from stagnation to improvement in life expectancy in the mid-1990s coincided with a decrease in the prevalence of major lifestyle risk factors: smoking, alcohol consumption, and sedentary lifestyle, which correspond to the changes seen in disease incidence. The obesity rate went up in the same time period, but only to a low level when compared with the United States. Denmark's generally positive development in lifestyle risk factors occurs despite a widespread reluctance toward "paternalistic policy" in the country. As an example, smoking was not prohibited in restaurants in Denmark until 2007. Also co-occurring with the change from stagnation to improvement in life expectancy in the mid-1990s, Denmark instituted what is called the "Heart Plan," which allocated substantial national funding to improve cardiovascular disease treatments.

The reason for the improvement in life expectancy in the early 1990s is mainly decreasing cardiovascular mortality, probably attributable to a better lifestyle profile for most Danes, more behavioral and medical disease prevention services, and better medical and surgical treatment.

REFERENCES

Andreev, K.F. (2002). *Evolution of the Danish Population from 1835 to 2000*. Odense monographs on population aging 9. Odense, Denmark: Odense University Press.

Brønnum-Hansen, H., and Juel, K. (2000). Estimating mortality due to cigarette smoking: Two methods, same result. *Epidemiology, 11*(4), 422-426.

Ekholm, O., Hesse, U., Davidsen, M., and Kjøller, M. (2009). The study design and characteristics of the Danish national health interview surveys. *Scandinavian Journal of Public Health* (in press).

EXPRESS Group. (2009). One-year survival of extremely preterm infants after active perinatal care in Sweden. *Journal of the American Medical Association, 301*(21), 2225-2233.

Jacobsen, R., Keiding, N., and Lynge, E. (2000). Long-term mortality trends behind low life expectancy of Danish women. *Journal of Epidemiology and Community Health, 65*, 205-208.

Jacobsen, R., Jensen, A., Keiding, N., and Lynge, E. (2001). Queen Margrethe II and mortality in Denmark. *Lancet, 358*, 875.

Jacobsen, R., Von Euler, M., Osler, M., Lynge, E., and Keiding, N. (2004). Women's death in Scandinavia—What makes Denmark different? *European Journal of Epidemiology, 19*, 117-121.

Jacobsen, R., Keiding, N., and Lynge, E. (2006). Causes of death behind low life expectancy of Danish women. *Scandinavian Journal of Public Health, 34*, 432-436.

Juel, K. (2000). Increased mortality among Danish women: Population based register study. *British Medical Journal, 321*(7257), 349-350.

Juel, K. (2004). *Mortality in Denmark During 100 Years. The Danes Are Living Longer, but Why 3-4 Years Shorter than Swedish Men and French Women?* Copenhagen, Denmark: National Institute of Public Health.

Juel, K. (2008). Middellevetid og dødelighed i Danmark sammenlignet med i Sverige. Hvad betyder rygning og alkohol? [Life expectancy and mortality in Denmark compared to Sweden. What is the effect of smoking and alcohol?] *Ugeskr Laeger, 170*(33), 2423-2427.

Juel, K., and Christensen, K. (2007). Kønsforskelle i dødelighed i Danmark 1840-2005. Kvinder lever længere end mænd, men der er sket store ændringer i de seneste 50 år. *Ugeskr Læger, 169*(25), 2398-2403.

Juel, K., Bjerregaard, P., and Madsen, M. (2000). Mortality and life expectancy in Denmark and in other European countries: What is happening to middle-aged Danes? *European Journal of Public Health, 10*(2), 93-100.

Juel, K., Sorensen, J., and Bronnum-Hansen, H. (2008). Risk factors and public health in Denmark. *Scandinavian Journal of Public Health, 36*(Suppl 1), 112-227.

Kesteloot, H. (2001). Queen Margrethe II and mortality in Danish women. *Lancet, 357*, 871-72.

Kramer, M.S. (2003). The epidemiology of adverse pregnancy outcomes. *Journal of Nutrition, 133*(5 Suppl 2), 1592S-1596S.

Kramer, M.S., Demissie, K., Yang, H., Platt, R.W., Sauve, R., and Liston, R. (2000). The contribution of mild and moderate preterm birth to infant mortality. Fetal and Infant Health Study Group of the Canadian Perinatal Surveillance System. *Journal of the American Medical Association, 284*, 843-849.

Liu, S., Joseph, K.S., Kramer, M.S., Allen, A.C., Sauve, R., Rusen, I.D., and Wen, S.W. (2002). Relationship of prenatal diagnosis and pregnancy termination to overall infant mortality in Canada. *Journal of the American Medical Association, 287*(12), 1561-1567.

Mortensen, L.H., Diderichsen, F., Arntzen, A., Gissler, M., Cnattingius, S., Schnor, O., Davey-Smith, G., Nybo Andersen, A-M. (2008). Social inequality in fetal growth: A comparative study. *Journal of Epidemiology and Community Health, 62*(4), 325-331.

Oeppen, J., and Vaupel, J.W. (2002). Broken limits to life expectancy. *Science, 296*, 1029-1031.

Pedersen, C.B., Gotzsche, H., Moller, J.O., and Mortensen, P.B. (2006). The Danish Civil Registration System: A cohort of eight million persons. *Danish Medical Bulletin, 53*(4), 441-449.

Petersen, C.B., Mortensen, L.H., Morgen, C.S., Madsen, M., Schnor, O., Arntzen, A., Gissler, M., Cnattingius, S., and Andersen, A.M. (2009). Socio-economic inequality in preterm birth: A comparative study of the Nordic countries from 1981 to 2000. *Paediatric and Perinatal Epidemiology, 23*, 66-75.

Peto, R., Lopez, A.D., Boreham, J., Thun, M., and Heath, C. (1992). Mortality from tobacco in developed countries: Indirect estimation from national vital statistics. *Lancet, 339*, 1268-1278.

Rasmussen, S., Abildstrøm, S.Z., Rosén, M., and Madsen, M. (2004). Case-fatality rates for myocardial infarction declined in Denmark and Sweden during 1987-1999. *Journal of Clinical Epidemiology, 57*, 638-646.

Søgaard, J. (2008). Har 35 års lavvækst I sundhedsvæsenet betydet større social ulighed i sundhed i Danmark? In J.G. Rasmussen and N. Döllner (Eds.), *Den tunge ende. Sandheden om ulighederne og uretfærdighederne i den danske sundhed* (pp. 175-191). Copenhagen, Denmark: Forfatterne og Dagens Medicins Bøger.

Specht, L.K., and Landberg, T. (2001). Kræftbehandling i Skåne og på Sjælland. Er forskelle i udredning og behandling med til at forklare danske kræftpatienters dårligere overlevelse? [Cancer treatment in Skane and in Sjaelland. Do differences concerning examination and treatment explain reduced survival among Danish cancer patients?] *Ugeskr Laeger, 163*, 439-442.

Wang, H., and Preston, S.H. (2009). Forecasting United States mortality using cohort smoking histories. *Proceedings of the National Academy of Sciences, 106*(2), 393-398.

Zhang, Z., and Vaupel, J.W. (2009). The age separating early deaths from late deaths. *Demographic Research, 20*, 721-730.

Biographical Sketches of Contributors

Dawn Alley completed her Ph.D. in gerontology at the University of Southern California, Davis, School of Gerontology, followed by postdoctoral studies as a Robert Wood Johnson Foundation Health and Society Scholar at the University of Pennsylvania. She is currently an assistant professor of epidemiology and preventive medicine at the University of Maryland School of Medicine, where her research focuses on obesity, biomarkers, and health disparities among older adults. Her work on obesity has appeared in the *Journal of the American Medical Association* and *Archives of Internal Medicine*.

Mauricio Avendano is assistant professor at the Erasmus University Medical Center and research fellow at the Center for Population and Development studies at Harvard University. His current research focuses on the role of national institutions and policies in shaping the pathways and magnitude of the socioeconomic status (SES) gradient in health in the United States and Europe. He has been awarded several grants to explore how social and economic aspects of life relate to health outcomes, and how these processes occur differently across various societies. He has been closely involved in the design, data collection, and analysis of the Survey of Health, Ageing and Retirement in Europe (SHARE). He is also involved in the European Global Burden of Disease Study, aimed at quantifying mortality attributable to SES. He has published in major epidemiological and medical journals, including *Lancet, American Journal of Public Health, Bulletin of the World Health Organization, American Journal of Epidemiology*, and *Stroke*.

James Banks is professor of economics at the University of Manchester and deputy research director of the Institute for Fiscal Studies, where he also directs the Centre for Economic Research on Ageing. His research focuses on empirical modeling of individual economic behavior over the life cycle, with particular focus on consumption and spending patterns, saving and asset accumulation, housing dynamics, and retirement and pension choices. Recent work has also begun to look at broader issues in the economics of aging, such as health, physical, and cognitive functioning and their association with labor market status; the dynamics of work disability; and the nature of expectations of retirement, health, and longevity. He is also coprincipal investigator of the English Longitudinal Study of Ageing and has become actively involved in designing economic measures for survey data. He holds a Ph.D. in economics from University College London.

Magali Barbieri has a joint position as an associate researcher at the Institut National d'Études Démographiques (INED) in Paris, France, and at the Department of Demography, University of California, Berkeley, where she is in charge of coordinating the Human Mortality Database project. She conducts research on a wide range of topics, including infant and child mortality in both developed and developing countries; changes in the structure of mortality by cause over time and across countries; and health in colonial Vietnam. Her most recent publications in English include a coedited volume on changes in the Vietnamese family after 20 years of socioeconomic reforms; a long coauthored article on 50 years of demographic trends in East and Southeast Asia; and an article on the mortality consequences of the 2003 heat wave in France.

Lisa F. Berkman is director, Harvard Center for Population and Development Studies and Thomas D. Cabot Professor of Public Policy, Epidemiology and Population and International Health within the Harvard School of Public Health. She is a social epidemiologist whose work is oriented toward understanding social inequalities in health and aging related to socioeconomic status, labor policy, and social networks and social isolation. She has recently started research on labor issues related to job design and flexibility. The majority of her work is devoted to identifying the role of social networks and support in predicting declines in physical and cognitive functioning, onset of disease, and mortality, especially related to cardiovascular or cerebrovascular disease. She has a Ph.D. in epidemiology from the University of California, Berkeley.

Carl Boe is research demographer with the Center on the Economics and Demography of Aging at the University of California, Berkeley. His research focuses on stochastic forecasting of mortality and population, biodemography, and life table calculations for the Human Mortality Database. He holds an M.A. in statistics and a Ph.D. in demography, both from the University of California, Berkeley.

Kaare Christensen is a professor of epidemiology at the Institute of Public Health, University of Southern Denmark, and a senior research scientist at the Terry Sanford Institute, Duke University, North Carolina. Christensen is the director of the Danish Twin Registry and the Danish Aging Research Centre, and he has conducted a long series of studies among twins and the oldest-old in order to shed light on the importance of genes and environment in aging and longevity. Furthermore, he has a longstanding interest in the relation between early life events and later life health outcome. He is engaged in interdisciplinary aging research combining methods from epidemiology, genetics, and demography. Professor Christensen received his Ph.D. at Odense University in 1994 and DMSc at the University of Southern Denmark in 1999.

Barney Cohen is director of the Committee on Population of the National Academies/NRC. His work at the NRC has encompassed a wide variety of domestic and international projects, including studies on fertility, morbidity, mortality, housing, urbanization, migration, aging, and HIV/AIDS. Currently, he is also serving as the liaison of the National Academies to the Academy of Science of South Africa and the Ghanaian Academy of Arts and Sciences as part of a larger project aimed at supporting the development of academies of science in Africa. Cohen holds an M.A. in economics from the University of Delaware and a Ph.D. in demography from the University of California, Berkeley.

Eileen M. Crimmins is AARP chair in gerontology and professor of gerontology and sociology at the University of Southern California (USC). She is also director of the USC/University of California, Los Angeles, Center on Biodemography and Population Health. Her research is on health trends, health change with age healthy life expectancy, and health differences in the population. She also examines how social, psychological, and biological factors affect health. Dr. Crimmins is a coprincipal investigator on the Health and Retirement Survey. She has served on a number of National Institute on Aging monitoring committees and on the board of counselors of the National Center for Health Statistics. She has a Ph.D. in demography from the University of Pennsylvania.

Michael Davidsen is a senior researcher at the National Institute of Public Health, University of Southern Denmark. His main topic is design and analysis of public health surveys with a special focus on health and morbidity.

Krista Garcia is currently a Ph.D. student at the University of Southern California (USC) Davis School of Gerontology whose research is done within the USC/University of California, Los Angeles, Center on Biodemography and Population Health. Her research focuses on cross-country comparisons in health outcomes and secondary prevention strategies.

Joop Garssen studied geography and non-Western demography at the University of Groningen, the Netherlands, and community health at the London School of Hygiene and Tropical Medicine. From 1978 to 1993, he was involved in demographic and health research in the South Pacific, and West and East Africa. Since 1993, he has been employed as editor and senior researcher at the department of demography, Statistics Netherlands.

Dana A. Glei is a senior research investigator at Georgetown University. Since 2001, she has worked on the Social Environment and Biomarkers of Aging Study (Taiwan). During 2001-2009, she also served as project coordinator for the Human Mortality Database project (http://www.mortality.org), a joint collaboration between researchers at the University of California, Berkeley, and the Max Planck Institute for Demographic Research. Her current research focuses on the effects of smoking on mortality and sex differences in mortality, the impact of stressors on subsequent health, and the role of bioindicators in mediating the relationship between psychosocial factors and health outcomes. She has an M.A. in sociology from the University of Virginia and a Ph.D. in sociology from Princeton University.

M. Maria Glymour is an assistant professor in the Department of Society, Human Development, and Health at the Harvard School of Public Health. Her research focuses on social determinants of cognitive aging; social inequalities in stroke; and adapting methodological innovations to overcome causal inference problems in social epidemiology.

Noreen Goldman is the Hughes-Rogers Professor of Demography and Public Affairs at the Woodrow Wilson School, Princeton University. She conducts research in areas of demography and epidemiology, and her current research examines the role of social and economic factors on adult health and the physiological pathways through which these factors operate. She has designed several large-scale health surveys in Latin America and Taiwan. She has been a fellow at the Center for Advanced Study in the Behavioral Sciences, served on the Institute of Medicine's Board on Global Health, the National Research Council's Committee on National Statistics, and the Population Research Subcommittee of the National Institute of Child Health and Human Development. She has a D.Sc. in population studies from Harvard University.

Jessica Ho is currently a graduate student in the Graduate Group in Demography at the University of Pennsylvania. Her recent research has focused on health and mortality. She holds a B.A. in economics and health and societies from the University of Pennsylvania.

Knud Juel received his Ph.D. from the University of Copenhagen in 1996. His field of research includes life expectancy, mortality, impact of risk factors on health, and smoking. He is currently the programme director of the Research Programme on Public Health in Denmark at the National Institute of Public Health University of Southern Denmark.

Ichiro Kawachi is professor of social epidemiology, and chair of the Department of Society, Human Development and Health at the Harvard School of Public Health. Kawachi received both his medical degree and Ph.D. (in epidemiology) from the University of Otago, New Zealand. He has taught at the Harvard School of Public Health since 1992. Kawachi has published widely on the relationship between stress and cardiovascular disease, as well as the broader social and economic determinants of population health. He was the coeditor (with Lisa Berkman) of the first textbook on *Social Epidemiology*, published by Oxford University Press in 2000. His books include *The Health of Nations* (The New Press, 2002) and *Social Capital and Health* (Springer, 2008). Kawachi currently serves as the senior editor (Social Epidemiology) of the international journal *Social Science & Medicine*, as well as an editor of the *American Journal of Epidemiology*. He has served as a consultant to the World Health Organization and the World Bank.

Jung Ki Kim is a research assistant professor at the Andrus Gerontology Center of the University of Southern California. She received a Ph.D. in gerontology/public policy at the University of Southern California and a dual master's in gerontology and social work. Her dissertation was on the effect of marital status on health outcomes among older people, particularly how different marital status, changes of marital status, duration of widowhood, and living arrangements affect health outcomes. She has done research on health and health-related issues in large national data sets. Her current and future research interests include work on socioeconomic status and biological risk, social support and health among older people, and cross-country comparison of health status.

Renske Kok is a consultant for Strategies in Regulated Markets (SiRM), a Dutch consulting firm with a major focus on health care. She uses econometric and epidemiological research techniques in cross-country comparisons of health and health care in Europe. Recent projects have dealt with evaluations of quality indicators and market analysis of curative care.

Previously she worked as a scientific researcher in the Department of Public Health at Erasmus University, where she was closely involved in the Survey of Health, Ageing and Retirement in Europe (SHARE), a comparative study of 15 countries. The project was designed to study the interaction between health and the social and economic dimensions of life in European countries. Kok was also part of the SHARELIFE project group, an extension of SHARE that aims to understand aging from a life-course perspective. Her current work involves the study of socioeconomic disparities in depression across European countries and the influence of reporting differences in these disparities. She has an M.Sc. in economics from Tilburg University and an M.Sc. in health economics from Erasmus University.

Anton Kunst is associate professor at the Department of Public Health, Academic Medical Centre (AMC), University of Amsterdam. Until 2009, he was also senior researcher at the Erasmus MC Rotterdam. His research focuses on geographic, socioeconomic, and ethnic inequalities in mortality, disability, diseases, and their risk factors including smoking and obesity. In addition to research focusing on the Netherlands, he has performed comparative studies at European and global levels. He has coordinated several European projects on socioeconomic inequalities in health, often with an emphasis on mortality. Currently, he also evaluates the population health impact of social policies at national and local levels. He has published on these topics in more than 150 papers in international journals.

Jennifer Lloyd is a doctoral student in the Doctoral Program in Gerontology at the University of Maryland, Baltimore. She currently works as a graduate assistant for the Peter Lamy Center for Drug Therapy and Aging, where she works with data from the Medicare Current Beneficiary Survey, and for the Department of Epidemiology and Preventive Medicine, where she works on a study related to caregivers of hip fracture patients.

Johan P. Mackenbach is chair of the Department of Public Health and Professor of Public Health at Erasmus University in Rotterdam, the Netherlands. He is also a registered epidemiologist and public health physician. His research interests include social epidemiology, medical demography, and health services research. He has coauthored about 350 papers in international, peer-reviewed scientific journals, as well as a number of books, and many book chapters and papers in Dutch-language journals. He is the editor in chief of the *European Journal of Public Health*, and he has coordinated a number of international-comparative studies funded by the European Commission. His current research focuses on socioeconomic inequalities in health, on issues related to aging and compression of morbidity, and on the effectiveness and quality of health services. He is actively engaged in exchanges between research and policy, among others as a member of several government advisory councils in the Netherlands (the Health Council, and the Council for Public Health and Health Care). He is a member of the Dutch Royal Academy of Sciences. He has both an M.D. and Ph.D. in public health from Erasmus University.

France Meslé was director of research at INED (National Institute for Demographic Studies in Paris) in the Mortality, Health, and Epidemiology research unit from 2003 to 2008. She was editor of the *European Journal for Population* from 2001 to 2005 and in charge of the INED web site in 1997-2000. Her research is mainly devoted to mortality and causes of death, especially long-term trends in causes of death, health crisis in Eastern Europe, and trends in mortality at old ages. She is leading a collaborative project on cause-of-death trends in the former USSR, which gathers several research teams from Russia, Ukraine, the Baltic countries, Armenia, Belarus, Georgia, and Moldova. She has an M.A. in demography from the University of Paris 1 and an M.D. from the University of Paris 6.

Laust H. Mortensen is a postdoctoral student at the unit of epidemiology at the University of Southern Denmark. He holds a Ph.D. in epidemiology from the University of Copenhagen.

Fred Pampel is professor of sociology and research associate of the Population Program at the University of Colorado, Boulder. He has served as sociology program officer at the National Science Foundation and associate vice chancellor for research at the University of Colorado, Boulder. His research focuses on cross-national patterns of tobacco use and on disparities in use by socioeconomic, gender, and race groups. He also examines the contribution of these smoking patterns to recent changes in the sex differential in mortality, widening of socioeconomic status disparities in health and mortality, and diverging patterns of mortality across developed and developing countries.

Samuel H. Preston is professor of demography, School of Arts and Sciences, the University of Pennsylvania. He has been a member of the sociology department since 1979. His research focuses on the causes and consequences of population change, with special attention to mortality. He is a member of the National Academy of Sciences and Institute of Medicine, as well as the American Philosophical Society. He is a fellow of the American Academy of Arts and Sciences, the American Association for the Advancement of Science, and the American Statistical Association. He holds a Ph.D. in economics from Princeton University.

Roland Rau is junior professor of demography at the University of Rostock, Germany, and research fellow at the Max Planck Institute for Demographic Research in Rostock, Germany. His research focuses on human mortality in highly developed countries. Before working for 2 years at Duke University's Population Research Institute as a research scholar, Rau received in 2006 the Otto-Hahn-Medal of the Max Planck Society for his doctoral dissertation on seasonal fluctuations in human mortality. He has a Ph.D. in demography from the University of Rostock, Germany.

Michelle Shardell is an assistant professor in the Department of Epidemiology and Preventive Medicine at the University of Maryland, School of Medicine. She received her Ph.D. in biostatistics from Johns Hopkins University, Bloomberg School of Public Health. Her research interests include the use of proxy data in studies of older adults, as well as determinants of health decline and recovery in older persons.

James P. Smith holds the RAND Chair in Labor Markets and Demographic Studies and was the director of RAND's Labor and Population Studies Program from 1977-1994. He has led numerous projects, including studies of immigration, the economics of aging, black-white wages and employment, wealth accumulation and savings behavior, the relation of health and economic status, the impact of the Asian economic crisis, and the causes and consequences of economic growth. Smith has worked extensively in Europe and Asia for 30 years. He currently serves as chair of the National Institute on Aging Data Monitoring Committee for the Health and Retirement Survey and was chair of the National Science Foundation Advisory Committee for the Panel Study of Income Dynamics. He has served as an international advisor on implementing health and retirement surveys in China, continental Europe, England, Korea, and Thailand. He was the public representative appointed by the governor on the California Occupational Health and Safety Board. He has twice received the National Institutes of Health MERIT Award, the most distinguished honor the National Institutes of Health grants to a researcher. He has a Ph.D. in economics from the University of Chicago.

Andrew Steptoe is British Heart Foundation professor of psychology at University College London (UCL). He graduated from Cambridge in 1972 and completed his doctorate at Oxford University in 1975. He moved to St. George's Hospital Medical School in 1977, becoming professor and chair of the department in 1988, where he remained until his appointment in 2000 to UCL. He is a past president of the International Society of Behavioral Medicine and of the Society for Psychosomatic Research. He was elected to fellowship of the Academy of Medical Sciences in 2008. He was founding editor of the *British Journal of Health Psychology*, an associate editor of

Psychophysiology, the *Annals of Behavioral Medicine*, the *British Journal of Clinical Psychology*, the *International Journal of Rehabilitation and Health*, and the *Journal of Psychosomatic Research*, and he is on the editorial boards of seven other journals. He is author or editor of 16 books, including *Psychosocial Processes and Health* (Cambridge University Press, 1994) and *Depression and Physical Illness* (Cambridge University Press, 2006). His main research interests are in psychosocial aspects of physical illness, health behavior, psychobiology, and aging. Steptoe joined the management group of the English Longitudinal Study of Ageing (ELSA) in 2008, and he is coprincipal investigator of the UCL ELSA group.

Jacques Vallin is emeritus research director at the Institut National d'Études Démographiques. His research interests include health transition, inequalities in death, causes of death, life expectancy and life span, population and development, consequences of global population growth, and population of the Maghreb. He is a coeditor of *Demography Analysis and Synthesis*, a four-volume treatise of demography recently published by Academic Press. He taught postgraduate courses at the Institut d'Études Politiques de Paris. He is honorary president of the International Union for the Scientific Study of Population, and he is also member of the Population Association of America, the European Association for Population Studies, and the Union for African Population Studies. He has a Ph.D. in demography from the University of Paris.

James W. Vaupel is the founding director of the Max Planck Institute for Demographic Research in Rostock, Germany, as well as director of Duke University's Population Research Institute. He oversees research projects in China, Denmark, Germany, Italy, Japan, Mexico, Russia, and the United States. He is best known for his research on mortality, morbidity, population aging, and biodemography (for which he received the Irene Taeuber Award from the Population Association of America), as well as for research on population heterogeneity, population surfaces, and other aspects of mathematical and statistical demography (for which he received the Mindel Sheps Award from the Population Association of America). He is a member of the U.S. National Academy of Sciences and the Max Planck Society for the Advancement of Science as well as a fellow of the American Academy of Arts and Sciences. He has a B.A. in mathematical statistics (with highest honors) and an M.P.P. and Ph.D. in public policy analysis, all from Harvard University.

Anna Wikman is a research fellow in the psychobiology group in the Department of Epidemiology and Public Health at University College London. She has a master's in health psychology (King's College London), and a master's in research methods (Goldsmith's College London). She completed her

Ph.D. in health psychology (University College London) studying patients' psychological reactions and adaptation following acute cardiac events, with a particular focus on the development of posttraumatic stress symptoms. Her current work involves working on the English Longitudinal Study of Ageing, investigating adaptation to chronic physical illness.

John R. Wilmoth is associate professor, Department of Demography, and researcher, Center on the Economics and Demography of Aging, University of California, Berkeley. In 2009-2010, he was a consultant to the World Health Organization to develop the United Nation's maternal mortality estimates. Prior to this, he worked for the Population Division of the United Nations in New York City (2005-2007). His research interests include causes of the historical mortality decline, future trends in human mortality and life expectancy at birth, exceptional longevity and possible limits to the human life span, and mortality differentials among social groups within populations. He is a member of the American Association for the Advancement of Science, the Population Association of America, and the Gerontological Society of America. He serves on the editorial boards of several journals including *Demographic Research* and *European Journal of Population*. He has a Ph.D. in statistics and demography from Princeton University.